Unity and Loyalty

The story of Chippenham's Red Cross Hospital

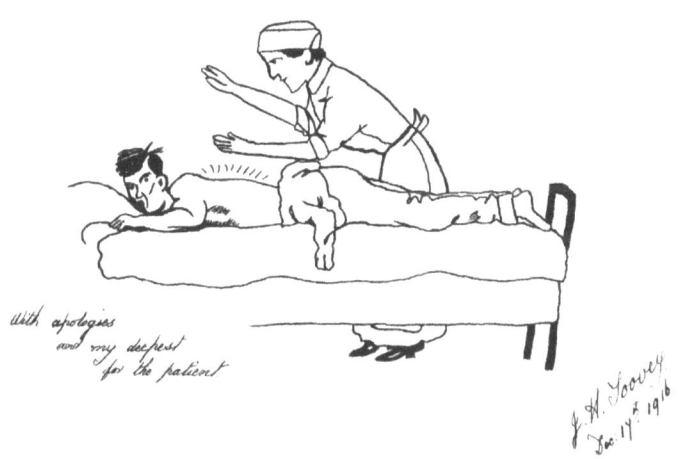

Chippenham Studies 5

Ray Alder

First published in the United Kingdom in 2021,
on behalf of Chippenham Museum, 9-10 Market Place, Chippenham SN15 3HF
www.chippenham.gov.uk/chippenham-museum
by The Hobnob Press, 8 Lock Warehouse, Severn Road, Gloucester GL1 2GA
www.hobnobpress.co.uk

© Ray Alder, 2021

All rights reserved. No part of this publication may be reproduced, stored in a retrieval system, or transmitted, in any form or by any means, electronic, mechanical, photocopying, recording or otherwise, without the prior permission of the publisher and copyright holder. The views expressed in this publication are those of the author, and are not necessarily endorsed by the publisher or Chippenham Town Council.

British Library Cataloguing in Publication Data
A catalogue record for this book is available from the British Library.

ISBN 978-1-914407-04-8
Typeset in 11/13 pt Octavian. Typesetting and origination by John Chandler

Chippenham Studies

1. *Bird's Marsh, Chippenham: an Unfinished Story*, Stephen E. Hunt, 2010
2. *Chippenham and the Wilts & Berks Canal*, Ray Alder, 2011
3. *Domesday to Demolition: A History of the Flour Mill in Chippenham, Wiltshire 1086-1957*, Kay S. Taylor, 2015
4. *An Appreciation of the life of Robin Tanner: Teacher and Etcher 1904-88*, Ernest Hird, 2018

Foreword

I'M DELIGHTED TO be able to provide the foreword for this book, which is the fifth in a series of Chippenham Studies books published by Chippenham Town Council. *Unity and Loyalty: the story of Chippenham's Red Cross Hospital* is based on the work of a team of wonderful, enthusiastic volunteers at Chippenham Museum, supported by some extremely knowledgeable and dedicated officers led by Melissa Barnett, the Town Council's Head of Heritage and Museum Services. Written by Ray Alder, *Unity and Loyalty: the story of Chippenham's Red Cross Hospital* is a magnificent addition to our understanding of the social history of Chippenham. Many people in Chippenham contributed to the war effort during the First World War. It really was one of Chippenham's finest hours, and it is therefore fitting that this book focuses on Chippenham's Red Cross Hospital which opened in 1915, treating those convalescing men who had been exposed to the injuries and horrors of war.

Chippenham Town Council is extremely proud to continue supporting this series of books.

**Mark Smith
Chief Executive,
Chippenham Town Council**

Acknowledgements

MY THANKS GO to the staff, volunteers and Friends of Chippenham Museum, both past and present, for their support in making this book a reality. In particular Melissa Barnett for her unfailing encouragement, Elaine Davis and Linda Gordon for their enthusiasm, especially making the Unity and Loyalty Exhibition come alive in 2015, and of course Ann Brinkworth, who spent so many hours sharing the research into the VAD albums and scrapbooks in the collection.

I would like to thank Chippenham Town Council for generously supporting the Chippenham Studies Series of which this book will be the latest addition. Further thanks also go to the staff of the Neeld Community and Arts Centre and the Town Hall for allowing me access behind the scenes of the VAD Hospital.

Unity and Loyalty

This book would not have been possible without countless contributions, including the personal memories, documents and photographs shared by families of those involved with the Hospital. Every anecdote helped tell how the people of the town came forward in the Great War to help the wounded men. I met so many people in the writing of this book, so please accept my apologies if I have inadvertently missed somebody, but my thanks go to:

Donald Barter, Betty Bird, Joan Blanchard, Christopher Boulton, Nick Burridge, Julian Carosi, Andrea Chilton, Simon Cray, Ron Crook, Chris Dallimore, Rosemary Devonold, Angela Frampton, Charles Fuller, Kevin Gaskin, Terry Gibson, Meg Goulding, George and Sally Gifford, Amanda and Philip Gregory, Debbie and Dave Gulley, Peter Hayes, Godfrey Hibberd, Rita Bullion Jackson, Jane Jordan, Paul Keen, Anna King, Andy Limbrick, Don Little, Richard McCormack, Alan Malpas, David Man, Stella Mann, Linda Newbury, Jeni and David Raby-Cox, David Robinson, Caroline Saye, Sue and Margaret Sorrell, Rosamund Spicer, Mike Stone, Kate Tayler, the Treweke Family, Margaret Troll, Bryant Vincent, Emilie Walker, Tony White, Avice Wilson and Doreen Wootten.

I am also grateful to the following who offered guidance, provided documents and gave permission to use images:

ArtCare at Salisbury District Hospital, the British Red Cross Society, Chippenham Civic Society Chippenham Museum, Corsham Community Group, Dundee Museum of Transport, the Joyce Dennys Estate, Stephen Flavin Corsham Collection, Glenside Museum Archive, the Imperial War Museum, Inver Museum Archive at Larne N. Ireland, Lacock History Society, the Don Little Collection, the National Archives, Ontario Genealogical Society, St Andrew's Church Chippenham, the Scout Association Archive, Trowbridge Museum, Wiltshire Family History Society, Wiltshire Museum, Wiltshire and Swindon History Centre, the Warden and Scholars of Winchester College and Jo Alder for his artwork.

My thanks are also due for the invaluable expertise and advice of John Chandler in the design and layout of the book. Finally, as Melissa Barnett will testify, this project grew beyond all expectations and I would like to thank my wife and family for their continued support, input and, most importantly, patience.

Ray Alder
March 2021

Contents

Introduction	1
Part 1 *The Scheme for Voluntary Aid*	9
1 1907 to 1909	10
2 1910 to 1912	24
3 1913	43
4 1914	49
Part 2 *War*	61
5 1914 – August	62
6 1915	90
7 1916	112
8 1917	138
9 1918	150
Part 3 *How Chippenham made the Wounded Welcome*	159
10 A Happy Home Hospital	160
11 Entertaining the Patients	166
12 Sport and Amusement	178
13 Fund Raising	185
14 Ambulances	191
15 Outings and Friendships	196
Part 4 *Peace and the Hospital Closes*	201
16 After the War – November 1918	202
17 Return to Peace – 1919	212
18 The VAD Hospital Closes	225
19 A New World for the VADs	235
The Final Word	245
Appendix 1 Staff and Volunteers at Chippenham Red Cross Hospital	247
Appendix 2 Work Parties in Chippenham Division	280
Bibliography	289
Index	291

Unity and Loyalty

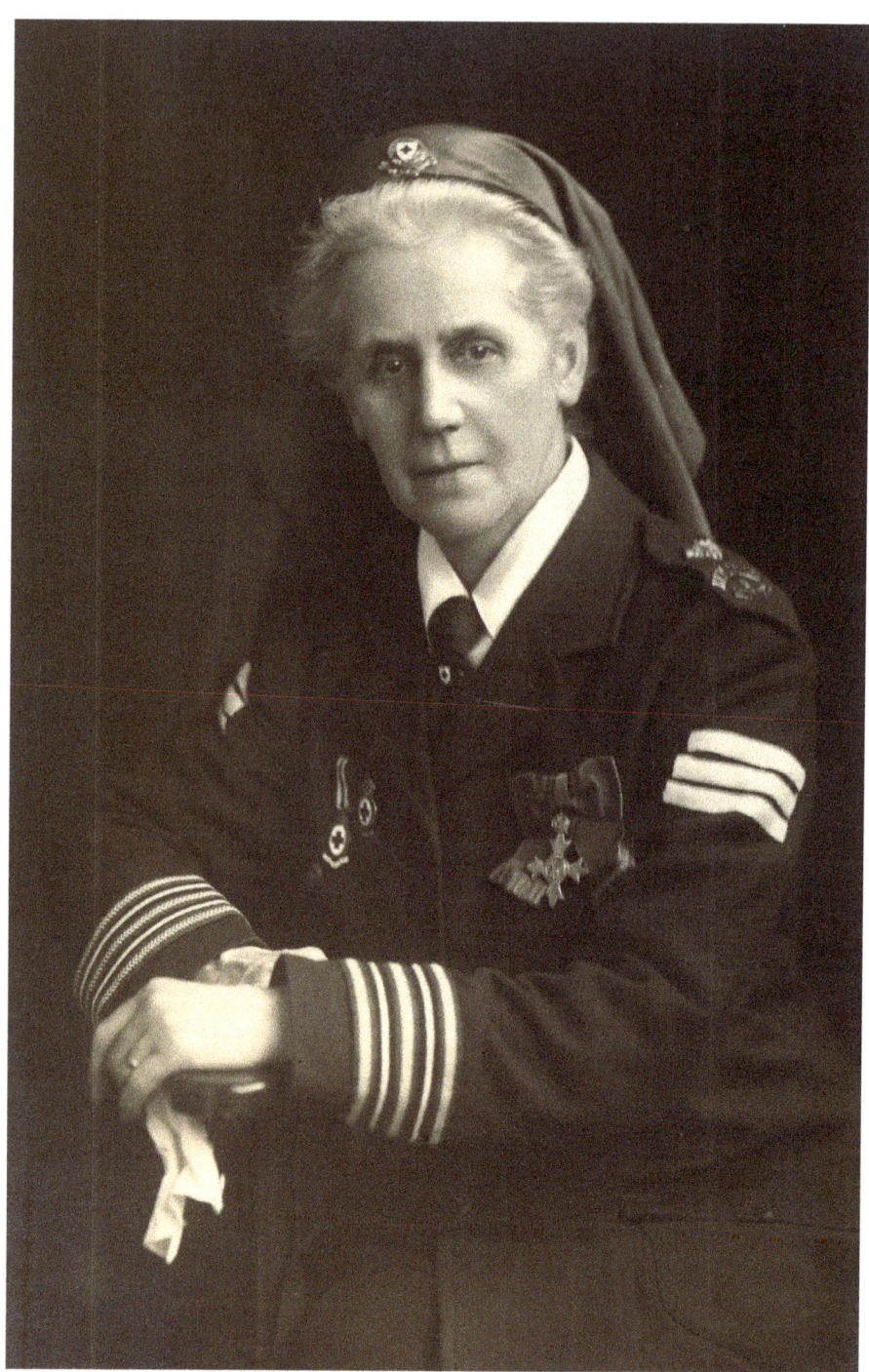

Helena Jane Wilson, 1858 - 1934. Commandant of Chippenham VAD Hospital

Introduction

THE IDEA FOR this book evolved in 2013 when Chippenham Museum was planning its exhibition programme to commemorate the centenary of the First World War. The fact the town had its own temporary Red Cross Hospital, treating wounded men, provided an ideal backdrop for an exhibition to tell a story of the War that related to the town. The inspiration for the design of the Museum's exhibition was a picture in its collection. A small, creased photograph showed everything that you could imagine in a hospital ward: the nurses, doctors, patients, wheelchairs and flowers. If the subject of the photograph could be recreated it would be the ideal vehicle to tell the story of how Chippenham was able to respond to the demands and hardships of the Great War.

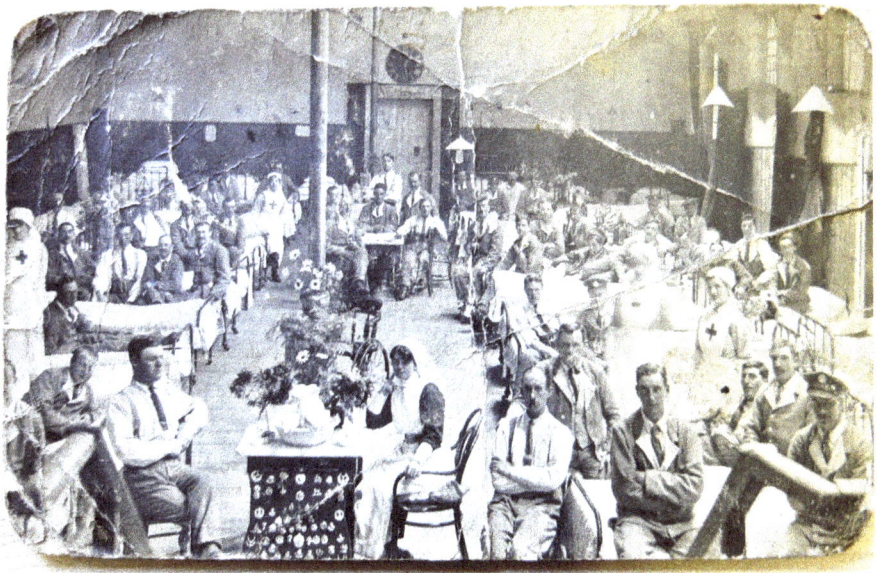

The photograph that inspired the exhibition at Chippenham Museum in 2015

The scene of recovering soldiers and nurses, grouped together in wards and the grounds of grand houses are familiar. Almost every district in the country had its own hospital in converted public buildings or stately houses and patients in their blue uniform became a common sight. The hospital in Chippenham was in the Town and Neeld Halls and was one of the many that treated convalescent men. These establishments were variously known as the VAD hospital, the Red Cross Hospital, the Auxiliary Hospital, the Convalescent Hospital or even the Temporary Hospital. Throughout this book all

Unity and Loyalty

these terms have been used to reflect the reporting of the time.

These hospitals, in towns like Chippenham, tend to warrant only a few paragraphs in accounts of the period. The military hospitals, particularly those overseas, where the horror of war was experienced at first-hand are documented in greater detail and have generated diaries and books published by nurses and soldiers that told of their experiences. The nurses in these hospitals were popularly known as VADS.

The VAD

THE OXFORD ENGLISH Dictionary describes the word VAD as *'Voluntary Aid Detachment, a British organisation of first-aid workers and nurses.'* Made up of either men or women. During the First World War the use of the term VAD was adapted to refer to a young volunteer nurse tending an injured soldier on the battlefield. This image was encouraged by Red Cross recruitment posters which included emotive slogans such as 'If I fail, he dies.'

The fascination of the VAD at war led to public lectures about heroic deeds which left the audience spellbound. Of particular interest was the work of British women in France and newspapers carried headlines about heroic and devoted service in temporary VAD stations and on hospital trains.

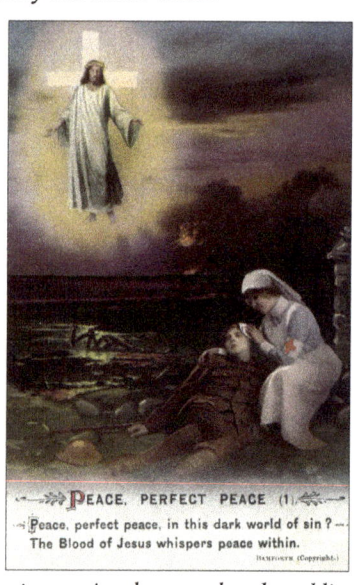

An emotional postcard as the public envisaged the VAD on the battlefield

There are many accounts of VAD bravery and well over a hundred VADs died in service. Thekla Bowser, a journalist who served with the VADs in France, wrote in 1917:[1]

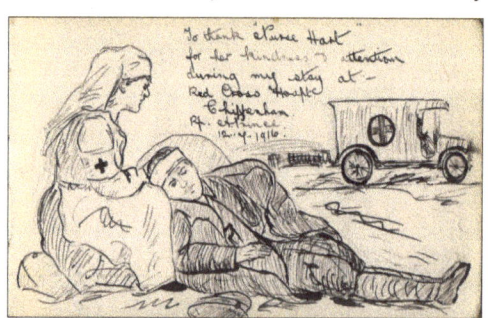

The VAD - Drawn by a patient at Chippenham with the inscription: To thank "Nurse Hart" for her kindness & attention during my stay at Red Cross Hospt Chippenham.

...those of us who have taken any active part in the service of the Red Cross know that wherever the task was hardest and the danger greatest there was always to be found a member of the Voluntary Aid Detachment.

Without doubt this picture of a VAD serving her country in the most difficult of conditions is well

1   *The Story of British VAD work in the Great War* - Thekla Bowser

The Story of Chippenham's Red Cross Hospital

deserved, but in reality, the majority of VADs, members of the Red Cross and Order of St John, served at home, with many volunteering at hospitals such as Chippenham. Their devotion was equal to that of their sisters closer to the battle, but perhaps not as stirring or as widely publicised.

The Museum's exhibition opened in November 2015 and was a great success, but there remained many unanswered questions about the VAD Hospital in Chippenham. Visitors volunteered tantalising snippets of information as they told of relations who had been involved, often supplementing their stories with photographs. The family of one of the cooks was able to tell about her reminiscences of the Hospital and they shared her recipe book which she used during the War. It even included details of some of the patients. The story behind the exhibition spread and information was offered, in some cases from other parts of the world.

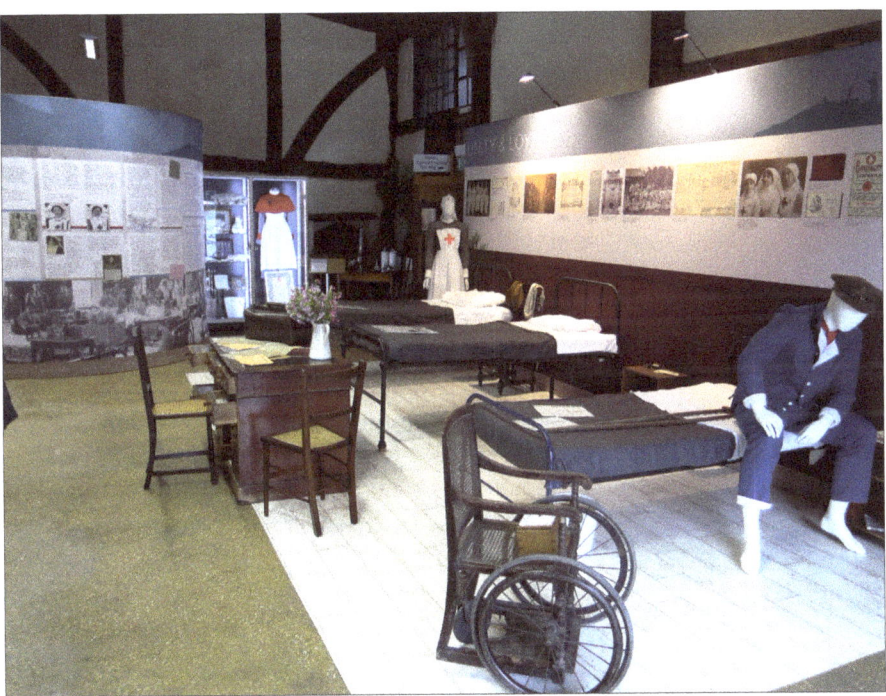

The Chippenham VAD Hospital Exhibition in 2015

A more personal picture of the Hospital was forming. Set against the hardship of war there were light hearted moments and fun, but equally it was well run and organised. The VADs were described as '*very efficient women*,' strong minded, who would take on the Authorities to do the best for their '*Boys in Blue*.'

The local newspaper archives revealed how the Hospital in Chippenham operated and how much it depended on the generosity of the whole town. One patient, a Sergeant, summed it up when he thanked the town for arranging an afternoon of entertainment for the wounded men:

Unity and Loyalty

> Wounded soldiers, whose lot it has been to be patients in Chippenham Red Cross Hospital have been left with a feeling of gratitude for the care and kindness bestowed upon them by the Commandant (Mrs Wilson) and her capable staff. The inhabitants too, have manifested their interest in the men in several ways and the 'boys' have frequently observed that Chippenham Hospital is really a 'home from home' and that they will always have pleasant recollections of their brief stay in the town. The work of the hospital has received sympathetic and generous support from all classes in the district.
>
> *Extract from Wounded Soldiers Entertained - Wiltshire Times 1 September 1917*

With so much new information, and help from many sources, the original idea of simply telling the story of the Red Cross Hospital seemed inadequate. The War and Hospital were the catalyst, the real story was how wonderfully a small North Wiltshire town stood up and selflessly cared for the strangers who arrived in their town during the War.

To tell this story of Chippenham, and it should be remembered that many towns around the country have similar stories to tell, it is important to understand what influenced those who joined the VAD, both before and during the War, and set this against the social and political scene both locally and nationally.

Therefore, this book is divided into four parts. The first tells of the fear of invasion, the resulting Voluntary Aid Scheme, introduced in 1909, and the growth of volunteers in Wiltshire. Part two continues with the outbreak of hostilities, its impact on Chippenham the opening of Red Cross hospitals in the area and how the volunteers organised. The third section tells of the hospital organisation and how the town pulled together with the community giving generously to maintain it. Most importantly it tells how the patients were made to feel welcome. The final part of the book considers the Hospital after the War, its closure in 1919 and how it influenced the future lives of the VADs, patients and people in the town.

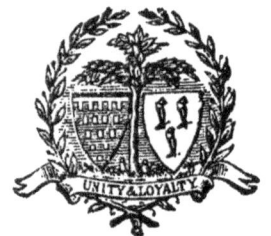

The town crest in 1916

Why call the book Unity and Loyalty? Unity and Loyalty is Chippenham's motto and features on the town crest. The names were adopted for the two large wards in the Hospital. It is clear it equally described the response of the people in the town when they worked with 'Unity and Loyalty' to help the wounded.

Chippenham

THE TOWN OF Chippenham, in North Wiltshire, can trace its history back to at least King Alfred and the Saxons, and like any other market town at the beginning of the twentieth century daily life was unremarkable. The population of nearly five and a

The Story of Chippenham's Red Cross Hospital

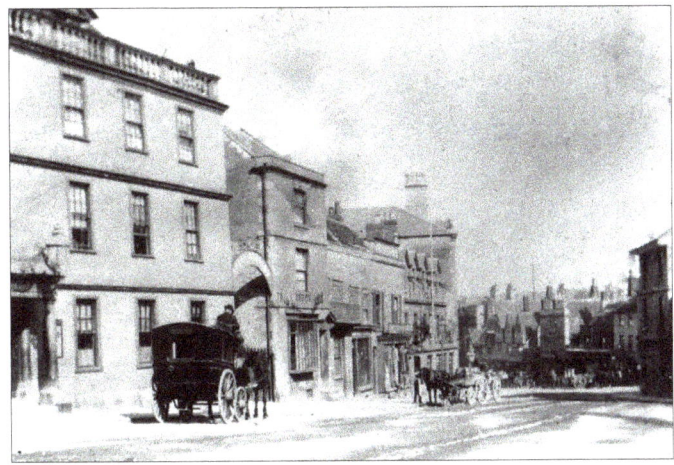

Chippenham Market Place looking toward the High Street. The building on the left is the Angel Hotel.

half thousand went about their daily business, as their forefathers had before them.

At the outbreak of the First World War the town was dependent on agriculture, food processing and engineering. The Great Western Railway and the Great West Road, now the A4, passed through the town. Frank Heath in his Wiltshire guide of 1911 described Chippenham as:

> A junction station on the Great Western Railway. The manufacture of broadcloth has not altogether deserted this famous Wiltshire town and other local industries are the making of cheese and condensed milk and bacon-curing on a large scale. There are also large engineering works where railway signals are manufactured, a tannery, wagon works and a gun and cartridge manufactory. The town is an important agricultural centre with regular cheese, corn and cattle markets.

The new Town Hall in Chippenham's High Street was built in 1833 by MP, Joseph Neeld.[1] Originally known as the Market House, it comprised a large meeting room with several side rooms built on the first floor above the covered market. Behind the Town Hall the Neeld Hall, which was opened in 1911, was described as the town's new public hall and boasted a stage and a number of dressing rooms with

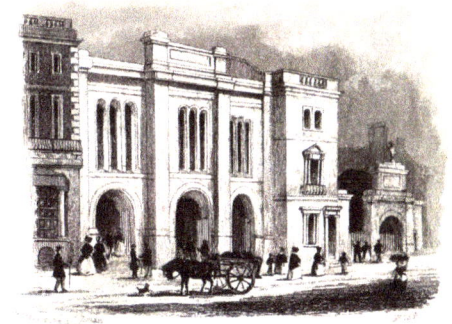

Mid 19C engraving of Chippenham Town Hall with the Market Hall below

1   *Bath Chronicle* – 1 August 1833

seating for a sizable audience.¹

The town had grown substantially in the first years of the twentieth century and in 1914 the borough Boundary was extended to reflect this expansion. The Borough Council correspondingly increased in size and comprised a mayor, six aldermen and 18 councillors.²

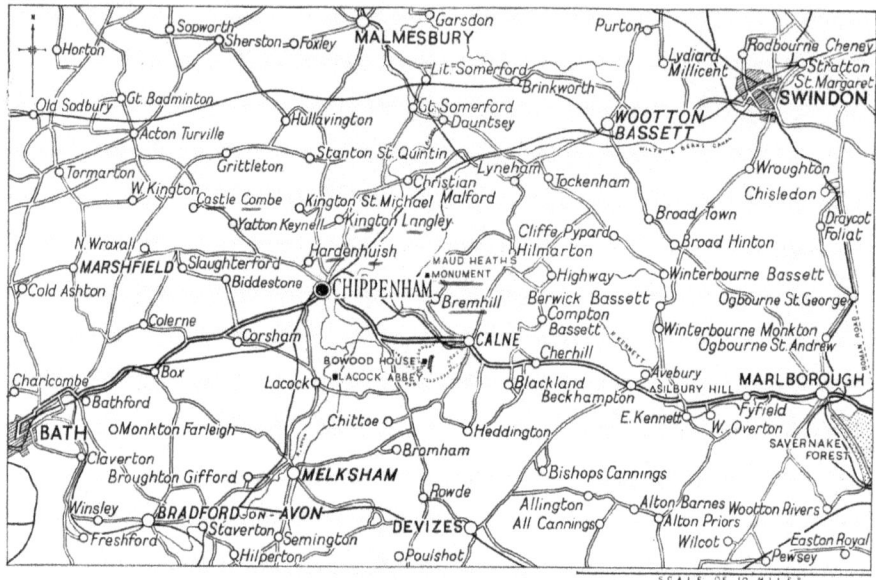

Map of Chippenham and the surrounding district

To further reflect the growth of the town the Cottage Hospital was opened in London Road in 1899 and in 1901 a new school, the Chippenham District Secondary School, was opened opposite the Railway Station.

Wages and prices

THROUGHOUT THIS BOOK wages and prices are quoted in pounds shillings and pence (£ s d). Twenty shillings equalled one pound and one shilling was made up of twelve pence.

Wages in agriculture before the War were less than a pound a week, a figure of 16s was quoted for the Wiltshire agricultural worker.³ To contrast the poor wages in agriculture the remuneration in the railway industry, which many of the men of the Ambulance Detachment belonged to, seemed relatively generous.

1 *Wiltshire Times* - 13 May 1911
2 *North Wilts Directory 1917*
3 *Hansard*-House of Lords debate 21 April 1914.

In 1914 a railway porter was earning between 20s and 26s, a train guard 25s to 30s and an engine driver 35s to 50s.

In 1919 wage rates were compared with those of 1914. Inflation during the war had increased average earnings, for example the engine driver in 1919 could expect wages of 68s to 83s per week.[1]

Although women went into the factories to continue war production, and did the same work as men, their wages were substantially less than those of a man. There were demands for equal pay and a committee was set up by the War Cabinet to examine the question of women's wages but this was only released after the War ended.

---

[1] *Hansard*-House of Commons debate 1 August 1919

Unity and Loyalty

Part 1
The Scheme for Voluntary Aid

Chapter 1
1907 to 1909

THE COUNTRY IS gripped by the fear of invasion. The Navy rules the waves but volunteers are recruited for a new Home Defence military unit to protect the nation. Voluntary Aid is introduced to provide first aid and emergency accommodation in the event of hostilities. Chippenham is chosen as one of the centres for Voluntary Aid and the ladies of the town come forward to do their patriotic duty.

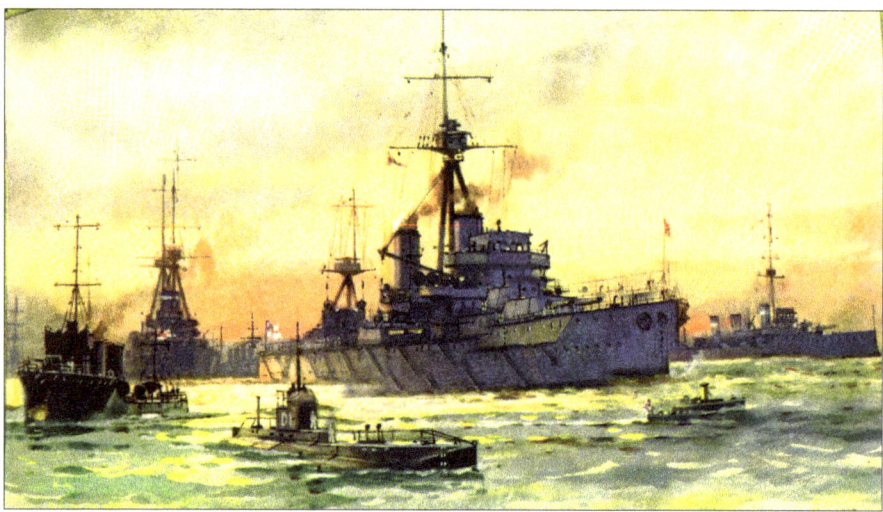

Postcard, painting of the fleet early twentieth century

The fear of invasion

THROUGHOUT HISTORY BRITAIN has planned for invasion. From the Armada to Napoleon there have been preparations to defend the nation's shores, with the building of coastal defences and local volunteer militia units raised to repel the invader. By the end of the nineteenth century there was increasing debate, both in the press and within Government, regarding the likelihood of invasion and the source of any likely aggressor. Germany was a formidable force in Europe. It had become an industrial powerhouse and was expanding its fleet, which threatened Britain's naval supremacy. The rate of this expansion caused alarm in Britain and by 1910 the arms race had escalated as the Government authorised the building of additional dreadnoughts.

At the beginning of the twentieth century Britain still ruled the waves, but it was clear the organisation of Home Defence, to protect the shores from invasion, was in need of review. Local militia units had developed piecemeal over the years meaning the organisation was disjointed with no central command and few plans to deal with the aftermath of an invasion: dealing with the inevitable injured and refugees fleeing from the battle.

To address these weaknesses Home Defence was included in a much-needed review of the whole of Britain's military structure. The South African Wars of 1899 to 1902 emphasised how inefficient the Regular Army was. It was cumbersome and expensive: relying on outdated tactics, some much as they were at Waterloo. South Africa also proved that Britain was not prepared for a prolonged overseas war, especially when confronted by the commando style tactics of the Boers.

As a result, Richard Haldane, the Secretary of State for War, instigated a series of radical reforms to improve efficiency and modernise the Army.

His reforms were not universally popular, but he introduced much needed modern training and a new structure, including a smaller, elite, well-trained force, prepared for overseas service at short notice. This became known as the British Expeditionary Force.

Haldane then turned his attentions to the second line, the Home Defence Force. He again found the organisation cumbersome and out of date and in need of total reform and

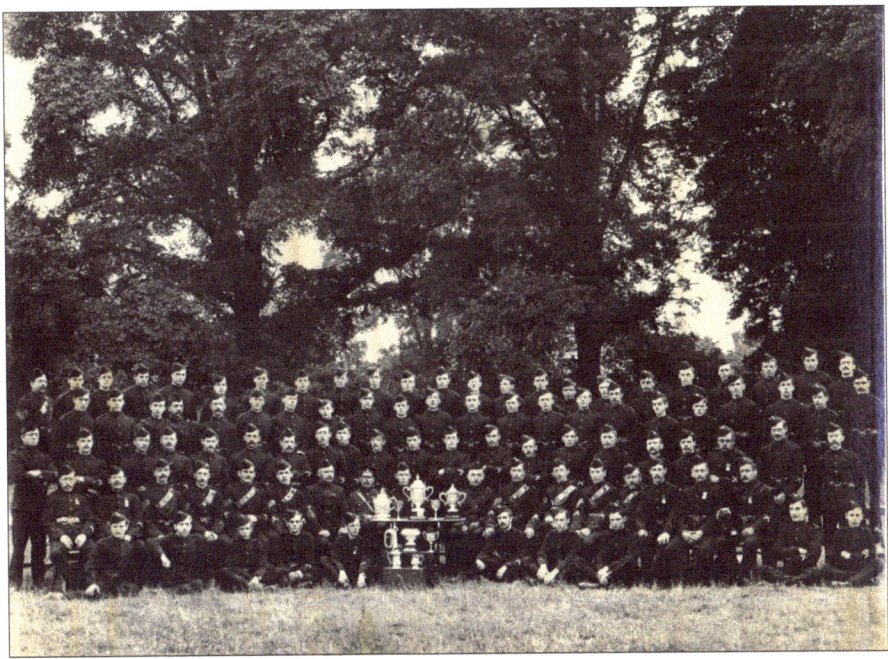

Chippenham Volunteers about 1900

Unity and Loyalty

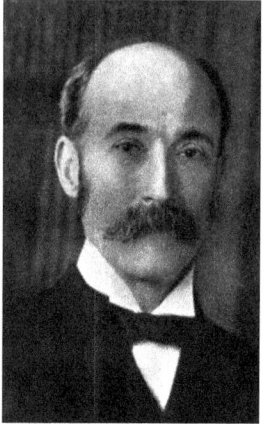

Lord Lansdowne

standardisation. To implement the changes to home defence, which was reliant on volunteers, he introduced the Territorial and Reserve Forces Act in 1907.

Since the eighteenth[1] century a diverse assortment of volunteer militia and yeomanry units had been raised to guard against invasion and deal with incidents of civil disorder. Haldane disbanded many of these units and replaced them with a new County organised military arm, the Territorial Force, also known as Haldane's Terriers. The Territorial Force remained a volunteer organisation but training standards were improved and aligned to the Regular Army. The administration was placed under the newly formed County Territorial Association, often under the leadership of the Lord Lieutenant, with responsibility to raise a well-trained fighting force, that the War Office could call on in time of emergency.

In Wiltshire the Lord Lieutenant, Lord Lansdowne of Bowood, called the inaugural meeting of the County Territorial Association in Trowbridge in November 1907.[2]

Attending the meeting were senior members of the County, gentry, officers of the local militia and representatives of the County and Borough Councils. The Earl of Radnor, who had seen active service with the 4th (Volunteer) Battalion in South Africa, was appointed Chairman of the Association and a committee was elected, renaming the group as The Wilts County Association. The Committee worked quickly and by February 1908 they had started to implement a programme of radical changes.

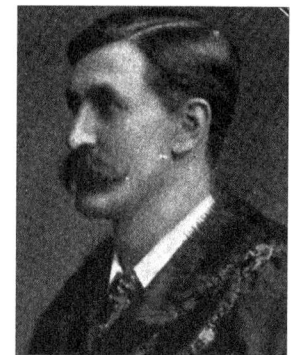

The Earl of Radnor, Jacob Pleydell-Bouverie

To align with the Territorial and Reserve Forces Act it was decided to disband the county's 2nd Volunteer Battalion. The remaining volunteer units in the county were amalgamated and strengthened into a new Territorial Battalion. This Battalion was attached to the county's regulars, the Wiltshire Regiment, and became the 4th Battalion, the Wiltshire Regiment, the Territorials.

This reorganisation was not popular as each of the Volunteer units in the county had a proud history, but by the end of the year the Wiltshire Territorial Force had been established.

In Chippenham the Territorials were designated as D Company and in December 1908 it was reported that the strength of the Company was 103 men: having transferred men from the old volunteers and recruited a further 22 men as a result of the new

---

1 *Militia Act 1757*. The Royal Wiltshire Militia was formed in 1758
2 The *Wiltshire Times* - 2 November 1907

The Story of Chippenham's Red Cross Hospital

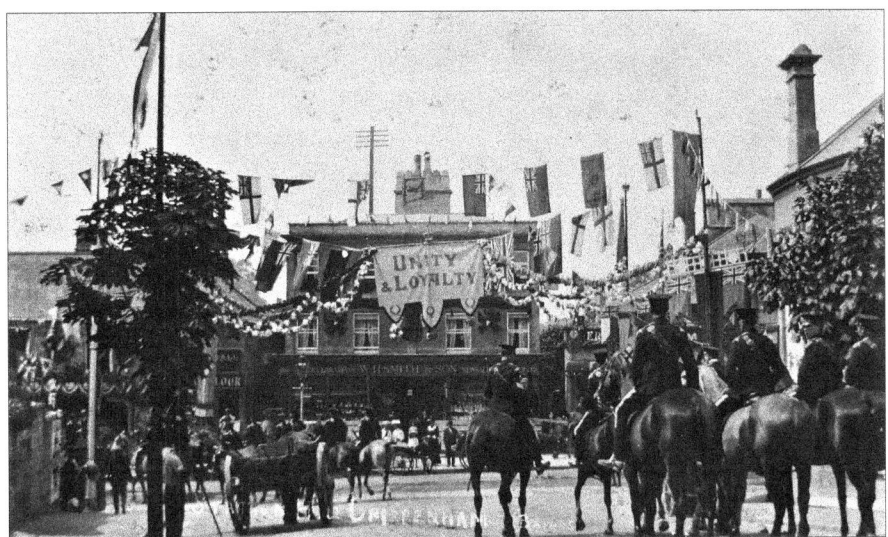

The Chippenham Squadron of the Wiltshire Yeomanry on parade in Chippenham, possibly a Royal visit.

organisation.[1] Their headquarters in the town was at the Yelde Hall in the Market Place, but as numbers of volunteers grew larger premises were needed and by 1911 plans were in place for the Company to move to the Little Ivy in Bath Road, which became known as the Drill Hall.

The Wiltshire Yeomanry, were also covered by the Act and they became part of the mounted section of the Territorial Force. Dating back to 1794 the Wiltshire Yeomanry was a volunteer cavalry regiment, traditionally drawing their recruits from the farming and landed classes and with officers from the local gentry. The Chippenham Squadron of the Wiltshire Yeomanry had its headquarters in the Butts with officers bearing well-known local family names such as Awdry, Methuen, Rooke and Fuller.

With Haldane's reform the Territorial Army was now better equipped and trained to deal with a hostile invasion. Those responsible for the central planning for the defence of the nation also took account of the inevitable military casualties and civilian disruption a conflict would bring. They anticipated that an invading force would result in large numbers of casualties and civilians fleeing the area. It was clear that medical support was needed to treat casualties and a network should be established to provide emergency food and shelter for civilian refugees.

To treat casualties the Regular Army had its own Army Nursing Service, later The Queen Alexandra's Imperial Military Service, which provided fully trained nursing staff[2] and had a heritage dating back to the Crimean War and Florence Nightingale. A corresponding reserve medical service was needed to support the Home Defence Force.

Lord Haldane invited twelve women, including his sister Elizabeth and matrons

1   *The Wiltshire Times* - 26 December 1908 - Report of Chippenham Prize giving.
2   In 1902 Queen Alexandra became the first President.

Unity and Loyalty

from London hospitals, to form a Territorial Nursing Council in March 1908. They proposed a volunteer nursing service should be established. Known as the Territorial Force Nursing Service, it was widely supported by the medical profession.[1]

The Royal Surgeon to Edward VII, Sir Frederick Treves, was a great advocate. Speaking at a meeting in his native Dorchester,[2] he described how an invasion on the Dorset Coast could lead to thousands of casualties and the urgent need for suitably trained men and women to deal with thousands of injured and evacuees forced to flee their homes.

Volunteers, who had to be fully trained nursing staff, came forward to join the Territorial Force Nursing Service. Men and women employed in hospitals and nursing homes around the country joined, giving a commitment to attend a number of training days and exercises each year with the Territorial Force.

Should an invasion take place the Army Council had arranged for existing hospitals and other suitable buildings to be converted into Territorial Force General Hospitals. This was usually in a large town where an agreement had been reached to release wards and operating theatres to the military at times of threat to the nation. Civilian patients and staff would transfer to nearby hospitals or establishments, such as, university buildings, lunatic asylums and even workhouses, which could be rapidly converted to temporary hospitals.

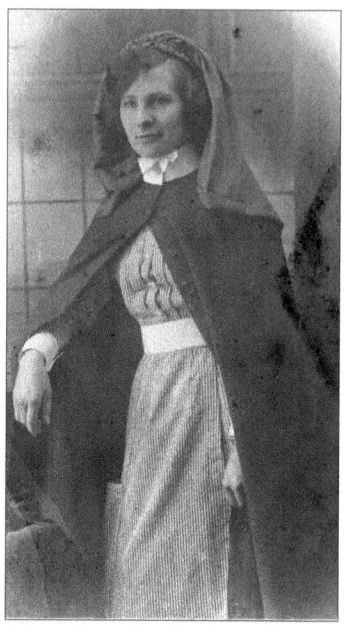

Mary Titcombe, daughter of Henry Titcombe, the landlord of the Pack Horse public house in Chippenham. She trained as a nurse and was a candidate for the Territorial Force Nursing Service

A nationwide network of Territorial Force General Hospitals would be brought into use in the event of invasion and the Territorial Force Nursing Service would be called to staff them. When war broke out in 1914 these became known as Military or Base Hospitals.[3]

Voluntary Aid

IT WAS POINTED out by the strategic planners that the Territorial Force General Hospital organisation could easily be disrupted by an advancing enemy force. They

1   *The Story of British VAD work in the Great War* - Thekla Bowser
2   *Bath Chronicle* - 14 July 1910
3   *The British Red Cross in Action* – Dame Beryl Oliver. Oliver used the term Base Hospital to describe the Military Hospital at Netley

The Story of Chippenham's Red Cross Hospital

were in large towns and relied on good rail links to evacuate wounded troops. Should the enemy take control of the transport infrastructure, or simply disable part of it, the hospitals couldn't be reached. To deal with this possibility it was decided there was a need to establish small, locally organised, groups of volunteers in towns around the country that, at short notice, could provide temporary medical facilities, even emergency wards set up in public buildings.

The members of the group would be sufficiently trained to administer emergency first aid until the wounded could be moved to military hospitals. They should also have the facilities to arrange for food and temporary shelter for refugees fleeing from the enemy.

The Army Council asked Sir Alfred Keogh, the Inspector General of the Army Medical Corps, to put forward proposals for a flexible volunteer body that could react at short notice to assist the Territorial Force Nursing Service.

His report became known as *the Scheme for the Organisation of Voluntary Aid in England and Wales* and was published in August 1909.[1] Keogh said that volunteers should be recruited as part of the County Territorial Association and work in small groups alongside existing bodies who had experience in first aid and the evacuation of injured. In most areas this would be the local branches of the Red Cross and St John Ambulance, who had experience of dealing with emergencies and provided training.

The Scheme for the Organisation of Voluntary Aid was approved and issued to the County Associations. The Times gave the following advice:

> ... a copy of a Scheme for the Organisation of Voluntary Aid in England and Wales was issued yesterday to Territorial County Associations throughout the country. It is hoped that the Associations will place themselves in communication with the council of the British Red Cross Society without delay, with a view to initiating the formation of Voluntary Aid Detachments

In 1907 the British Red Cross Society had re-organised[2] its structure, setting up branches at County level, often under the leadership of the wife of the Lord Lieutenant. These branches agreed to take responsibility for recruiting and training volunteers for Voluntary Aid and in October 1909 the agreed syllabus[3] of instruction for Voluntary Aid was issued by the Red Cross in conjunction with St John Ambulance Association.

Col. Sir Herbert Perrott, Chief Secretary of the St John Ambulance Association

---

1. *The Times* - 17 August 1909 gave a comprehensive summary of the scheme
2. At a meeting at Buckingham Palace on 17 July 1905 Queen Alexandra said 'It has been on my mind ever since the South African War to try and re-organise the Red Cross Society on a more practical and sounder basis. This new organisation should be based upon Membership and Association. The Members and associates shall be recruited from all classes.
3. *The Times* - 15 October 1909. The syllabus was published in the paper.

Unity and Loyalty

confirmed their support to the scheme saying it was essential for volunteers to come forward '*...to be prepared to provide work required for adequate aid to the sick and wounded in case of invasion.*' Prominent people wrote letters of support for the scheme. Locally the Duke of Beaufort at Badminton, wrote how important it was to help the Red Cross Society to fulfil its pledge to the nation:[1]

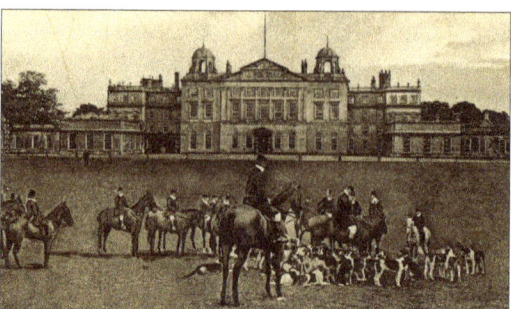
Badminton House, the home of the Duke of Beaufort

> If our civilian soldiers are patriotic enough to give their leisure in time of peace and in case of war to risk their lives in defence of their country, it is only the bare duty of those of us who cannot actually fight to so prepare ourselves now, that we may be enabled to take our place—properly trained and equipped —behind the fighting line should the necessity, unhappily, ever arise. This movement is not a temporary one. It is entirely non-political and non-sectarian, and is definitely a part of the Territorial scheme. I appeal to everyone who can assist either by subscribing as a member or associate, or giving personal service as a member of a voluntary aid detachment, to communicate with the vice-president of his or her district.

It soon became clear there was no shortage of women interested in volunteering. The Western Daily Press reported:[2]

> The Red Cross Society continues to receive large numbers of letters from ladies curious to join the new organisation of nurses in connection with the Territorial Army. In many cases mothers have written offering their own services and those of their daughters.

Such was the enthusiasm that the London headquarters of the Red Cross was soon overwhelmed with enquires and volunteers were asked to contact the secretary of their County Branch directly to seek advice about their local detachments and make arrangements to join.

The women who came forward were predominantly 'society', the middle and upper middle classes and included a number of young women of title.[3] Within a few months of the publication of the Scheme for the Organisation of Voluntary Aid the first detachments were established and training courses were underway.

In Wiltshire the Scheme for the Organisation of Voluntary Aid was

1 *Gloucester Journal* - Saturday 20 November 1909
2 *Western Daily Press* - 24 August 1909
3 *The Lamp and the Book* - Gerald Bowman

The Story of Chippenham's Red Cross Hospital

enthusiastically adopted. The two organisations, the Wilts County Association and the Wiltshire Branch of the Red Cross, agreed they should work together to establish Voluntary Aid in the County. The two bodies were respectively led by Lord and Lady Lansdowne, which ensured the scheme was given every opportunity to succeed.

In September 1909, at a meeting of the two organisations, it was decided to form the Wilts Joint Voluntary Aid Committee who took responsibility to establish Voluntary Aid Detachments throughout the County. The Western Gazette reported on the meeting:[1]

The Marchioness of Lansdowne presided at a meeting of Wiltshire ladies, at which a scheme for the formation of a county branch of the Red Cross Society, to work in conjunction with the County Territorial Association was approved. A joint committee has been appointed, the members of which include the Earl of Radnor, chairman of the County Association, and the Duke of Somerset.

Others on the Committee representing the Red Cross were a number of influential Wiltshire people including, Mr and Mrs Basil Hankey of Stanton Manor, Mrs. Money-Kyrle of Whetham House, near Bowood, Lady Neeld of Grittleton and Lady Margaret Spicer of Spye Park.

A few weeks later, at a public meeting in Calne, Lady Lansdowne described the role of the Joint Voluntary Aid Committee in Wiltshire and explained the work Voluntary Aid Detachments would be asked to perform. She went on to say that she fully expected meetings to be held in the near future where those interested in volunteering for the scheme could put their name forward.

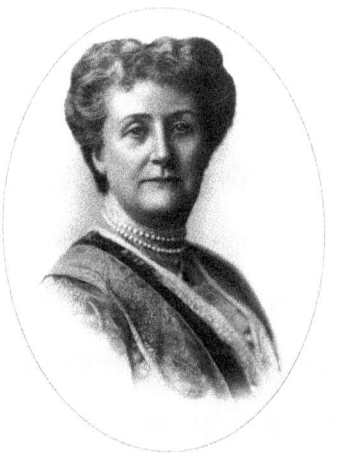

Lady Lansdowne, President of the Wiltshire branch of the Red Cross

Although the Wiltshire Joint Voluntary Aid Committee was pressing ahead it needed to ensure the work it was doing was aligned to official plans. Every County was to be allocated to a Territorial Military Command. Wiltshire, Somerset and Gloucestershire were allocated to the Second Southern Military Hospital Command in Bristol under the leadership of Colonel Bush[2] of the Territorial branch of the Royal Army Medical Corps.

J. Paul Bush was a surgeon at the Bristol Royal Infirmary, which gave him an advantage when negotiating with the governors of the hospital. By February 1911 he had reached an agreement that should there be an invasion the Bristol Royal Infirmary would be available to the military authorities.[3] This was a paper agreement: a plan only to

1   *Western Gazette* - 17 September 1909
2   James Paul Bush 1857-1930 Consulting Surgeon to the Bristol Royal Infirmary. He was often known as Paul Bush.
3   *Western Daily Press* - 5 August 1914.

be implemented should there be an invasion. This meant that when the Territorials were mobilised for annual exercises both hospital and patients saw little disruption.

Under the initial plans devised by Colonel Bush, the task of evacuating civilian patients from Bristol would fall to the newly organised Voluntary Aid Detachments and it was estimated the three counties, Wiltshire, Somerset and Gloucestershire, should prepare to accommodate a total of 500 beds for the transfer of civilian patients and also be prepared to provide convalescent beds for injured men.

In Wiltshire the Joint Voluntary Aid Committee decided, to meet the Colonel's plans, five areas in the county were identified where the Voluntary Aid Detachments could arrange accommodation for the sick and wounded. These were Salisbury, Swindon, Chippenham, Devizes and Westbury[1] chosen primarily for their proximity to important railway junctions, and in the case of Devizes, the link with Bristol by the Kennet and Avon canal.

The First Wiltshire Detachment

In December 1909 the Committee arranged the first meeting in the county with the purpose of raising a Voluntary Aid Detachment. The Wiltshire Gazette announced:

A public meeting to consider the raising of a Voluntary Aid Detachment consisting of men and women in Chippenham and the neighbourhood in connection with the medical service of the Territorial Army, and to invite applicants for the same.

On 16 December 1909 Chippenham Town Hall was packed with an audience keen to hear the speakers from the Joint Voluntary Aid Committee.

Those present were a 'who's who' of Chippenham Society including the Mayor, William Crofts and Reverends Maxwell H Smith and Livingstone representing the churches of Chippenham; from the Territorials Sir George Helme,[2] who had seen service in the South African wars, and Captain Ashley Phillips, commander of the Chippenham Company, Mrs Clutterbuck of Hardenhuish House represented the local aristocracy, while Lady Dickson Poynder and Lady Neeld both sent their apologies, but wanted the meeting to know they were great supporters of the scheme. They would both play an active part in the future of the organisation.

Business leaders were amongst those in the audience; men like Frederick Hake and Joseph Lane, managers of the Wilts and Dorset bank; Mr Hathaway, the butter churn manufacturer; George Gillett, general secretary to the bacon factory; Percy Stops, the manager of the brewery and Lionel Marshall a Land Agent who lived in St Mary Street.

One of the speakers during the evening said '*I need to make an appeal to those present to support the movement to the utmost in their power*': a message to the

---

1 *Devizes and Wiltshire Gazette* - 23 December 1909
2 In 1922 George Helme took the surname Mashiter under royal licence. When war broke out he was the recruiting officer for Chippenham.

The Story of Chippenham's Red Cross Hospital

businessmen in the town that financial and practical help would be needed to establish these units. The Marchioness of Lansdowne chaired the meeting and asked Mr H. Herbert Smith to take the stage and explain why it was proposed to raise a Detachment in the town.

Henry Herbert Smith was the land agent for Lord Lansdowne and lived on the Bowood estate. He was also the County Director of the Red Cross and a member of the Joint Voluntary Aid Committee. He opened his presentation by outlining the Red Cross in Wiltshire and the work of the Territorial Force saying the Red Cross would perform a vital function: [1]

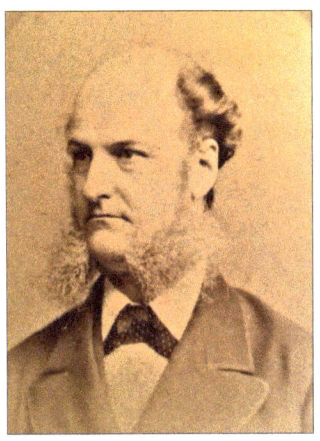

Joseph Lane, manager of the Wilts and Dorset Bank, was a keen supporter of the Scheme for Voluntary Aid. His daughter, Florence, would go on to lead a sewing party during the war.

...a large portion of the medical organisation already exists in the Territorial Force. Thanks to the energy and patriotism of the medical and nursing professions they had the medical organisation at the front. For the fighting troops, they had the doctors and nurses and managers for 23 large hospitals, which would be opened as important centres from the North of Scotland to the South of England. But there was nothing between the fighting force in the front and the hospitals in the rear. The work which had to be done could be done by their un-enlisted fellow countrymen. They proposed to rely upon the assistance of the people who did not form part of the fighting force.

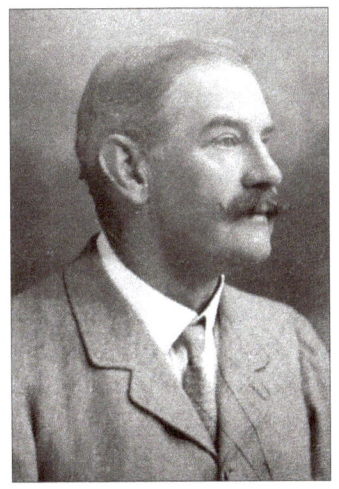

Henry Herbert Smith

He went on to say that the Red Cross were seeking both men and women members to form a Detachment and he felt certain that people would come forward as members, associates or subscribers pledging donations. He was also confident that Chippenham would be able to raise a full Detachment, as he knew that it was a town '*always at the front*'.

Mr H. Herbert Smith then told the audience that a suitable Commandant needed to be appointed to oversee the recruitment and training. He announced that Lionel Marshall had offered his services and was considered an ideal candidate as he was well known as a member of the Cottage Hospital Committee and former mayor. Doctors Briscoe and Wilson, both of the Cottage Hospital, gave their support to Mr Marshall

1   *Devizes and Wiltshire Gazette* – 23 December 1909

by offering to arrange suitable training classes for the volunteers.

In reply Mr Marshall said it now only remained for volunteers to come forward, and for first aid and ambulance classes to start without delay.

Many of those who showed an interest in Voluntary Aid were supporters of the town's Cottage Hospital. Built at the end of the nineteenth century, as enlightened legislation and medical advances saw standards of sanitation and healthcare improve, this was part of a growing movement towards small local hospitals with a few beds, run by general practitioners.

Normally found in rural areas, these units provided local care and avoided long journeys to the County Hospital. In Chippenham a site in London Road was allocated and work started in November 1897. The Cottage Hospital opened in 1899, financed by donations and subscriptions, and managed by a committee of volunteers. The President of the Committee was John Dickson Poynder, MP for Chippenham, and amongst the committee were Reverend Maxwell Smith, William Burridge, Daniel Collen, Francis Belcher and Lionel Marshall: names that would play a major part in the organisation of Chippenham's Voluntary Aid Detachment in the coming years.

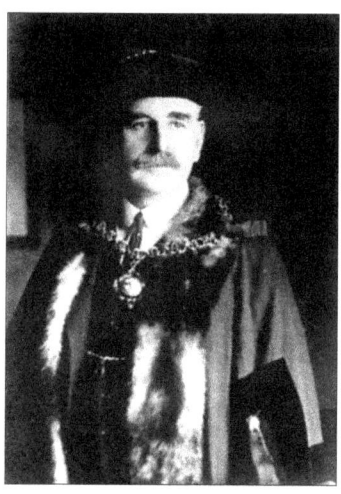

Lionel Marshall in his mayoral robes. He became Chippenham Detachment Commandant in 1909.

To support the call for volunteers at the Chippenham meeting Sir George Helme, of the Territorial Force, took to the stage and gave a robust speech about the military situation. In his opinion the need for home defence was now at its greatest:

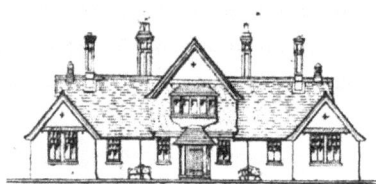

THE PROPOSED CHIPPENHAM COTTAGE HOSPITAL.

Design for the Cottage Hospital 1897

At a time like this, when we read how foreign nations were adding to the strength of their navies and their armies, a Voluntary Aid society of this sort would be of considerable help to the Territorial force, ...when military experts like Lord Roberts had said that he thought it was not only possible but probable that an invasion will take place,— we could scarcely disregard such a warning, and it behoved us more than ever to be prepared.

The Story of Chippenham's Red Cross Hospital

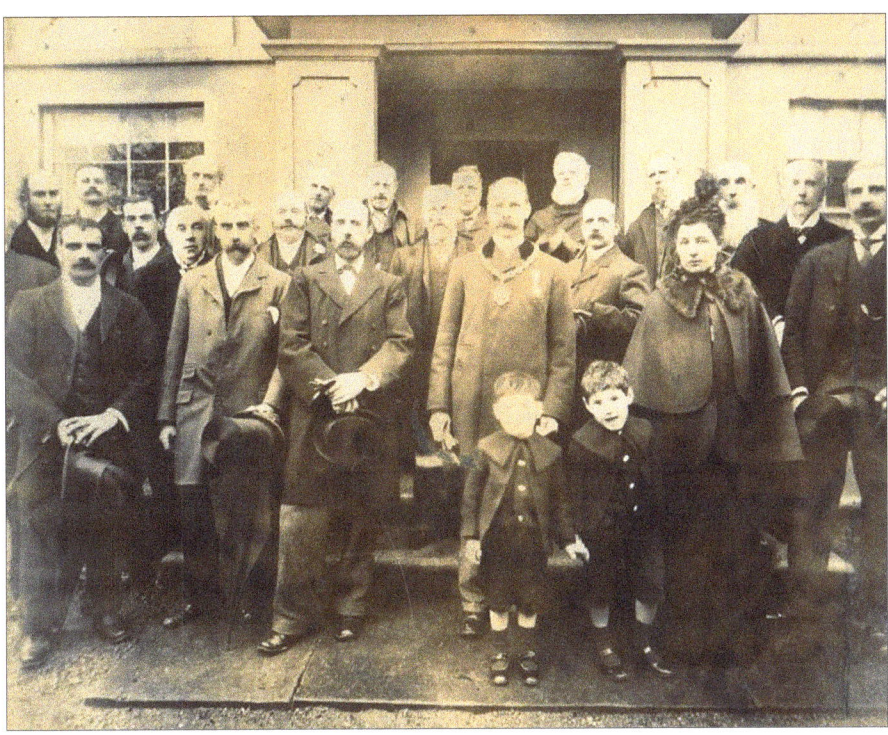

The Hospital Committee at the opening of the Cottage Hospital. Many of those present became involved with Voluntary Aid in Chippenham

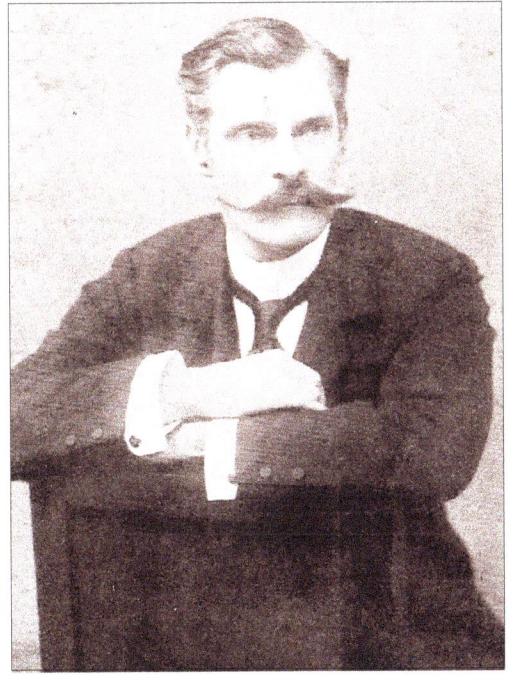

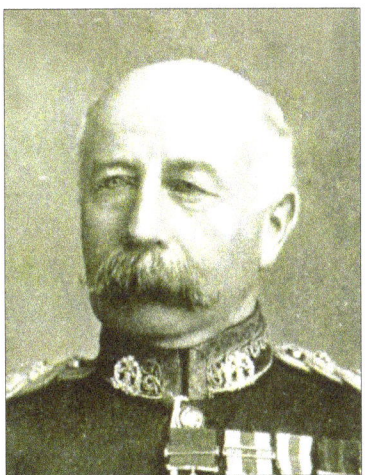

(left) John Dickson Poynder. President of the Cottage Hospital Committee (above) Sir George Helme

Lord Methuen of Corsham was equally convinced that invasion was imminent. Addressing the Chippenham Volunteer Militia in December 1898:[1]

> When invasion came it would come in a different way to what it did in former days. When it came now, on account of electricity and steam, it would come like a hurricane and it would come heavily.

He was clearly referring to Germany, whose rapid industrialisation and increasing naval power was seen as a threat to the nation. Baden Powell, well known and respected for his military service and founder of the Scout Movement, spoke out about invasion, calling Germany our *'natural enemy'*.

However, there were those who disagreed that invasion was inevitable and that Germany was not such a threat. This led to debate throughout the country and political camps known as the 'Blue-Water' School and 'Bolt-from-the-Blue' School were established. Simply put, the Blue-Water was the naval view that a strong fleet maintained the command of the sea and therefore an invasion would be of little consequence and should be dealt with by a small Home Defence Force. The counter, the Bolt-from the Blue, reflected the army view that a surprise attack while the Navy was distracted was quite feasible and an adequate second line of defence was needed. The popular press were keen to tell of German spies about to take over the country.

Public opinion was mixed in 1909. Some agreed that that conflict with Germany was inevitable, while others worked towards improving relations and two years later, in 1911, the Anglo German Friendship Society was formed under the patronage of the Duke of Argyll.[2]

To counter this goodwill the Agadir crisis in 1911 saw tensions between the two countries escalate. Patriotic zeal was fuelled when Lloyd George made a statement warning Germany against any acts of aggression.

The threat of invasion was a regular topic of conversation. German spies were seen everywhere although the truth was that between August 1911 and July 1914 only ten suspects were arrested for spying.[3]

Such was the fascination with invasion that it inspired popular fiction: the book 'The Battle of Dorking' by George Tomkyns Chesney told of the conquest of Britain following a surprise attack. On the stage there were dramatic productions: in February 1909 the play, 'The Invasion of England' included scenes described as *'The awe inspiring spectacle of London in flames'* and *'a night attack on a volunteer encampment'*.[4] Young boys, who a few years later would volunteer to fight the Germans, were reading ripping yarns where the enemy, who inevitably had German or South African sounding names, were swiftly dealt with, often with the help of the Boy Scouts.

1 *Bristol Mercury* - 23 December 1898
2 *The Times* - 19 January 1911
3 The National Archives - Spotlights on History- Espionage. www.nationalarchives.gov.uk
4 *The Era* – 6 February 1909

For those who attended the Voluntary Aid meeting in Chippenham there were mixed feelings. For some, despite the speech by George Helme, invasion was the threat that would never happen. The German Kaiser was the bogey man to frighten the children, but equally Germans were part of everyday life. There were many trading links. Chippenham's Saxby and Farmer had won sizable contracts to install signalling on the Prussian railway and German companies such as Bosch and Siemens did so much business that they opened factories in Britain.

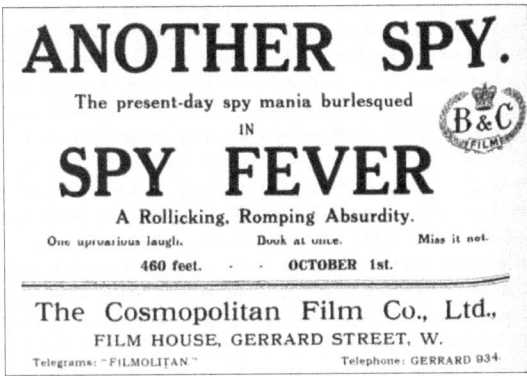

The film Another Spy, mocking the nation's fixation with spies

Thousands of Germans were living and working in Britain. It was said that most of the waiters in London were German and in fact, many estates in Wiltshire employed German staff. Clara Wilhem, from Berlin[1] was employed as a Governess at Hartham Park, the home of John Dickson Poynder. Also popular for their music, visiting German bands travelled the country giving concerts in towns and villages. Edith Bull remembered the excitement when the German bands arrived in her village of Aldbourne and the pleasure of their lively tunes.[2] A group of German musicians had lodged in Chippenham a few years earlier[3] and had provided entertainment around the area.

This was the situation at the end of the first decade of the twentieth century. The military men were predicting an imminent invasion while others were not so sure. Germany was the candidate to lead the invasion, but they were also friends in business and on a personal level the Germans weren't such bad types. In Chippenham the meeting for Voluntary Aid had raised considerable interest, particularly amongst the ladies of the town. This was an opportunity to join an organisation that offered some independence and perhaps a little excitement.[4] It was their patriotic duty to join the scheme, but perhaps the talk of invasion was exaggerated. Being prepared meant invasion would never happen.

---

1   *1911 census*
2   From the *Dabchick*, the Aldbourne village newsletter in the 1960s. (A village in North East Wiltshire.)
3   *1871 Census*
4   *Women and the Great War* – Joyce Marlow. This book discusses women's role before the War and the excitement of joining the VADs.

Chapter 2
1910 to 1912

THE SCHEME FOR Voluntary Aid proves to be very popular with women of the middle and upper classes. In Wiltshire a number of women's detachments are raised and First Aid and Home Nursing training is arranged for the volunteers. It proves difficult to attract men to join the detachments. A dispute between the Red Cross and The Order of St John of Jerusalem means the planned joint working of the two organisations for Voluntary Aid does not materialise.

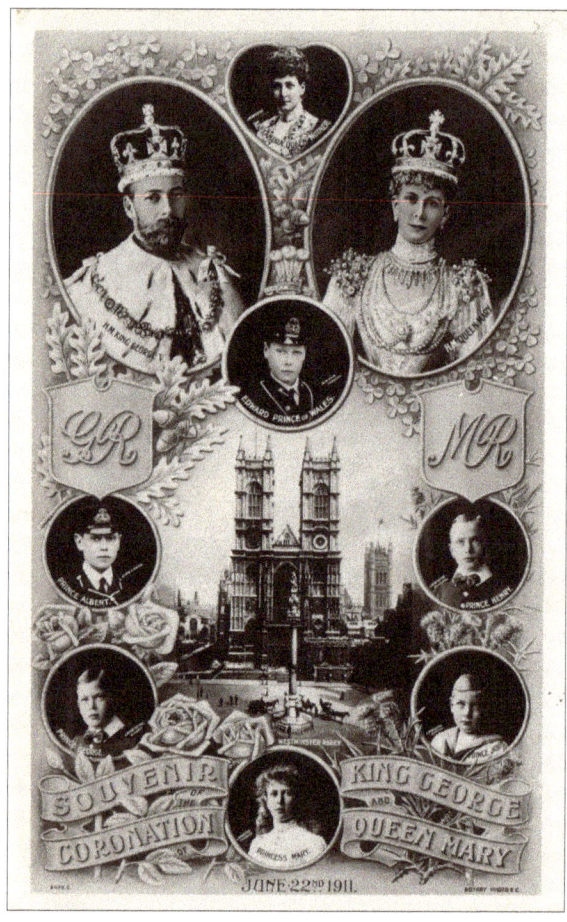

Commemorative post card of the coronation in 1911

The coronation of George V and Mary of Teck takes place at Westminster Abbey on 22 June 1911. In April 1912 news is received of the sinking of the Titanic.

Registering Voluntary Aid Detachments

THE FIRST WILTSHIRE recruiting meeting at Chippenham Town Hall in December 1909 had proved to be a success and the newly appointed Commandant, Lionel Marshall, received numerous enquiries from the ladies in the town about joining the Detachment.

Two months later, in February 1910, Mr H. Herbert Smith was at the Council Chamber in Salisbury seeking support for the Scheme for Voluntary Aid in the south of the County. He was able to tell the meeting that Chippenham had registered enough volunteers to form a women's Detachment.

In April he was in Devizes telling an interested audience about Voluntary Aid and such was the enthusiasm throughout the county that the Joint Voluntary Aid Committee was asked if they would allow detachments in towns, additional to the five locations originally chosen.

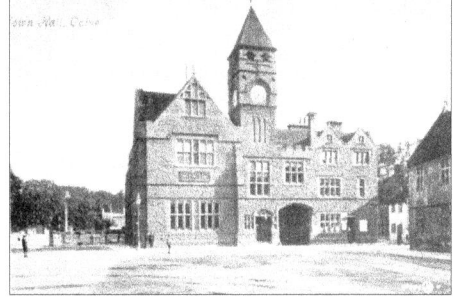

Calne Town Hall. Lady Lansdowne agreed that a Detachment should be raised in the town

The ladies in Calne, some who had attended the meeting in Chippenham, were keen to raise a group in their town.[1] When the Marchioness of Lansdowne met them in March 1910 she agreed they continue and said how pleased she was to think how patriotically Calne had risen to the occasion by raising a Voluntary Aid Detachment.[2] In May 1912, it was reported there were six fully trained detachments registered in Wiltshire, with a number of others undertaking training and soon to be registered. Two years later the number of detachments in the county had risen to twenty-one.[3] Unfortunately very few men came forward and it proved impossible to raise corresponding male units.

This enthusiasm was reflected nationally, In October 1910 there were 202 detachments undertaking training, with a membership of over six thousand.[4] By 1 July 1914 the War Office announced that the number of registered detachments was 2,390 representing a total strength of 71,147 members, of whom about two-thirds were women.[5]

Amongst the first ladies to register in Chippenham Voluntary Aid Detachment

1 *Salisbury and Winchester Journal* – 26 February 1910
2 *Western Daily Press* - 31 March 1910
3 *Devizes and Wiltshire Gazette* – 4 June 1914.
4 *The British Red Cross in Action* – Dame Beryl Oliver
5 *Western Morning News* - 28 July 1914

(VAD) was May Ennis, the wife of William Ennis, the Manager of the Capital and Counties bank.[1] She was soon promoted to Quartermaster responsible for supplies and equipment. Kate Hinton, wife of Frederick Hinton, the headmaster of Ivy Lane School, also decided to join the VAD in 1910.

Others who joined were Sarah Mackness, wife of Frederick, who owned the wagon works in the Causeway, and Katherine Spencer, whose husband's music shop was in the Market Place. Sisters Dora and Evelyn Belcher joined in June 1910. They were daughters of Frank Belcher, who owned a successful drapery business in the Market Place and was also director of the Chippenham Sanitary Laundry.[2] Mr Belcher was respected for his voluntary work for the town: a Governor of the secondary school, a churchwarden, on the committee of the Cottage Hospital he

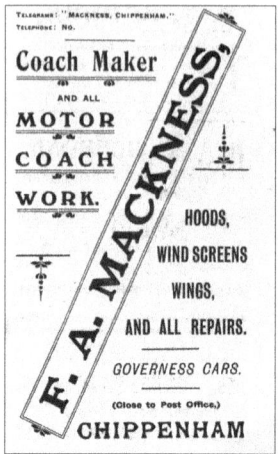

Advertisement for Frederick Mackness Wagon Works

was also a member of the Lansdowne Lodge of Unity. The whole Belcher family were supporters of the Red Cross and the VADs and it is thought that a third daughter, Muriel, was a member until she died in September 1914.

Dora and Evelyn typified the young woman who joined the VAD. They were active in a number of organisations in the town, leaders of the Girl Guides, members of the Cottage Hospital fundraising committee and energetic in the Operatic Society.

Friends, of the Belcher sisters, some from school days,[3] joined the VAD over the following months. The sisters

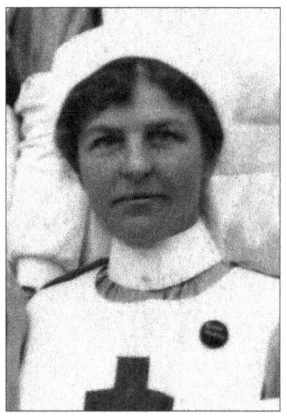

above: Sarah Mackness one of the first ladies to join the VAD

right: Advertisement for Belcher's drapery store

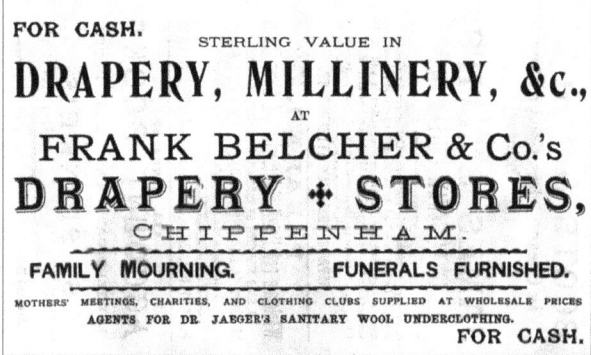

1 Kelly's Directory 1911.
2 Chippenham Museum - *Garlick Scrapbooks*
3 A History of the Chippenham Grammar School 1896-1956 A Platts. They attended the girls school in the Temperance Hall in Foghamshire and by 1913 were members of the VAD.

The Story of Chippenham's Red Cross Hospital

no doubt told of the interesting work they were doing with the Red Cross. Amongst those who registered were Ethel Brinkworth, Nettie King, Daisy Spinke and Elsie Hickling - all daughters of businessmen in the town.

In 1913 Olive and Ivy Gladstone joined Chippenham VAD. They were daughters of Sir John Gladstone of Bowden Park and members of Wiltshire Aristocracy. Sir John became the fourth Baronet of Fasque and Balfour and was a nephew of the late Prime Minister William Ewart Gladstone.

The criteria for establishing a Voluntary Aid Detachment were based on Territorial Force standards set by the War Office and they were subject to inspections by the Military. A Detachment could only be registered when it could be shown 70 percent[1] of the complement had enrolled and were undertaking suitable training. This was achieved in Chippenham by February 1910.

Once registered, the War Office allocated a unique number within the County command: women's detachments were registered with even numbers and male detachments with odd numbers. Chippenham was registered as Wilts 6 VAD. Where a full detachment could not be raised a smaller section could be assigned to a neighbouring organisation. This was particularly the case with men's units where only a few volunteers came forward. It is thought a small section of men were initially assigned to Wilts 6 VAD and later joined men from nearby Corsham, registered as Wilts 3 VAD.

The structure was also strictly prescribed by the War Office.[2] When the Army Council published the Scheme for Voluntary Aid in 1909 it specified that a women's detachment should consist of 23 qualified members:[3]

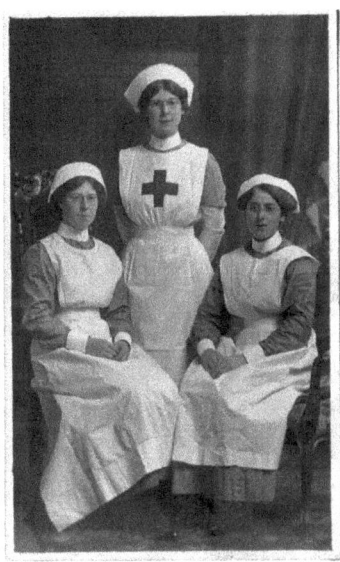

Whole families would join the Red Cross. The three Hunt sisters from Calne all became VADs.

A Commandant (Man or Woman)
Quartermaster (Man or Woman)
Lady Superintendent (A trained nurse)
Twenty women, of which four should be qualified in cooking.

Male detachments were far larger, consisting of 56 members:[4]

---

1 *The Story of British VAD work in the Great War* - Thekla Bowser
2 The British red Cross Society – Information sheet: *Volunteering during the First World War*. The only relaxation was for a short time in August 1914, when uncertified, untrained, members were accepted as 'special service probationers.'–.
3 *The Story of British VAD work in the Great War* - Thekla Bowser
4 *The Story of British VAD work in the Great War* - Thekla Bowser

Unity and Loyalty

A Commandant
Medical officer
Quartermaster
Pharmacist
Four section leaders
48 orderlies (4 sections of 12 men)

Initially members were free to make their own decision regarding the wearing of a uniform. Some chose a military style, while others a nursing style. A number of detachments decided against a uniform as it was felt the cost would deter less well-off members from joining. In March 1911 the Red Cross Council decided it was unacceptable to continue with this unstructured approach and prescribed a uniform, where the members could be easily recognised, but would not appear too military in style.[1]

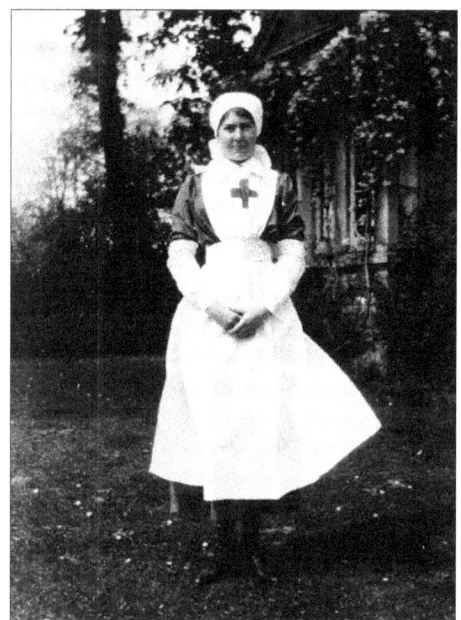

A Chippenham VAD in indoor uniform

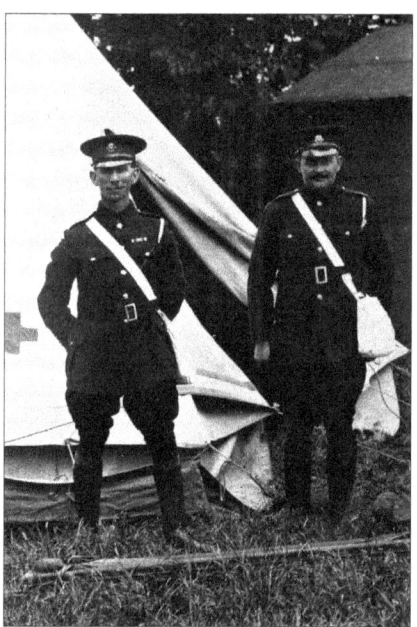

Men's Detachment uniform

The standard uniform consisted of:

Women's Detachments
Dark blue rough serge overcoat
Dark Blue peaked cap, with badge
Light blue dress in oxford material, dark blue for Quartermaster and trained nurses, red for Commandant

1   *The British Red Cross in Action* – Dame Beryl Oliver.

The Story of Chippenham's Red Cross Hospital

White linen collar and cuffs
Sister Dora cap
Apron with pockets and Red Cross on bib (it appears this was not always worn)
Black belt

The standardisation of uniform also differentiated the Red Cross from the Order of St John, who also had units in the area. The ladies of the Order of St John Nursing Division could be recognised by their uniform of light grey dresses.[1]

Men's Detachment
Dark Blue service cap with badge
Dark Blue serge Norfolk Tunic with belt
Strap and buckle, breeches and puttees

The VADs in Society

IN AUGUST 1909, when the Scheme for Voluntary Aid was announced, the Red Cross was inundated with enquiries from women wishing to join the VAD far exceeding the expectations of the County branches. The reasons for this enthusiasm are many, but may in part be explained by the social and political attitudes of the early twentieth century.

Most of the women who were interested in joining the VAD were the wives and daughters of men in business and the professional classes. They had a relatively leisured but ordered life,[2] not that much different to that of their Victorian grandmothers. They were expected to support their husbands and run the household. Mrs Beeton's Household Management, first published fifty years earlier, still gave advice on manners, how the household should be run and how to deal with servants. The guide 'Etiquette and Entertaining' by Lucie Heath Armstrong in 1913 gave strict advice for the mistress of the house on how to entertain and behave, even dictating when it was appropriate to visit friends.

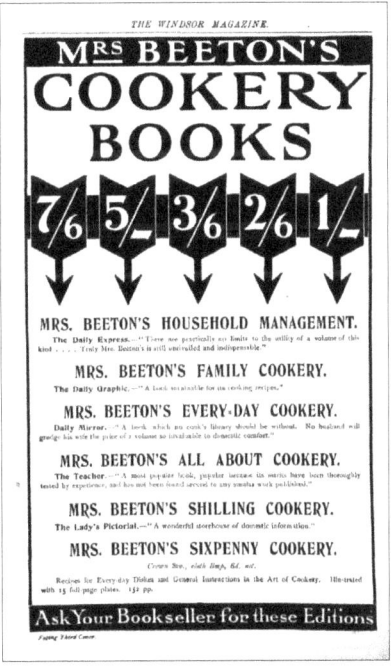

Mrs Beeton's Household Management advertised in 1910 telling the reader Mrs Beeton's is still unrivalled and indispensable

1   *The Story of British VAD work in the Great War* - Thekla Bowser
2   *Great War Britain, The First World War at Home* – Lucinda Gosling

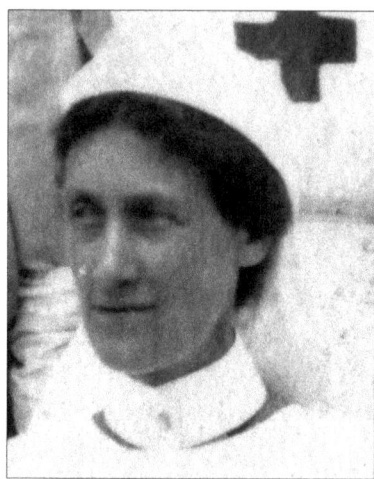
Kate Hinton

Married women were not expected to work, but it was usual that they should be involved in benevolent works and sit on boards of charitable organisations, such as, the Church Missionary Society and the Waifs and Strays Society. Some women in Chippenham were interested in the Cottage Hospital and became members of the Ladies Committee, raising money and organising fetes.

The Scheme for Voluntary Aid was an interesting alternative for those who were keen to step out of their routine lives. Voluntary Aid was socially acceptable and seen as 'good work'. At the same time it offered an element of independence and the opportunity to train and gain qualifications. Some ladies even talked of voluntary aid being their work.

For those with an interest in medicine this was an opportunity to get involved. Nancy Briscoe and Helena Wilson were both the wives of doctors and had some medical knowledge. Kate Hinton, the wife of the headmaster of Ivy Lane School, held a lifelong ambition to become a nurse, but her family had persuaded her it was not appropriate. Joining the Detachment fulfilled her ambition and when the Red Cross Hospital opened in 1915, with several years' experience in the VAD, she was appointed a Staff Nurse.[1]

Emma Hulbert, the wife of Francis Hulbert, a successful builder and plumber who employed a number of workers in the town, joined the VAD in 1910.

The Hulbert's employed a servant, a young woman called Margaret Tanner who looked after the household and the children enabling Emma, who had been a District Nurse before she married, to devote her time to VAD work. In 1915 she became a Ward Sister and later Assistant Superintendent.

The VADs offered excitement at outdoor camps, particularly when on exercise with the Territorials, and the opportunity to train in useful skills, although some didn't take it as seriously as they might and saw voluntary aid simply as part of their social calendar. Vera Brittain, in her book Testament of Youth describes how representatives of 'the set' would attend classes but only came to listen to gossip.

VADs and Politics

VOLUNTARY AID WAS also an opportunity to show a patriotic spirit and a number of political groups championed this new role for women.

[1] *Wiltshire Family History Society magazine July 2003* Article by Susan Mole about her Grandmother Kate Hinton

The Story of Chippenham's Red Cross Hospital

The Women's Local Government Society[1] was founded by a group of liberals and suffragettes, who believed that women should be allowed to play a greater part in political life. The Society had gained many influential supporters including Lady Frances Balfour, sister in law of MP Arthur Balfour, and the author Elizabeth Haldane, sister of the Secretary of State for War. Elizabeth Haldane was also a member of the Territorial Nursing Council.

In June 1910 the Society held a Women's Congress where a whole day was dedicated to General Nursing and Voluntary Aid.

The speakers included the Duchess of Montrose, President of the Scottish Branch of the Red Cross Society and Vice-President of the Advisory Committee of the Territorial Nursing Society. Mrs Bedford Fenwick, Chairwoman of the Matrons Council and Editor of the British Nursing Journal and Lady Helen Munro Ferguson,[2] who spoke fervently about the Scheme for Voluntary Aid saying: '... the Red Cross Society offered women the only opportunity they could have to take an effective part in national defence'.

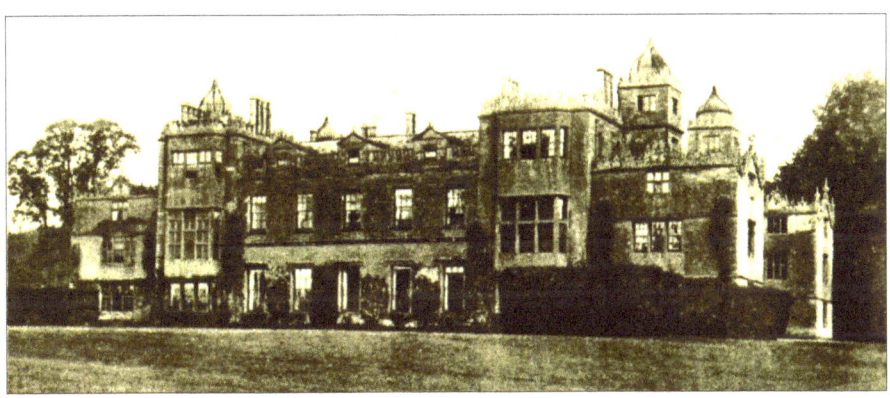

Charlton Park, near Malmesbury, home of the Earl of Suffolk, where a VAD recruiting meeting was held in 1913

In 1913 Lady Suffolk of nearby Charlton Park opened her home to the Red Cross recruiting meeting for a detachment in Malmesbury. One of the speakers said:[3] 'It is the first time in the history of England that women had been asked openly to take their share in this great work in defence of the nation'.

The introduction of the Scheme for Voluntary Aid in 1909 coincided with growth of the Suffrage movement. In June 1908 a demonstration, organised by the National Union of Women's Suffrage Societies, in Hyde Park was attended by 250,000 people from around Britain, one of the largest-ever political rallies in London.[4] For some who

1 The Women's Local Government Society (also called the Society for Promoting Women as County Councillors) was founded in the late 1880s by Annie Leigh Browne.
2 Founder of the Australian branch of the Red Cross.
3 *Devizes and Wiltshire Gazette* - 20 February 1913
4 British Library- Collection resource - *Votes for Women* www.bl.uk/votes-for-women

Unity and Loyalty

joined the Scheme for Voluntary Aid there was some empathy with the emancipation movement. Certainly, there were VADs who were also members of the Suffrage Movement. At a suffrage camp in Weymouth some of the members, who were also VADs, used the skills they had learned in open air cookery and tent pitching to give classes to the suffragettes.[1]

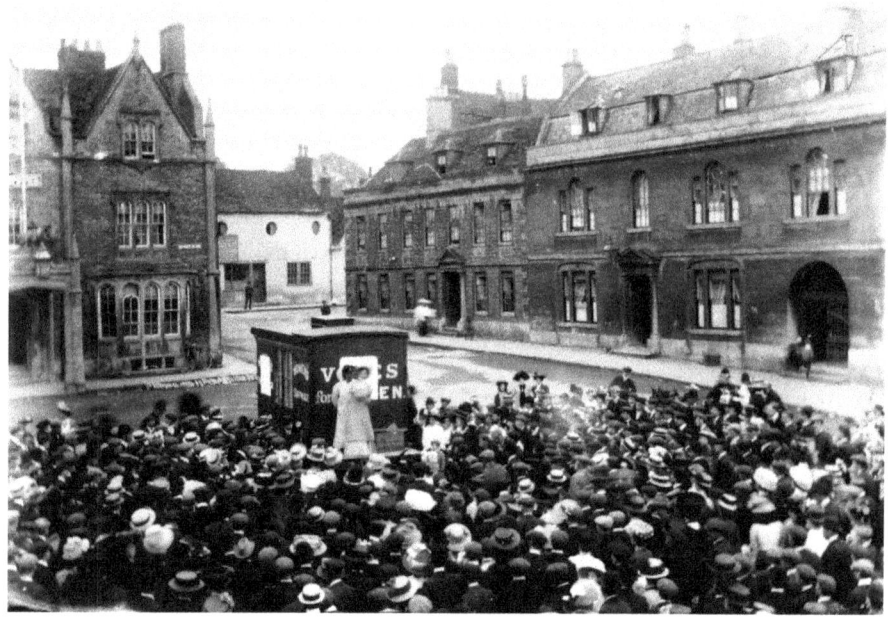

Suffragettes in Chippenham Market place

The Red Cross response to the Suffrage Movement, particularly activists, varied around the country. Sympathy relied on the view of the County Committee. In 1912 a question was put to the Secretary of State for War asking why, in one Detachment a lady guilty of a minor crime in support of the Women's Social and Political Union[2] was struck off the Red Cross register, while elsewhere a lady who had been arrested six times and imprisoned three times remained an active member of her Detachment.[3]

Locally Maud Hardiman, the daughter of Chippenham VAD Ellen Hardiman, was accused of criminal damage in Corsham in support of the Suffrage Movement.[4]

The opinion of those in the Chippenham area are not known, but there are reports of suffragettes not being welcomed in the town and escorted by the police from the meeting halls, whereas in neighbouring Corsham there was a warmer welcome.

1 *Wiltshire Times* – 13 June 1914
2 Emmeline Pankhurst and her daughters Christabel and Sylvia had founded the Women's Social and Political Union (WSPU) in Manchester in 1903.
3 *Hansard* - House of Commons debate 05 August 1912
4 Information from Peter Hayes, grandson of Maud Hardiman

The Working Class

THE SCHEME FOR Voluntary Aid naturally appealed to ladies from the middle and upper social classes: women who had time to take part in training and could afford to buy their own uniforms.

There were attempts to attract the wife of the working man. At recruiting meetings, it was pointed out that the commitment in time and money was relatively small and initially uniform was optional. To further attract the lower classes concessions were offered, for example, in 1911 the Vice President of the Bath and District Red Cross wrote to the local paper:[1]

> It is proposed to start first aid classes as soon as sufficient numbers of volunteers are enrolled. They will be arranged to suit the candidates in afternoon or evening classes and will be followed by home nursing classes. It is calculated that each course will cost from 5s to 8s a head, but it is hoped that those who cannot afford this will not be prevented from offering their services, as Red Cross funds are available to help.

Despite this, very few working-class women came forward. The idea of a servant working alongside her mistress as an equal was unthinkable and the working-class woman with a home and family had plenty enough to do without considering voluntary work.

The Scheme for Voluntary Aid assumed an invasion could disrupt transport links. Voluntary Aid Detachments needed to be prepared to use improvised farm carts and railway wagons as emergency transport and modify buildings as temporary shelters and hospitals.[2] The ideal candidate was the working-class man, especially builders, carpenters and engineers who had the skill and experience to take on the challenges asked of him. Despite this explanation and the clear link to the defence of the nation most men rejected the Scheme for Voluntary Aid.

For the working man there was a more exciting opportunity to show his patriotism, he need only look at the Territorials to see a proper uniform that gained respect and the excitement of shooting practice and military training. There was a further reason why men rejected Voluntary Aid. Doubts were being raised about the value of the Scheme and there was a growing suggestion the men and women of the detachments, were wasting their time.[3]

Ridicule and doubt about Voluntary Aid

KATHERINE FURSE, A leading member of the VAD movement wrote in 1917 that in the early days of the movement men and women volunteers were all faced with a good

---

1   *Bath Chronicle*-25 November 1911 letters to the editor.
2   *The Times* - 15 October 1909.
3   *The Story of British VAD work in the Great War* - Thekla Bowser

Unity and Loyalty

deal of ridicule and chaff from friends. She said members were always being asked why they prepared for what would never come, referring to the debate regarding the likelihood of invasion.

Even Lord Radnor, the chairman of the County Territorial Association, speaking in 1911 at Wilton, near Salisbury, raised doubts about the continuing need for a Territorial Force after the Admiralty announced the Territorial Force was not needed as an invasion would never happen.[1]

Equally, Voluntary Aid was not popular with the medical profession. It was suggested that those joining the Voluntary Aid Detachment simply wanted an excuse to wear a uniform and take part in parades and socialise. Some said voluntary aid was playing at nursing and ambulance work and would be of no help to the sick and wounded and, worse, be a hindrance should there be an invasion. A typical letter to the British Journal of Nursing in 1910 commented:[2]

> The fact of having five lectures on First Aid and a similar number on Home Nursing, however well given, will be of little value to the people without the special knowledge necessary for the management of temporary hospitals in time of war

For middle and upper class women this ridicule and doubt was ignored and they continued to come forward to form detachments.

The Order of St John of Jerusalem

TO ATTRACT MEN in Chippenham the Commandant, Mr Marshall, turned to groups of workers in the town who already received first aid training as part of their employment.

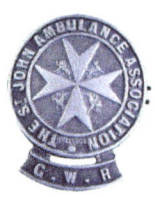

St John Ambulance badge worn by trained GWR workers

Since the late 1870s the Order of St John of Jerusalem Ambulance Association had been providing first aid training in the railway, engineering and mining industries.[3] These were dangerous environments and there was great emphasis, especially on the railways, to have well trained and prepared workers to deal with accidents. In Chippenham both Great Western Railway and the engineering company of Saxby and Farmer had a First Aid Training Programme and Ambulance Units: these men were considered ideal candidates for voluntary aid work as they had practical and engineering skills.

In February 1910 Mr Marshall was a guest at a Great Western Railway, Ambulance Award ceremony held in the first-class waiting room at Chippenham Station.

---

1 *Exeter and Plymouth Gazette* - 20 February 1911
2 *The British Nursing Journal* - 16 April 1910
3 *The Order of the Hospital of St. John of Jerusalem* - H. W. Fincham

The Story of Chippenham's Red Cross Hospital

Following the presentations, he gave a speech congratulating the recipients and explained how he hoped to raise a Voluntary Aid Detachment in the town that would be ready to help the territorial forces. He told the railwaymen:[1] 'I would be pleased to enrol all the men present and with their help Chippenham Detachment would be as good as any in the country'.

Some months later, in November 1910, there was a further award ceremony at the railway station where George Terrell, the Member of Parliament for Chippenham, presented certificates to the railway workers. He pressed the point that what they had studied as part of their employment would be equally useful should there be an invasion:[2]

...this ambulance work is one of many branches of voluntary work. The St John Ambulance Association proved its value in times of peace where its members rendered practical help in cases of accident and in time of war to help the wounded and distressed.

Minutes of the Great Western Ambulance Committee, July 1913. Ambulance training was provided by St John Ambulance

Very few railwaymen came forward, but amongst those receiving certificates that day were railway porter Edwin Duck and ticket collector Walter Archard, who five years later would volunteer for ambulance duty when the first injured men arrived in Chippenham.

The local constabulary were also approached to support Voluntary Aid Work. Constables were fully trained in first aid and had practical experience of dealing with injured members of the public. Regular St John Ambulance classes were held in at the police station in New Road, where Dr Briscoe presented the lectures.

Superintendent Henry Moore, of Chippenham Police, was particularly interested in Voluntary Aid and early in 1910, possibly after attending the Red Cross meeting in the

1   *North Wilts Herald* - 23 February 1910
2   *Devizes and Wiltshire Gazette* - 3 November 1910

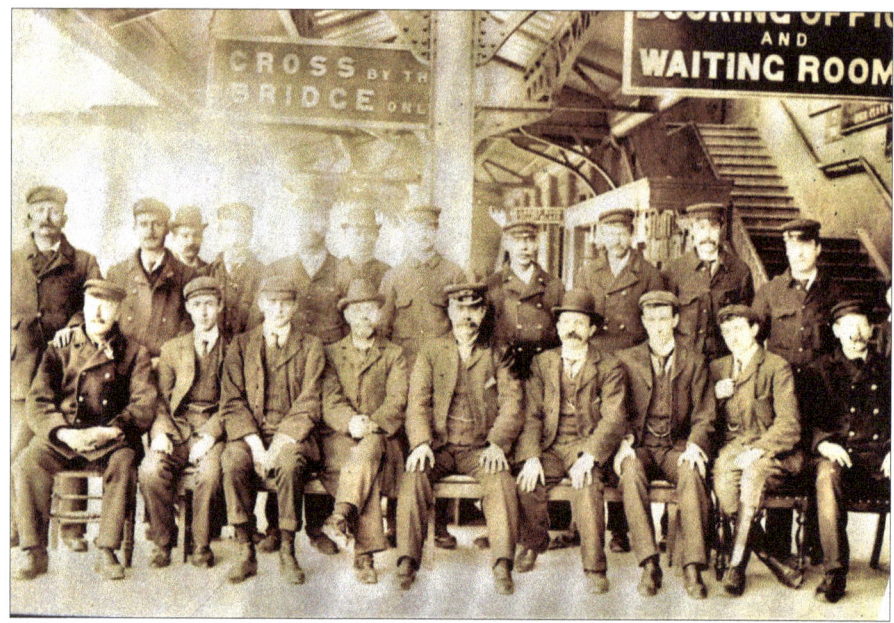

Group of railway workers at Chippenham Station

Town Hall, he opened a public subscription to purchase an ambulance for the town.

Outside of London it was left to the police, the fire brigade or the patient's family to deal with the sick and injured and transport them to a hospital. The public subscription raised £17.16s, sufficient to purchase, from the St. John Ambulance Association, a two wheeled hand propelled stretcher, known as an Ashford Litter. [1]

In October 1910 Lady Muriel Coventry of Monkton House presented the ambulance at the police station in Chippenham.[2] It bore a brass plate with the inscription —'*This ambulance was purchased by the Chippenham Police for use in the Borough of Chippenham from funds raised by public subscriptions*'.

The ambulance was used regularly by the police in the town and used by VADs in their training exercises.

Despite Mr Marshall's efforts to gain members for a men's detachment there was little response. This was reflected in other towns and in April

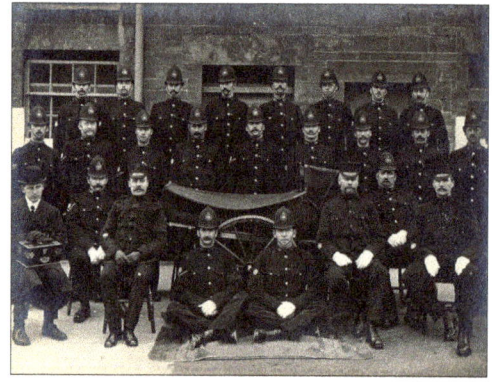

Police First Aid class with the Ashford Litter. Dr Briscoe who arranged the class is sat on the left wearing a bowler hat

1   Invented by John Furley of the St John Ambulance Association in the late nineteenth century.
2   *Devizes and Wiltshire Gazette* - 3 November 1910

The Story of Chippenham's Red Cross Hospital

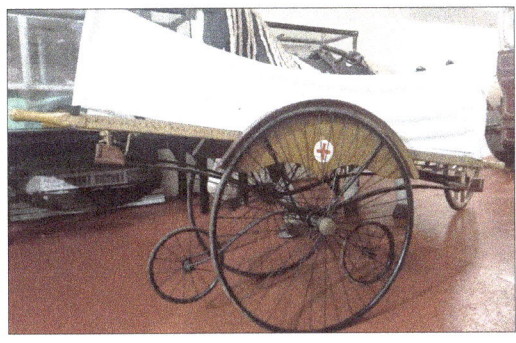
An Ashford Litter

1913 it was agreed that it was proving impossible to attract sufficient numbers of men for the needs of the County and the matter was referred to the County Territorial committee.[1]

Wiltshire wasn't alone in failing to attract men. Sir Edward Ridsdale, the Red Cross Chairman, appealed to prospective male volunteers. He spoke at a number of meetings throughout the country, where he highlighted to the prospective recruits, '....the knowledge acquired would be the greatest use to them in the ordinary accidents of civil life'.[2]

When the Scheme for Voluntary Aid was introduced in 1909 it was anticipated men already trained with St John Ambulance Association would come forward. Col. Sir Herbert Perrott, the Chief Secretary of the Association was fully in support of joint working with the Red Cross, he wrote in October 1909:[3]

> I have the pleasure to inform you that the Ambulance Department of the Order of St John of Jerusalem has made an arrangement with the War Office, and with the British Red Cross Society, that the St. John Ambulance Association should afford the preliminary instruction in first aid and home nursing to the Voluntary Aid Detachments.

This meant both organisations would work side by side and raise their own detachments. The St. John Ambulance Association, with their experience would take the lead forming Ambulance Detachments and the Territorial Ambulance Service. Men working on the railway and in industries, who had trained with the Order of St. John, would be encouraged to volunteer.

A few months later, in the spring of 1910, the Order of St. John distanced itself from the Territorial organisations and the Scheme for Voluntary Aid following increasing disagreement regarding standards of First Aid and Ambulance Training. This gulf between the two organisations was so significant a threat to Voluntary Aid that it was debated in the House of Lords. The Western Daily Press reported:[4]

Lord Lucas, (replying to the Earl of Dartmouth), said no one regretted more sincerely than the War Office that the St. John Ambulance Association had seen fit to express their inability to be further formally connected with the Voluntary Aid Scheme published by the War Office in 1909.

1   *Devizes and Wiltshire Gazette* - 1 May 1913
2   *Lichfield Mercury* - 9 May 1913, one of a number of speeches at county meetings.
3   *Western Daily Press* - 5 October 1909
4   *Western Daily Press* - 17 June 1910

The Wiltshire branch of the St John Association echoed this dispute in their Brigade Orders of 30 June 1910 which noted:[1] 'St John have withdrawn from the VAD scheme but will continue to provide training. Instead St John Ambulance companies to be organised to carry out transport of wounded'.

This meant that the St John Association would set up independent groups with no connection to the War Office organisation. The need to resolve the dispute was summed up by the Duchess of Devonshire[2] in October 1910 when she spoke to the Derbyshire branch of the Red Cross. 'It is very desirable that anything approaching friction between two such excellent institutions as the St John Association and the Red Cross Society should be avoided.'

Thekla Bowser, in her book the Story of the British VAD,[3] likened the two organisations to two great rivers, the Rhone and the Arve, 'flowing side by side for many miles without mingling'.

Within a year the friction between the organisations had moderated, but the damage had been done. In October 1912 the Wiltshire St John Brigade Orders[4] instructed that branches should once again use War Office numbering to align with the Voluntary Aid Scheme, but instructed that they remain independent and should not take part in Red Cross training exercises. There was some reconciliation when Miss Gorst, representing the Order of St John nursing division at Castle Combe, was invited to attend the Red Cross Wiltshire Voluntary Aid Organisation committee meeting in May 1913 at Trowbridge,[5] but the two organisations remained independent until October 1914.

Training

TRAINING WAS THE cornerstone of Voluntary Aid. The War Office had agreed a training syllabus with the Red Cross and the St. John Ambulance Association, but from 1910, after the disagreement between the societies, all training for Voluntary Aid Detachments was arranged through the Red Cross. The minimum standards for VADs, both men and women were a certificate in First Aid and Home Nursing.

In Chippenham training classes for women in First Aid and Home Nursing were presented by Doctors Wilson and Briscoe at various locations in the town, including the Drill Hall in Bath Road. Advertisements were placed in local papers giving dates for

---

1   Wiltshire and Swindon History Centre 2611/13 *Wilts St John Records Brigade Orders* 30 June 1910.
2   In 1914 the Duke of Devonshire offered the ground floor of Devonshire House in Piccadilly to the British Red Cross. It became the organisation's wartime headquarters.
3   *The Story of British VAD work in the Great War* - Thekla Bowser
4   Wiltshire and Swindon History Centre 2611/13 *Wilts St John Records Brigade Orders* October 1912
5   *Devizes and Wiltshire Gazette* - 1 May 1913

classes, a typical one in February 1913:[1]

> RED CROSS VAD (WOMEN) CHIPPENHAM. Classes commencing this month will be held on Wednesday afternoon and Thursday evening. Candidates must apply for information to the Commandant.

The VADs were encouraged to practise bandaging and Scouts were invited to join the classes and act as injured. Sometimes the VADs got over enthusiastic with their bandages and the boys were wrapped so tightly they couldn't move.

Detachments were also offered the opportunity to observe basic medical procedures and some were even given practical experience in wards. At the Royal United Hospital in Bath training sessions for VADs took place regularly. To protect the sensibilities of the ladies physical contact was kept to minimum and certainly when dealing with wounded men they were told:[2]

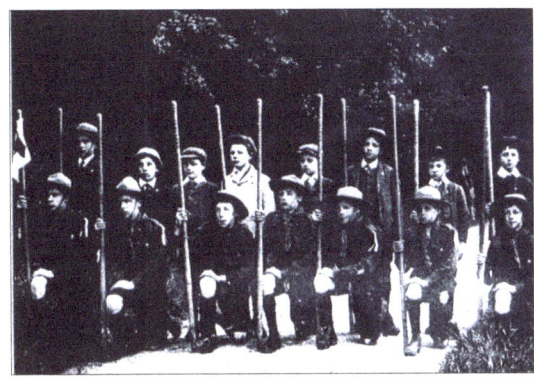

A Scout troop from Castle Combe

> ... your ministrations to soldiers would be restricted to hands and feet only.

In addition to First Aid and Home Nursing the VADs needed to learn about cooking, laundry and cleaning, particularly the importance of maintaining sanitary conditions when establishing temporary accommodation for hospitals.

The Scheme for Voluntary Aid described the skills in which the VADs needed to be proficient:[3]

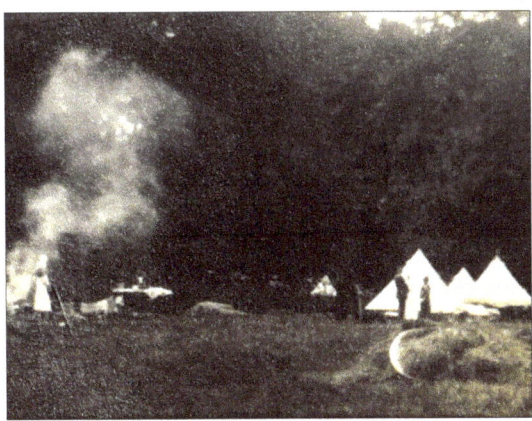

Wiltshire VAD camp. Training included cooking over open fires.

cooking suitable for the sick and wounded, improvising cooking facilities in temporary rest stations in the field and sewing and mending of soldier's clothes and hospital bedding.

1   *Devizes and Wiltshire Gazette* -13 February 1913.
2   *The Royal United Hospital 1747-1947* – Kate Clarke
3   *The Times* - 15 October 1909

For many of the ladies of the middle and upper classes these were totally new subjects. They had spent their lives relying on servants to look after daily domestic chores. One VAD summed it up when she wrote in her diary:[1]

I was much interested in the work and, having three servants, I could devote much of my leisure to practise.

Joan Money–Kyrle, who lived at Whetham near Calne, in a house with eight servants, described in her diary of 1914[2] how she took classes in bandaging and found learning domestic chores fascinating: 'I went up to the laundry and helped Mrs Street iron. She taught us all about it. Such fun! '

The preparation of food for wounded men or homeless refugees was an essential part of VAD work and classes were part of the curriculum. Matilda Talbot, of Lacock Abbey, was a professional and highly qualified cookery instructor and gave cookery classes to VADs. In her book about her life at Lacock[3] she describes how she trained young women in the art of cooking. She said there were young girls who had obviously never been inside a kitchen in their lives. One particular girl, when asked to clean and prepare potatoes, asked for some soap to wash them.

The quality of training for cooks varied greatly between detachments, as did the interpretation of a qualified cook. To ensure an acceptable standard in food preparation the Red Cross published the booklet 'Cooking notes for V A Cooks' in February 1913.

The booklet recognised the shortcomings of many members in its introduction: 'In very few cases can it be said that Detachment Cooks are competent to perform the highly responsible duties which might be theirs in the event of mobilisation'.

It went on to specify the criteria expected for a qualified cook and gave instruction on diet and menus. It also reminded cooks that they should be prepared to improvise, including adapting for work in the field using a primus stove or open fire.

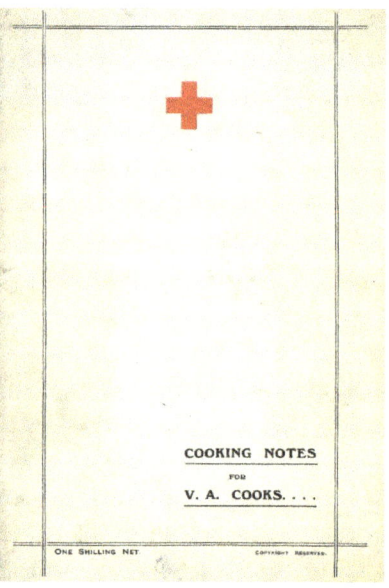

Cooking Notes for VA Cooks

---

1. *East Anglian Daily Times* - 14 April 2014. An article about VADS and Woodbridge Grammar School in 1913.
2. Wiltshire and Swindon Archive - 1720/720 *Diaries of Joan Money-Kyrle*
3. *My life and Lacock Abbey* – Matilda Talbot

The Story of Chippenham's Red Cross Hospital

Territorial exercises

HAVING UNDERTAKEN THE requisite training, the Chippenham ladies were eager to make use of their new-found skills. During the summer months they joined the men of the Territorials to act out sham battles at the practice ground at Westmead. VADs would set up tents and use farm wagons as makeshift hospital wards to treat the wounded and Boy Scouts were recruited to act as injured.

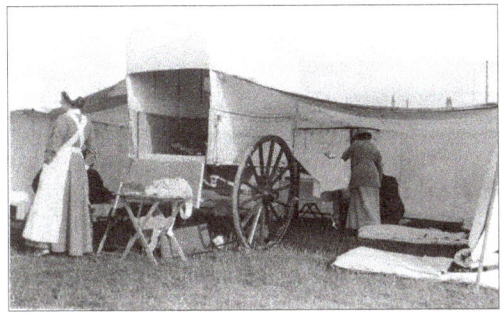

A typical VAD camp at a training exercise

The Territorials also arranged larger exercises with neighbouring units. The South Midland Artillery Brigade and the Bristol Battalion of the Gloucester Regiment visited Chippenham on a Saturday afternoon in February 1914 for a tactical exercise.[1] No doubt the local VADs were mobilised to practise their field kitchen skills and provide refreshments.

The War Office arranged exercises for Territorial troops on Salisbury Plain. In August 1911 the Wiltshire Times[2] reported that several Voluntary Aid Detachments from the area had joined the Territorials. Regiments from around the country took part in a series of mock battles over a number of days and the VADs were camped at Tidworth to deal with the wounded.

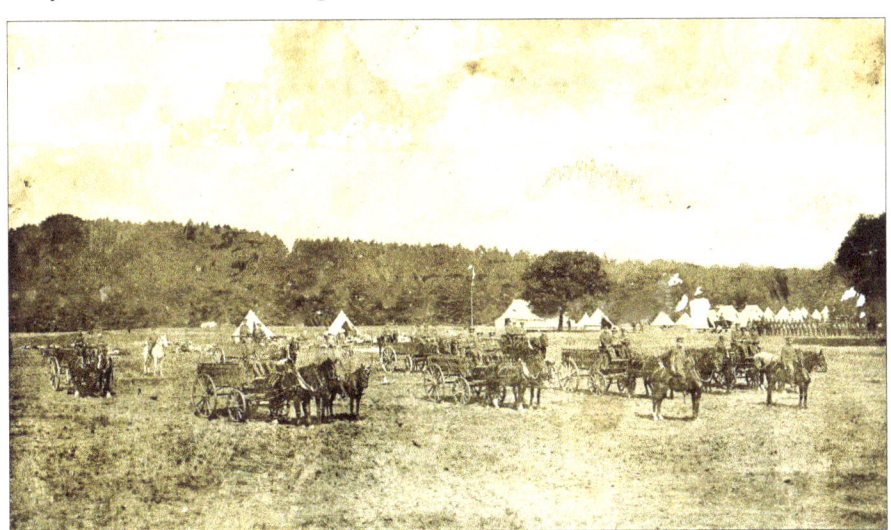

Wiltshire Territorials on Salisbury Plain

1   *Western Daily Press* – 23 February 1914
2   *Wiltshire Times* - 12 August 1911

Unity and Loyalty

To make the battle as realistic as possible for the VADs there were *'instructional displays'* creating wartime scenarios.[1] One such session included transporting sick and wounded, using improvised farm wagons, to the nearest railway station at West Lavington, near Devizes, where a specially prepared GWR carriage was ready to receive wounded.

Camps were essential training for the VADs and were thoroughly enjoyed by the members. Thekla Bowser wrote about detachments in the years before the War:[2]

Detachments would make tremendous efforts to go into camp for a week or a fortnight during the summer, when they lived the real camp life, cooking in field kitchens, building their own field incinerators and improvising hospital and transport equipment out of the most unpromising material.

The VAD training was tested at Easter 1912 when a member of one of the Wiltshire detachments used her first aid knowledge to save a life.

Sixteen year old Walter Giffard, the son of magistrate Henry Giffard, of Lockridge House near Marlborough, was out shooting pigeons when he stumbled and the gun discharged. Luckily, he was with one of his sisters who had recently undertaken a course of ambulance training as a VAD. She was able to treat the injury and stem the bleeding until surgical aid was available.[3] Unfortunately, Walter's foot could not be saved, but the surgeons said his sister's actions saved his life.

May Giffard continued as a VAD and when war broke out she served at a hospital in Kent. In 1916 she transferred to the Military Hospital in Egypt, where she remained as a nurse until April 1919. She was mentioned in dispatches for her service during the War.[4]

1 *Devizes and Wiltshire Gazette* - 20 February 1913.
2 *The Story of British VAD work in the Great War* - Thekla Bowser
3 *Western Daily Press* - 12 April 1912
4 The British Red Cross Society - VAD index card record

Chapter 3
1913

THE LADIES OF Wiltshire gather at Bowood House for a Red Cross Rally where they test their skills should an invasion occur. Boy Scouts are recruited to help with ambulance duties as there is a serious shortage of men interested in taking part in Voluntary Aid. There are complaints about the organisation of the Red Cross in Wiltshire and changes are proposed.

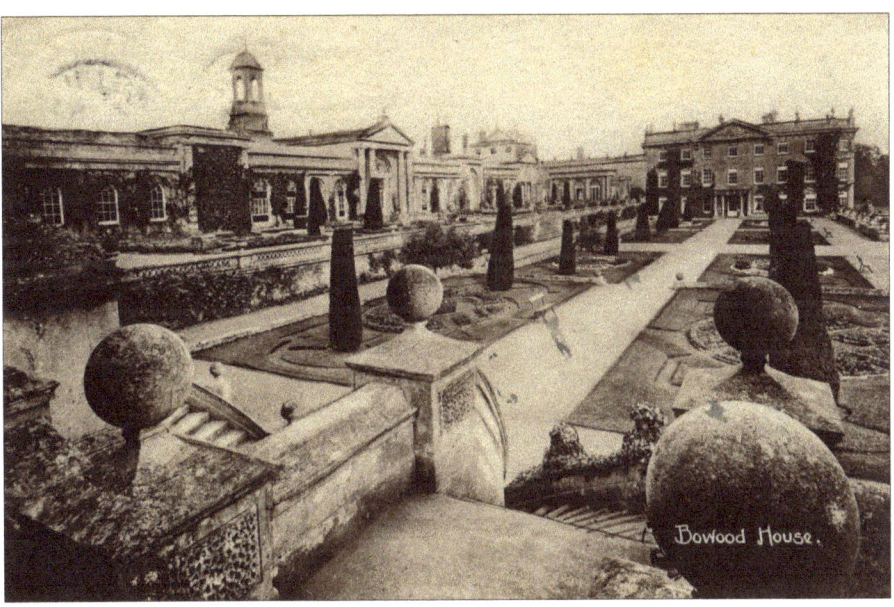

Bowood House the home of Lady Lansdowne the President of the Wiltshire Red Cross

Musical entertainment

THE YEAR 1913 opened in Chippenham with a production of Gilbert and Sullivan's HMS Pinafore by the Chippenham Amateur Operatic and Dramatic Society.[1] A few weeks later the Chippenham Sports, Operatic and Dramatic Society[2] gave a performance

1   *Wiltshire Times* - 25 January 1913
2   *Wiltshire Times* – 19 April 1913

Unity and Loyalty

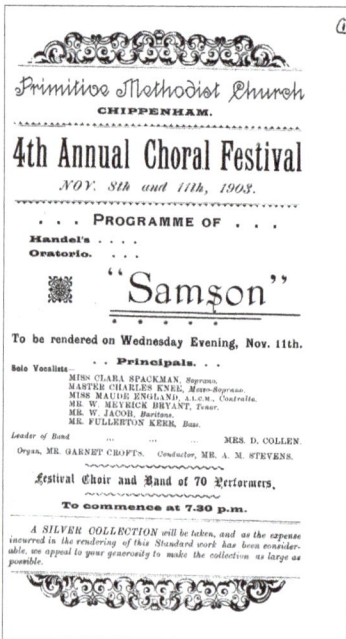

A Choral Festival in Chippenham in 1903. Florence Collen, the leader of the band and Mr Bryant's wife both joined the VAD

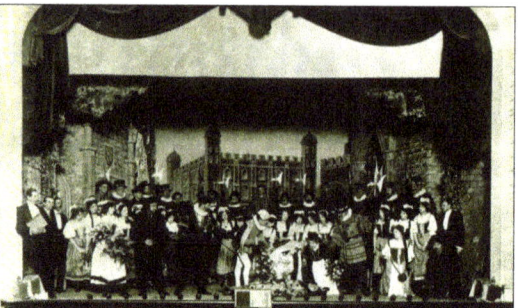

A production of the Yeoman of the Guard performed in Chippenham

of the Yeoman of the Guard. The proceeds from the shows were donated to local causes, often to the Cottage Hospital.

These amateur theatrical productions and musical events such as Choral Festivals were extremely popular. The performers were local people and some, like Elinor Davis, the wife of the head postmaster in the town, were extremely accomplished musicians who were in great demand around the district.

A number of ladies from the musical societies were also members of the Voluntary Aid Detachment. Performing alongside Elinor Davis was Evelyn Belcher an accomplished pianist and the secretary of the Operatic and Dramatic Society.[1] The cast of the musical Snow White and the Three Bears in 1912[2] included the Shipp family, the Hiscock sisters and Nellie Pike. All these ladies were associated with the Red Cross and became workers at the Hospital after it opened in 1915.

The calendars complemented each other, musical productions and rehearsal tended to be for the autumn and winter and with the better weather VAD practice, often outdoors took place. Of course, this wasn't a strict division and VAD meetings were also held in the in the winter where they practised bandaging and took first aid classes.

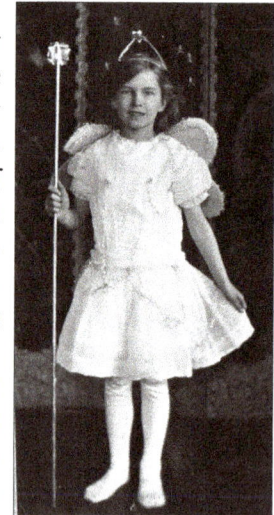

One of the Hiscock sisters in costume. Several years later they would entertain the wounded at the hospital.

1   Chippenham Museum - *Garlick Scrapbooks*
2   *Wiltshire Times* – 12 February 1912

Red Cross Rally

With the Chippenham Detachment established, Lionel Marshall stepped down from his role as Commandant and Maud Long, wife of Major Robert Long, replaced him. Her tenure was short lived and by the end of 1912 she had also stepped down.

To replace her Helena Wilson, the wife of Doctor Mervyn Wilson, the medical officer for Castle Combe and Chippenham, was appointed as Commandant at the beginning of the 1913.

Helena Wilson was well qualified for the role: she was well known in Chippenham and for many years had administered her husband's medical practice. Her knowledge of medical matters and her administration skills would prove invaluable for the smooth running of the Detachment in Chippenham.

Mrs Wilson, with other commandants in the County, realised that the VADs needed to test their skills in a realistic setting. The territorial exercises had been useful, but often the VADs were used merely to provide refreshments for the men training for battle.

The members of the detachments needed their own exercise to prove their skills and therefore the Wiltshire Red Cross Committee decided to arrange a rally; where the Voluntary Aid Detachments could be inspected and demonstrate their proficiency in a realistic battle environment.

In August 1913 the Marchioness of Lansdowne opened her Bowood House home to the Calne, Chippenham, Devizes, Pewsey and Marlborough Detachments.

Representatives of the Royal Army Medical Corps (RAMC) and the County Red Cross Committee were invited to inspect and judge the competitions.[1]

Mr H Herbert Smith was in charge of proceedings and had arranged for the grounds of the house to be set as the scene of a fictional battle between invading forces and defending Territorials. To add to the realism a number of tents had been erected to receive

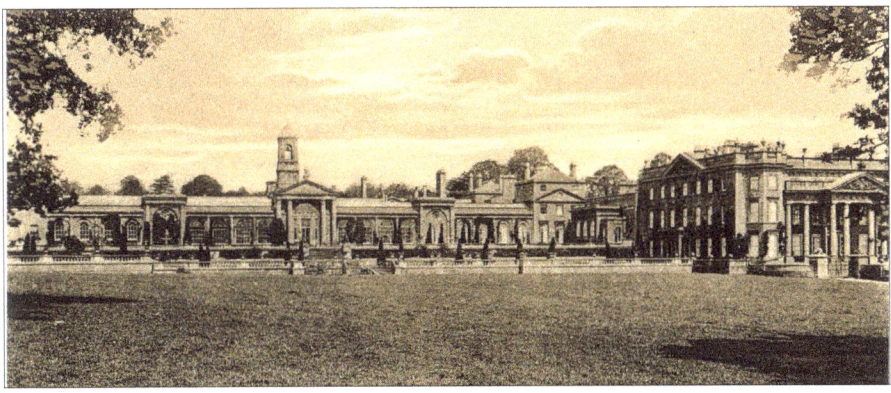

The House and grounds of Bowood where the VADs treated wounded during a mock battle

1   *Wiltshire Times* - 9 August 1913

the wounded with the stables and outbuildings of the estate serving as a temporary Base Hospital, which included facilities for a makeshift operating theatre.

The VADs and guests arrived during the morning and at midday 130 people were served a meal of stew prepared by Devizes Detachment who, in keeping with the spirit of exercise, cooked outdoors over open fires. Following the meal the volunteers paraded in their detachments and were inspected by Lady Lansdowne and Captain Ainsworth of the RAMC.

In the afternoon the imaginary battle started and hostilities were described as raging fiercely with the injured, in reality inmates drawn from the Devizes Workhouse, stretchered from the battlefield. Pewsey was the only group who could muster a male section for ambulance service on the day and 26 men reported for duty. This was too few to deal with numbers of casualties on the battlefield and the local Boy Scout troops were also invited to join in.

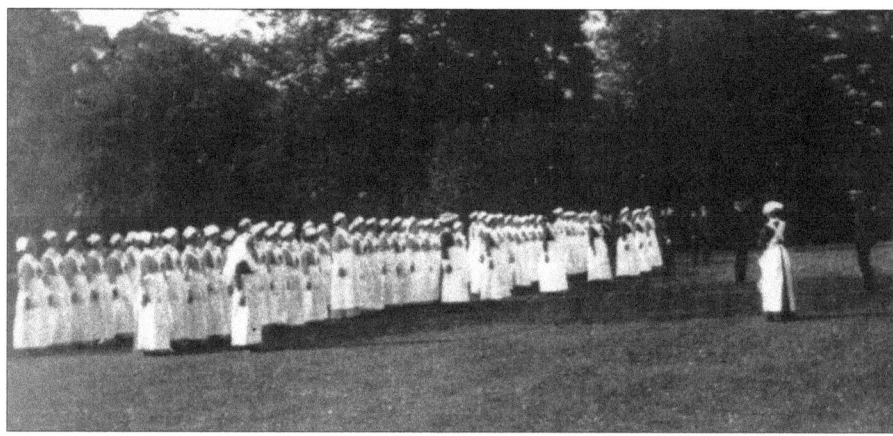

VADs on parade, though to be at Bowood. Chippenham Detachment are in the centre

The Boy Scouts, who were considered part of the Defence Force, were first aid trained and would regularly assist at Red Cross VAD demonstrations. At Bowood the Chippenham troop, under Scoutmaster Spinke,[1] took on stretcher duties and had designed an ingenious vehicle for transporting stretchers using bicycles.

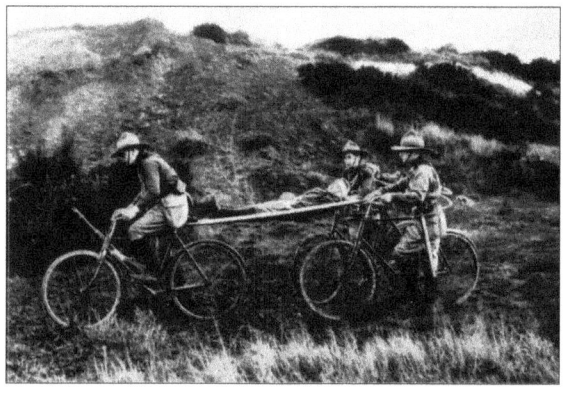

Scouts transporting a patient

1   Thought to be 27-year-old William Spinke, brother of Daisy and Beatrice who were members of the Voluntary Aid Detachment.

The Story of Chippenham's Red Cross Hospital

Several of the detachments were assigned to the outbuildings of Bowood House, where the medical and surgical wards received a steady flow of injured from the field station. Chippenham were allocated to one of the field stations: a series of tents, where as well as assessing and treating wounds they were responsible for preparing the more seriously injured for evacuation. Amongst the ladies from Chippenham were Mrs Wilson, the Commandant, Miss Green the Lady Superintendent and Dorothy Brinkworth who in October 1914 would serve at Corsham Hospital as Quartermaster.

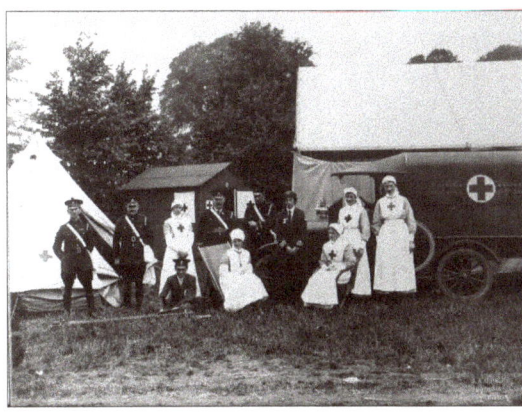

A typical field station

As well as tending to wounds, the Chippenham Detachment were responsible for feeding the patients as they waited. Cooking was carried out under canvas, following the guidelines set out in the pamphlet *Cooking Notes for VA Cooks*. The four cooks for the day were Mrs Shipp, of Cadenham Manor, Foxham; Mrs Sarah Hetherington, whose husband owned a tailoring business in the High Street in Chippenham; Mrs Isobel Garne of Lanhill in Chippenham, who like Dorothy Brinkworth would see service at Corsham Hospital; and Miss Ellen Cornish of The Comedy at Christian Malford.

At the end of the day's proceedings Lady Lansdowne provided tea in a marquee in front of the house where prizes were given and speeches were made declaring the event a complete success and that it was gratifying to see such a display which showed the public how beneficial the work was for the nation.

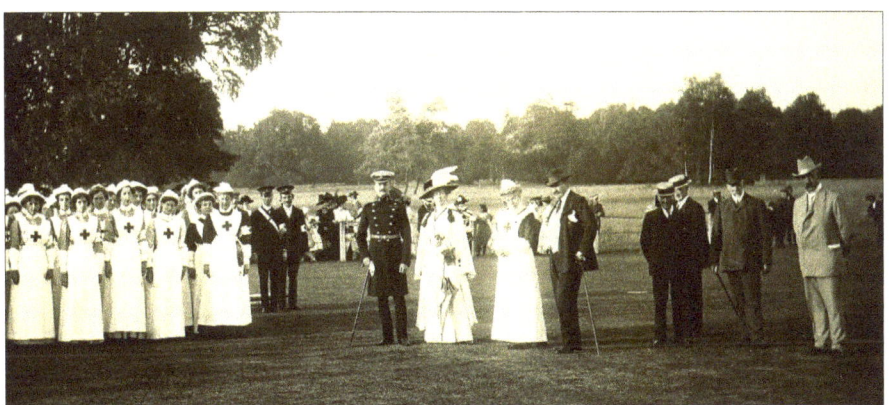

A prize giving and inspection at a Red Cross VAD exercise

Unity and Loyalty

Interest in Voluntary Aid declines

ALTHOUGH THE BOWOOD day was seen as a success the number of new detachments being registered in the county by 1913 was described as disappointing. Since the initial eagerness in 1910 interest had gradually waned and it was reported that Wiltshire was falling behind other counties.[1]

To reinvigorate interest a meeting of the Red Cross Director and Commandants of the Wiltshire detachments was held in Trowbridge. The positive note from the Commandants was that training courses were going well, but the enthusiasm of new members had faltered and many had either not completed their training or decided to leave the Red Cross.

There were a number of reasons why new volunteers felt disillusioned with the Red Cross and Voluntary Aid. One complaint was the lack of equipment and the inadequate funds allocated by the County Committee. In some detachments the members had to buy their own bandages and splints to complete their training.

A further issue was the confused instructions and procedures given to volunteers in the county. There was no handbook to guide the members and each detachment set its own standards.

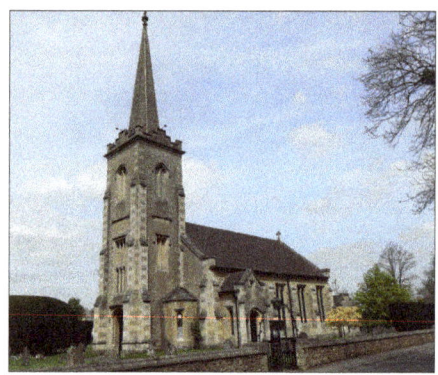

Derry Hill Church

The biggest problem, however was that much of the day to day organisation and decision making was left to the County Director. A new County Director, Colonel Fletcher, appointed during 1913, stated at a Red Cross County meeting that he did not have the time and energy to fully support the organisation. He simply had too much work to do. As a result it was agreed that changes to the Wiltshire Red Cross procedures and organisation were urgently needed to retain volunteers and share the work in the county more evenly.

Colonel Walter Fletcher[2] had taken over as County Director earlier in the 1913, when Mr H Herbert Smith stood down due to ill health and took on lighter duties as the secretary to the Chippenham and Calne Detachments.

Henry Herbert Smith's health had been failing for some time and he died at his home, Buckhill on the Bowood Estate, on 19 October 1913.

The Joint Voluntary Aid Committee, the County Red Cross Committee and Chippenham and Calne Detachments all said what a good and faithful friend the Red Cross had lost. The funeral took place at Derry Hill and Chippenham and Calne VAD attended in full uniform.[3]

1   *Western Gazette* - 28 November 1913
2   Colonel Walter Blunt Fletcher, also secretary to Wiltshire Territorial Force Association.
3   *Devizes and Wiltshire Gazette* – 30 October 1913

Chapter 4
1914

IMPROVEMENTS ARE MADE in the organisation of the Red Cross in Wiltshire and more volunteers come forward. An inter- Detachment competition is held in Trowbridge. During the summer the VADs continue to practise First Aid and Home Nursing, little realising that war clouds are gathering, and they would soon be called to use their skills.

Nationally the Government is dealing with domestic problems and the increasing fear of Civil War in Ireland.

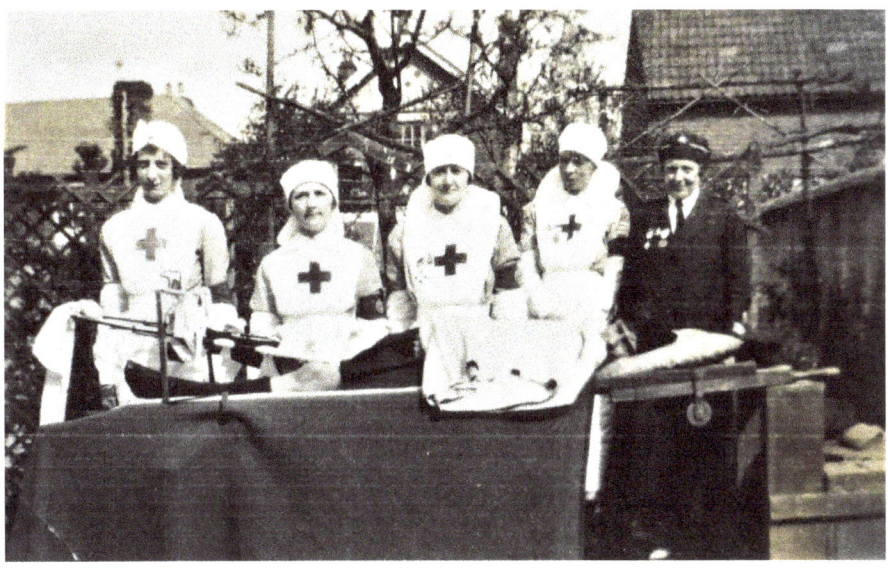

Wiltshire VADS training

Domestic Affairs

As 1914 OPENED the Government struggled with a number of domestic affairs. Suffragette agitation was becoming increasingly forceful and had escalated to acts of violence and damage to properties.

Unity and Loyalty

There was increasing militancy and industrial action by workers seeking better conditions and pay, including in June 1914, strikes by miners and transport workers. The Workers Union visited Chippenham in 1913 and held a recruiting meeting. Amongst those who joined was twenty year old Florence Hancock, who a few years later would take an active part in industrial action in the town to support two men who had been unfairly dismissed.[1]

Overshadowing both the Suffragettes and union activity was the increasingly controversial subject of self-government for Ireland. By 1914 tensions were such that both the Unionists and Nationalists in Ireland had raised military style units and political deals were being negotiated to avoid the very real fear of a Civil War.

The Wiltshire Gazette of July 1914 commented on the constantly changing situation in verse:[2]

> One page hints of Civil War, the next one speaks of peace.
> As it is all as clear as mud we then our reading cease
> Despite our angry protests, the papers aren't to blame
> It's simply due to Asquith who plays a shuffling game
> 'Wait and see' The Premier cries. He's a patient man forsooth.
> Ignoring us poor readers, who vainly seek the truth.

The Government of Ireland Act 1914, the Home Rule Bill, was passed and given Royal Assent on 18 September 1914, but due to the War was immediately suspended.[3]

In Chippenham sanitary conditions had been a priority for the Borough Council for some years. There were slum areas in the town and the drinking water was thought to be responsible for disease. A reservoir was built to provide improved water quality and new waste treatment works constructed.[4] In February 1914 the Town Clerk applied for a loan of £2460 to buy land in Wood Lane and erect 12 workmen's cottages to provide improved living standards.[5]

Red Cross improvements in the County

THE YEAR 1914 saw changes in the County Red Cross organisation. Following the meeting at Trowbridge in 1913, where the Red Cross Director and the Commandants of the Wiltshire detachments met to discuss necessary improvements, a number of recommendations were made to the County Committee to increase recruitment and

1 Chippenham Civic Society - *Dame Florence May Hancock 1893 – 1974*. Article by Donald Little.
2 *Devizes and Wiltshire Gazette* - 23 July 1914
3 www.parliament.uk – Living Heritage *Parliament and Ireland*.
4 *A History of Chippenham AD 853-1946* - Arnold Platts
5 *Chippenham Town Council minute book 8* - 3 February 1914

The Story of Chippenham's Red Cross Hospital

standards in the Voluntary Aid Detachments. A year later, in April 1914, the Director, Colonel Fletcher, was able to say the proposals had been adopted and gave a positive report to the County Committee.[1]

He said that, following discussion with the Central Committee of the Red Cross regarding the allocation of funds it was agreed the County were to retain a percentage of all subscriptions. This meant he could award grants to detachments and had already been able to help Malmesbury, Chippenham and Calne to buy equipment.

The question of setting common instructions had also been dealt with. A County Handbook had been issued that gave consistent guidance to members regarding training levels, frequency of meetings and the organisation of the Detachment. For new members an introductory pamphlet had been produced giving an outline of the Voluntary Aid Movement. Wiltshire was not alone in having suffered mixed standards between detachments. This was a national problem the War Office questioned the efficiency of Voluntary Aid Detachments in a number of districts around the country. Thekla Bowser in her book, The Story of the British VAD in the Great War told how:

Some Commandants were exceedingly up to date and earnest over their work... Other Detachments were content to meet occasionally for a medical lecture and scrape through the yearly inspection insisted upon by the War Office.

A report for the inspection of a Devon detachment in October 1913 highlighted the result of the lack of training when the inspector said:[2]

I was rather disappointed with regard to several members not knowing matters appertaining to the general organisation for carrying sick from the battlefield to the temporary hospital.

In Wiltshire, with the recent improvements to the organisation, Colonel Fletcher was able to tell the County Committee that he had received a report in April 1914 from the military saying that all recent inspections in the County were positive and a number of new detachments had successfully registered with the War Office.

He went on to say that to maintain standards and test the detachments a County Competition was to be held later in the year in Trowbridge. Lady Lansdowne had offered a challenge cup for the most efficient unit.

The Division

ANOTHER POLICY AIMED at maintaining standards and relieving the pressure on the Director was the introduction of an additional management tier between detachments and the County Committee: The Division.

The Division grouped a number of neighbouring detachments under the

1   *Wiltshire Times* - 25 April 1914
2   *The Devon and Exeter Gazette* – 9 October 1913

command of a Red Cross Vice President. Some of the administrative functions, such as finance, moved to divisional committees, meaning the Commandant of each detachment reported to a Vice President rather than, as previously, directly to the County Director. The Vice President was also able to improve efficiency by arranging shared training courses and enabling volunteers to move between detachments in the division.

At a meeting, in April 1914, Lady Ethel Methuen of Corsham explained that she had been appointed Vice President of Chippenham Division.[1] She said her Division was made up of three neighbouring detachments;[2] Chippenham formed in 1910, and now under the leadership of Helena Wilson; Derry Hill under Commandant Lady Walter Hervey; and Corsham led by the Honourable Christian Methuen, the daughter of Lady Methuen.

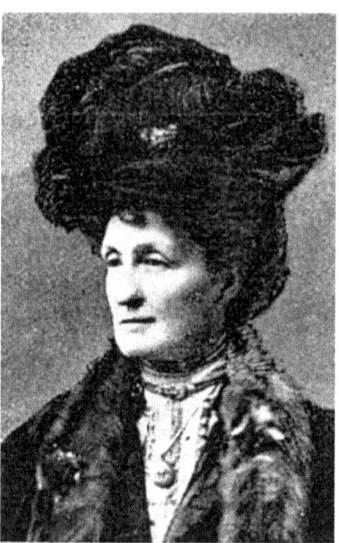

Lady Mary Ethel Methuen

The hierarchy in the Red Cross organisation reflected the county social structure and Vice Presidents were appointed as much for their influence as their knowledge of Voluntary Aid. Lady Methuen admitted she knew little about Voluntary Aid until the County Director explained it to her.

Nine Divisions were established in Wiltshire with vice presidents appointed in eight of them:[3]

> *Malmesbury* - Vice President the Countess of Suffolk of Charlton Park.
>
> *Swindon* (also known as North Wilts) - Vice President Emily Calley of Burderop Park.
>
> *Marlborough* (also known as East Wilts) - Vice President Louisa Newman Rogers of Rainscombe, Oare near Pewsey.
>
> *Trowbridge* - Vice President Maud Long of West Ashton, previously Commandant for Chippenham Detachment.
>
> *Salisbury* - Vice President Countess of Pembroke, Wilton House.
>
> *Devizes* - Vice President Edward Colston JP of Roundway Park, Devizes.

---

1   *Wiltshire Times* – 4 April 1914
2   *Western Daily Press* - 10 July 1914
3   *Wiltshire Times* - 25 April 1914

The Story of Chippenham's Red Cross Hospital

Warminster - Vice President Lady Heytesbury of Heytesbury.

Tisbury – In 1914 a Vice President had not been appointed and Tisbury was under the command of the Countess of Pembroke at Wilton.

Chippenham – Vice President Lady Ethel Methuen of Corsham Court, succeeded by Lady Margaret Spicer of Spye Park in early 1915.

The three detachments of Chippenham Division met at the Neeld Hall at the beginning of July 1914 to test their first aid and domestic skills. A competition was organised and it was decided the winner of the inter-detachment contest would represent the Division in the Lady Lansdowne Challenge Cup at Trowbridge.[1]

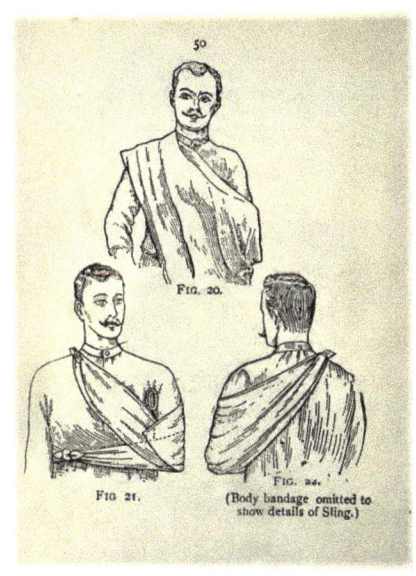

First Aid handbook. The VADs in Chippenham Division would have studied it in readiness for their inspection

The VADs had spent weeks preparing to ensure they performed at their peak, especially as there were added pressures because the competition was combined with the annual inspection.

Following demonstrations by each detachment and after much deliberation by Major Maurice of the RAMC, the inspecting officer, first place was awarded to the Chippenham Detachment, with Derry Hill second and Corsham third. In his summing up he said the work he had seen that afternoon was equal to any detachment in that part of the Country.

The County Competition

On 18 July 1914 the ladies of the Chippenham Voluntary Aid Detachment arrived at Trowbridge Town Hall to take part in the County Competition,[2] joining Detachments from Marlborough, Heytesbury, Sopworth, Malmesbury, Crudwell, Calne and Devizes to compete for the Lansdowne Cup. While the men who represented Salisbury, Devizes, Malmesbury and Crudwell were in competition for the Suffolk Cup presented by the Countess of Suffolk of Charlton Park.

The Town Hall was turned into a battlefield hospital with medical supervision

1 *Western Daily Press* - 10 July 1914
2 *Devizes and Wiltshire Gazette* - 23 July 1914

provided by Miss Butler, the Matron of Trowbridge Cottage Hospital and the judges for the day were four officers from the RAMC. The Boy Scouts acted as the wounded and presented all manner of injuries for the VADs to deal with. Chippenham Detachment were represented by May Ennis, who at the time was Deputy Commandant and nurses Kate Hinton, Sarah Mackness, Miss Belcher and Miss Maddock. The cooks were Mrs Shipp and Mrs Craig. The judges gave them a series of nursing tasks and asked questions on the transport of wounded. The competition ended with the cooks taking part in a field cooking competition.

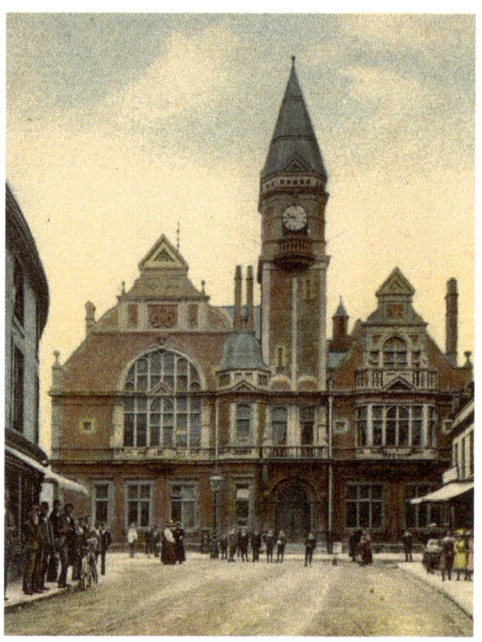

The Town Hall Trowbridge.

When the results were announced three points separated the first four detachments. Marlborough ladies were awarded the Lansdowne Cup, with 192 points, out of 200, while Chippenham and Devizes shared second place, with 191 points, and Heytesbury achieved a credible fourth place.[1]

The public were invited to watch the proceedings in Trowbridge and a few days later Colonel Fletcher chaired a meeting in the town to recruit volunteers. Twenty-five volunteers came forward interested in establishing a detachment and there was sufficient interest from people in nearby Melksham, Westbury and Bradford on Avon to consider raising further detachments in those towns.

Temporary Hospitals

IN ADDITION TO raising detachments of trained volunteers the County Red Cross Branches were also responsible for identifying public buildings, such as schools and town halls that could be prepared as rest stations or temporary hospitals to deal with the injured and homeless. The Voluntary Aid Scheme:[2]

> County Associations should either themselves or through the British Red Cross Society proceed to select the necessary buildings in consultation with administrative medical officers, officers commanding the general hospitals, and sanitary officers of their

1   *Wiltshire Times* - 25 July 1914
2   *The Times* - 17 August 1909

The Story of Chippenham's Red Cross Hospital

territorial division and plans should be drawn up showing how the buildings will be arranged for hospital purposes the organising matron also being consulted regarding these.

Following the County Competition it was clear the Town Hall in Trowbridge was ideally suited as emergency accommodation and the Vice Presidents and Commandants were instructed to seek agreement with their local authorities that similar public buildings may be released to the Red Cross at short notice in times of crisis.

In Chippenham the Town and Neeld Halls were considered suitable for the purpose and, having gained the support of the County Committee, Mrs Wilson wrote to Chippenham Borough Council to ask for their agreement to release the buildings to the Red Cross should the need ever arise.

Mrs Wilson's letter was debated on 7 July 1914 and with little discussion the Borough Council agreed to her request. The minutes recorded:[1]

> The Town Clerk read a letter from Mrs M S Wilson, Commandant of the Chippenham Division of the British Red Cross Society, making Application for the use of the Town and Neeld Halls and the Market Yard, in the event of war in the immediate neighbourhood and on the proposition of Mr Councillor Stevens seconded by Mr

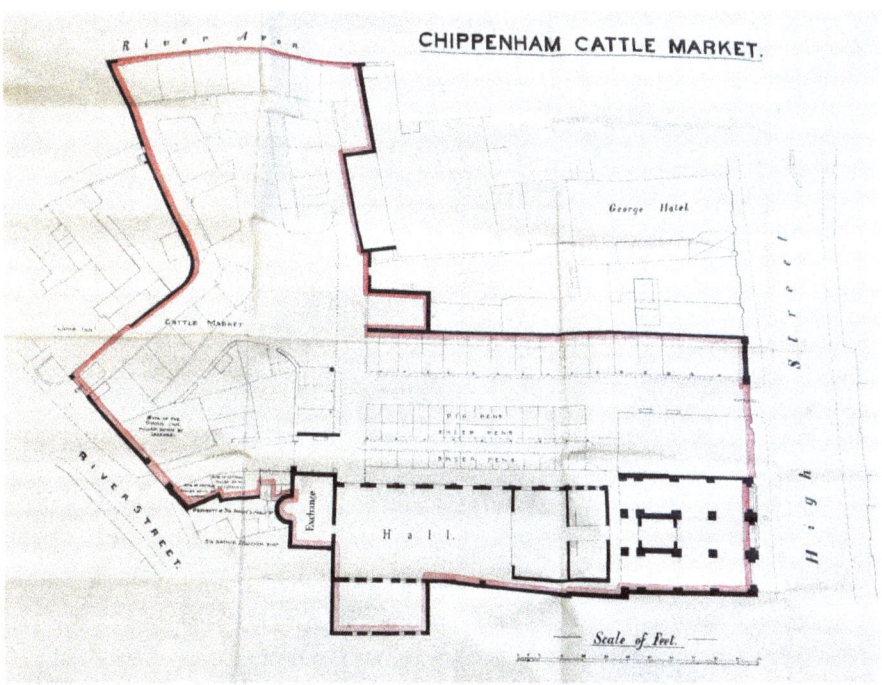

Plan of Market Yard, Neeld Hall and Town Hall. This plan is dated 1924.

1   *Chippenham Town Council minute book 8*

Unity and Loyalty

Alderman Neale the Application was granted.

It appeared that Mrs Wilson had gained the full support of the Borough Council to hand over the halls to the Red Cross should there be an invasion. In reality Mrs Wilson's request was granted because it was considered by the Borough Council that the likelihood of invasion was now so improbable that it deserved little debate.[1]

Peaceful relations with Germany

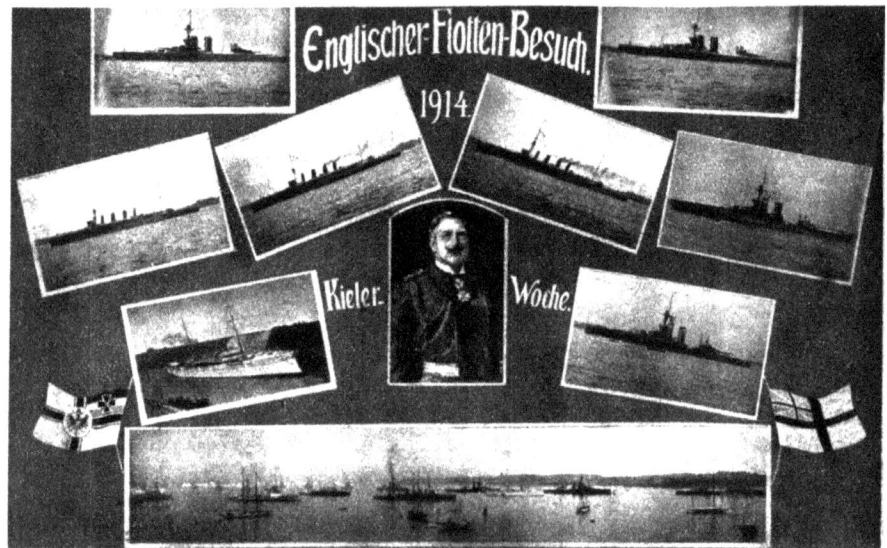

A German postcard celebrating the British Navy visit to Kiel week in June 1914.

EUROPEAN RELATIONSHIPS HAD much improved over recent years and for most people the fear of invasion had lessened. In Europe peace was on the political agenda following the ending of the Balkan wars. In 1907 there had been an initial Peace Convention between nations[2] and by 1913 there was an increasing willingness to seek arbitration with a further Peace Conference planned at The Hague at the end of 1914.

The newspaper headlines in August 1913 were 'Peace Nearer, Rumania and Bulgaria come to terms'[3] and later in the month they reported the opening of the Palace of Peace in The Hague:[4] a forum for nations to air their disputes. The Tsar of Russia spoke

---

1. *North Wilts Herald* - 10 July 1914. The newspaper reported the Town Clerk joked about Mrs Wilson's request.
2. 1907 Convention for The Pacific Settlement of International Disputes
3. *Pall Mall Gazette* – 4 August 1913
4. The Hague Conventions of 1899 and 1907 included both Britain and Germany

The Story of Chippenham's Red Cross Hospital

of the Peace Palace, describing a new bond between nations willing to arbitrate.[1]

The Government had even questioned[2] the cost of home defence as German aggression seemed to be a thing of the past. The Kaiser had extended the hand of friendship and invited a squadron of British warships to visit the German High Fleet in Kiel where the officers and men of both navies fraternised as comrades. The Daily Telegraph reported:[3]

> It was very pleasant to see the cordial comradeship that existed between the British and German sailors and the evidently friendly feelings towards the former that prevailed among the crowd.

The Kaiser was invited to visit the British flagship and the newspaper went on to say: 'The Kaiser, who wore the uniform of a British Admiral[4] of the Fleet made a thorough inspection of every part of the ship'. In a further act of friendship naval squadrons of the two nations met and sailed together off the coast of Mexico.

By the summer of 1914 the shift of opinion regarding threatened aggression was reflected in VAD recruiting meetings. Although invasion and war work were mentioned the emphasis for VADs was beginning to turn to being prepared to deal with accidents in the community and the home. Even at the Trowbridge competition in July 1914, where a war scenario had been assumed, the only reference to hostilities referred to civil war in Ireland:

> The element of realism was intensified by the thoughts of the warlike clouds which hover over a certain agitated province of the British Isles, and one frequently heard the proceedings associated with the scare created by the doings of a Volunteer Army in the Emerald Isle.

The Red Cross Voluntary Aid organisation had proved its usefulness in the community; one Detachment had treated airmen after a crash at an airshow, and VADs were becoming a regular sight at fetes and shows where they treated minor injuries.

In October 1913 at a disaster at Senghenydd Colliery in Glamorgan a massive underground explosion resulted in 439 deaths and hundreds injured. The scale of the catastrophe meant that local Detachments were called to help and they put their training to the test setting up a temporary hospital to assess and deal with the injured. Such was the professionalism of the VADs the British Medical Journal said about the Red Cross Voluntary Aid Detachments:[5] '...this is a movement which is likely to be of great service in giving first aid in cases of national disasters'.

Volunteers in detachments around the country would have been encouraged by

---

1 *Pall Mall Gazette* – 30 August 1913
2 *Hansard* - House of Commons debate. 25 February 1914
3 *Daily Telegraph* - 26 June 1914
4 Queen Victoria had made the Kaiser an honorary Admiral in 1889
5 *The British Red Cross in Action* – Dame Beryl Oliver.

Unity and Loyalty

this: hearing how their work and training had a real purpose and was recognised by the medical establishment.

This acknowledgement by the medical profession of the value of VADs was no doubt emphasised when the Red Cross held a VAD recruiting meeting at the end of July 1914 at Melksham, just a few miles from Chippenham. Interest had been shown in Voluntary Aid and the ladies of the town were invited to meet the VADs from Chippenham Division and hear about Voluntary Aid.[1]

Vice President, Lady Methuen, gave a speech at the meeting expressing her desire to raise a full Detachment in Melksham to join those in Derry Hill, Chippenham and Corsham as part of her Division. She then gave some background to the Scheme for Voluntary Aid: how it was part of the Defence Force raised in 1909, but since that time the threat of invasion had abated and it was her hope that invasion would never be the case.

Another speaker in support of raising a Detachment in Melksham was Canon Edwin Wyld, the vicar of Melksham. He continued Lady Methuen's theme that, even if VADS were not needed in war, it was his experience that knowledge of first aid in ordinary civilian life was extremely valuable as accidents could occur at any time. The meeting closed with a number of ladies expressing an interest in joining.

Incredibly the Melksham meeting, that emphasised the peaceful role of the VADS, took place less than a week before the declaration of war. Events in Europe were to escalate rapidly.

The Clouds of War gather

THE SUMMER OF 1914 had been warm dry and sunny[2] and by July people were looking forward to the August Bank Holiday, which fell on Monday 3 August. For several weeks they had been planning how to enjoy the weekend. Employers in Chippenham arranged day trips for their workers and the Great Western Railway offered excursions to the coast. A favourite destination being Weston Super Mare.

For those who stayed in Chippenham an afternoon of entertainment was planned at Hardenhuish Park with the Pipers of the Highland Light Infantry, a military gymnastics team from Aldershot and a Horse Show. The Chippenham Town Silver Band played popular music during the afternoon.

Little thought had been given to the increasing tension in Europe, in fact, most people remained oblivious to the mounting danger. Many words have been written about the rapid decline to war. David Lloyd George wrote in his War Memoirs:[3]

How was it that the world was so unexpectedly plunged into this terrible conflict? Who was responsible? Not even the astutest and most far-seeing statesman foresaw in the early summer of 1914 that the autumn would find the nations of the world interlocked in

1   *Wiltshire Times* - 1 August 1914
2   Meteorological Office - *Monthly weather report*
3   *War Memoirs of David Lloyd George* - 1933

The Story of Chippenham's Red Cross Hospital

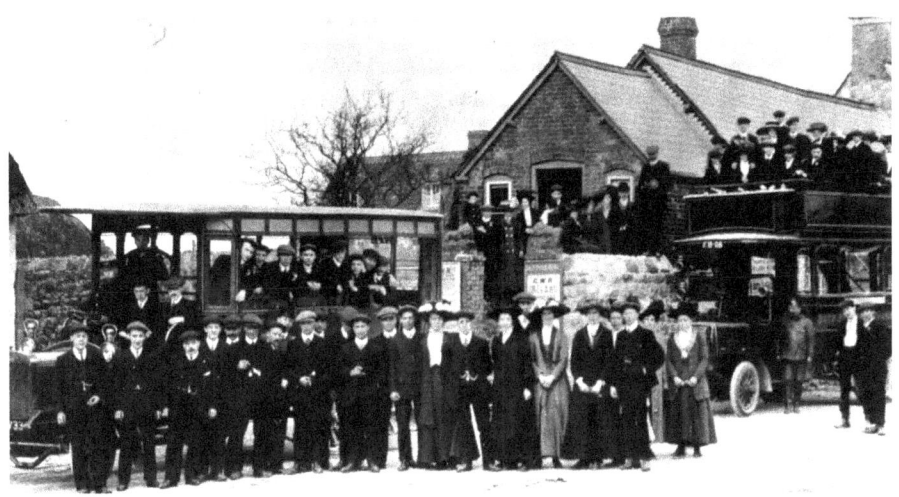

Chippenham workers on an outing to the seaside in 1912

the most terrible conflict that had ever been witnessed in the history of mankind; and if you came to the ordinary men and women who were engaged in their daily avocations in all countries there was not one of them who suspected the imminence of such a catastrophe. Of those who, in the first weeks of July, were employed in garnering their hay or corn harvests, either in this country or on the Continent of Europe, it is safe to say that not one ever contemplated the possibility that another month would find them called to the Colours and organised in battle array for a struggle that would end in the violent death of millions of them, and in the mutilation of many more millions. The nations slithered over the brink into the boiling cauldron of war without any trace of apprehension or dismay.

Bank holiday entertainment in Chippenham

News in June 1914 that Archduke Franz Ferdinand of Austria had been assassinated in Sarajevo was of no more than passing interest to the people of Chippenham. The British Government sent their sympathies to Austria, *'expressed their abhorrence of the crime',* but then continued with their own pressing domestic business.

Nobody anticipated the swift turn of events that put the country on course for war as the European crisis escalated and threatened to involve Britain. On 29 July the Government agreed to invoke the Official Precautionary Period. This meant the Services were put on alert and should prepare to mobilise. Regular soldiers were recalled from leave, Territorial units were put on standby and the fleet was sent a warning telegram.

The Government, however, remained undecided about taking any further action and it was hoped a

Unity and Loyalty

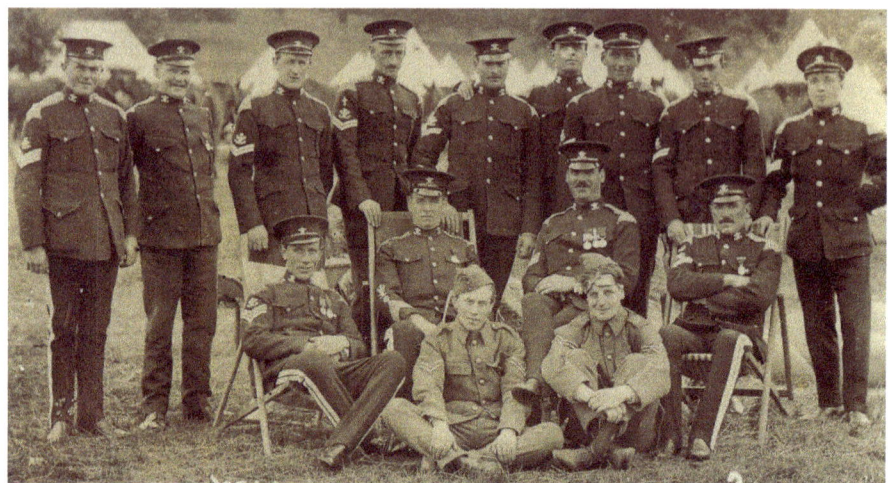

A group of Wiltshire Yeomanry, on exercise. At the beginning of August 1914 they were instructed to mobilise at the Butts in Chippenham.

peaceful solution could still be achieved. Some newspapers as late as the fourth of August still posed the question, is it too late for peace?

By the beginning of August members of the Territorial Force, who had been on standby, were instructed to report for duty and the Regular Army were despatched for guard duty at strategic locations around the country.[1] Troop trains passed through Chippenham carrying men ready to guard coastal towns. In Weston-Super-Mare, where Chippenham holiday makers were making the most of the weather, armed soldiers patrolled the area protecting the important Atlantic Telegraph Cable[2] that came ashore near the town.

The public continued to enjoy themselves over the Bank Holiday, most remaining unaware of the increasingly serious nature of the situation.[3] In London the Foreign Secretary, Sir Edward Grey, spoke to a tense House of Commons on 3 August, starting his speech by saying:[4] 'Today events move so rapidly that it is exceedingly difficult to state with technical accuracy the actual state of affairs'.

He told the house he felt the situation was extremely grave and reminded them of Britain's obligation to stand by France and Belgium should Germany enter those countries.

The following day it was announced that Germany had invaded Belgium. This brought a realisation that the threat of war was a reality and holiday makers in London joined the crowds gathered at Buckingham Palace and Whitehall to await an official announcement.

1   *Illustrated London News* - 8 August 1914
2   North Somerset Museum. Weston Super Mare was heavily guarded to protect the Atlantic Telegraph Cable station. www.cial.org.uk
3   Imperial War Museum. Article – *Voices of the First World War*
4   *The Story of Twenty Five Years* – W J Makin

Part 2
War

Chapter 5
1914 – August

WAR IS DECLARED and there is great enthusiasm to take on the Germans. The War will be over by Christmas and the Government tells the nation it is 'Business as usual'. The VADs rely on their training and prepare to treat the expected wounded. Groups of women start knitting and sewing to provide comforts for the troops. By the end of the year the British forces in Europe have suffered setbacks and the realisation dawns the War will continue for much longer than anticipated.

Declaration of War

THE ANNOUNCEMENT CAME just after midnight on the fifth of August when the Foreign Office released the following statement:[1]

> Owing to the summary rejection by the German Government of the request made by his Majesty's Government for assurances that the neutrality of Belgium will be respected, his Majesty's Ambassador at Berlin has received his passports and his Majesty's Government have declared to the German Government that a state of war exists between Great Britain and Germany as from 11 pm on August 4th.

Public opinion responded with almost unanimous approval to the Government's action. The crowds outside Buckingham Palace were jubilant and started to celebrate in the streets. The popular belief was this would be a short war and the Germans would be defeated within three months seeing the victorious army home by Christmas.[2]

There were some who doubted the prospect of a short war. Lord Kitchener, who became Secretary of

Your King and Country Need You.

Will you answer your Country's Call? Each day is fraught with the gravest possibilities, and at this very moment the Empire is on the brink of the greatest war in the history of the world.

In this crisis your Country calls on all her young unmarried men to rally round the Flag and enlist in the ranks of her Army.

If every patriotic young man answers her call, England and her Empire will emerge stronger and more united than ever.

If you are unmarried and between 18 and 30 years old will you answer your Country's Call? and go to the nearest Recruiter—whose address you can get at any Post Office, and

JOIN THE ARMY TO-DAY!

The call for volunteers to join the army

---

1 *The Times* - 5 August 1914
2 Lloyd George in his memoirs suggested the slogan Over by Christmas was maintained to retain public opinion.

Chippenham VAD Hospital

State for War, was amongst those who predicted a protracted conflict, perhaps a number of years, but these voices were dismissed as being over pessimistic.

Sir Edward Grey, the Foreign Secretary, reflected on the length of the coming war and how it would change the world when he famously said:[1] *'The lamps are going out all over Europe, we shall not see them lit again in our lifetime.'*

Eager young men came forward in their droves to 'Rally Round the Flag' and volunteer to catch a slice of the action before it was all over. A young Wiltshire woman and her mother were left to run the family farm when both her brothers left to join the Wiltshire Yeomanry. As they left, they confidently told her not to worry about the farm as they would soon be back, she recalled them saying *'Well it won't be long, we shall soon be home again'*.[2]

Lord Kitchener called for all unmarried men between 18 and 30 to attend their nearest recruiting office. Joan Money-Kyrle of Whetham near Calne wrote in her diary on 8 August about the numbers of men being recruited at home and around the Empire saying:[3] *'Lord Kitchener is at the War Office and has asked for an extra 100,000 men. Canada promised 20,000 and Australia ditto, Newfoundland 8000 and all the navies.'*

Chippenham at War

IN CHIPPENHAM THE declaration of war saw a flurry of excitement. Large crowds gathered at the Post Office in the Market Place where the proclamation of war was posted and it remained the centre of celebration until late in the evening, with bands playing patriotic music and the crowds bursting into spontaneous singing of God Save the King.

A temporary recruiting office was opened using the offices of the Chippenham Brewery Company and within 24 hours forty men had come forward.[4] The town was suddenly full of activity and men in uniform were seen everywhere. The Chippenham Squadron of the Wiltshire Yeomanry was cheered as they marched towards their headquarters in the Butts.[5] Many of the squadron had come from the surrounding villages and were billeted at local hostelries as they waited for orders to move to their war station at Winchester. The Territorial battalion of the Wiltshire Regiment had also gathered at the Drill Hall in Bath Road and was awaiting orders to move to Salisbury Plain. Full time, regular, soldiers arrived in Chippenham and the surrounding area with orders to guard the railway.[6] There were armed guards at Box Tunnel[7] and bridges were protected by troops to avoid German activists blowing them up.

1   The National Archive Blog - *The lamps are going out all over Europe*
2   *Wiltshire Within Living Memory* – Wiltshire Federation of Women's Institutes.
3   Wiltshire and Swindon Archive - 1720/720 *Diaries of Joan Money-Kyrle*
4   *Devizes and Wiltshire Gazette* - 6 August 1914
5   *Wiltshire Times* - 8 April 1914
6   *The Great War Chippenham Soldiers* – Richard Broadhead –Private Idle a regular soldier from Bolton was killed in an accident on the railway and is buried at Hullavington.
7   *Bath Chronicle* - 5 September 1914

Unity and Loyalty

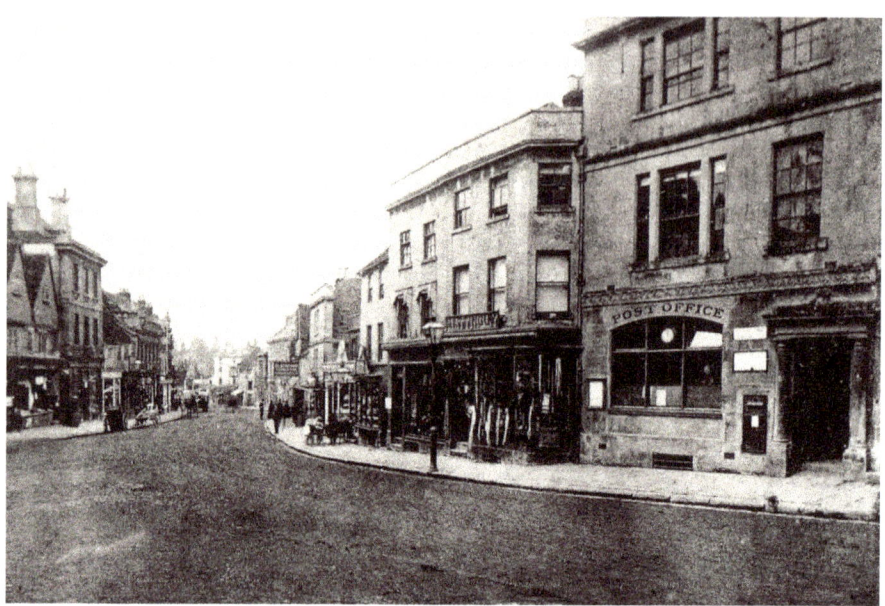

The Post Office in the Market Place where the crowds gathered as war was declared

The normally peaceful High Street suddenly became a busy highway as convoys of military vehicles carrying supplies and troops were seen heading for the ports of Avonmouth and Southampton to embark for France.[1] Vehicles came from all parts of Britain, many having been requisitioned at short notice. Vans from Waring and Gillow, the London Furniture store, were seen transporting men and equipment, while vehicles from the Johnny Walker distillery in Scotland were still going strong as the Scottish troops paused at Chippenham.[2] The Edinburgh paper told how the people of Chippenham provided the men with buttered bread, tea, cheese and fruit to eat on their journey.[3] Ambrose Neate, who grew up in Chippenham, had joined the Black Watch in August 1914 at Perth. He visited relations in the town as his regiment stopped on route to Salisbury plain.

The Chippenham Borough Surveyor wrote in 1915 that in two days at the beginning of the War he estimated nearly 700 vehicles passed through Chippenham.[4]

The uncertainty in Europe during the weeks leading up to the outbreak of war threatened a banking crisis. To avoid a run on the financial institutions after the Bank Holiday the Government announced the holiday was to be extended to include the Tuesday, Wednesday and Thursday, the 4 ,5 and 6 August. When the banks finally reopened the Treasury removed gold coins from circulation and replaced them with ten-shilling and £1 notes.

1   *Wiltshire Times* - 8 August 1914 describes vehicles heading for Avonmouth.
2   *Commercial Motor magazine* - 13 August 1914 www.archive.commercialmotor.com
3   *Edinburgh Evening News*- 10 October 1914
4   Wiltshire and Swindon Heritage Centre - G19/130/4 *Chippenham Borough Council Letter Book*

Chippenham VAD Hospital

Edith Olivier, of Salisbury, wrote:[1] *'On August 8th, we saw for the first time paper currency, we accepted them as one of the unpleasant things, which as patriots, we were bound to endure in our country's time of stress.'*

Despite the outbreak of war, and to manage business confidence, the Government told the country to expect little change and announced it would be business as usual.

In Chippenham, traders such as the draper W H Wheeler, placed advertisements in the local papers:[2] *'England's Motto - Business as usual. Our customers may rely upon us that no advance will be made in prices until the markets absolutely compel us.'*

The Chippenham and District Chamber of Commerce placed similar notices:

> The Committee of the Chamber earnestly hopes that in this time of National stress the general public will assist the traders of the town to keep business running as usual, thus enabling them to retain their full staff of employees.

They went on to give advice to the public to continue to shop as normal and settle accounts promptly. The fear for businesses was that the War would cause uncertainty with a resulting fall in trade and ultimately unemployment.

These messages were also given in response to a period of panic buying during the first days as the hint of economic uncertainty and the rumour of shortages of food resulted in hoarding. The Wiltshire Times gave suggestions for practical patriotism and provided the following advice to the public:[3]

> Keep your heads. Be calm. Go about your ordinary business quietly and soberly. Do not indulge in excitement or foolish demonstration. Do not store goods and create a scarcity to the hurt of others.

The Government passed legislation allowing the seizure of hoarded food and gave a further assurance to traders that it would be business as usual. They also introduced the Defence of the Realm Act (DORA) that gave greater powers to support the war effort.

Good horses were in great demand by the Army and around the district farms were visited to provide a supply of horses. Mr Barsted's yard in Langley Road became a horse depot to receive animals commandeered in the district for war service.[4] The Duke of Beaufort wrote a letter to the Western Daily Press:[5] *'Owing to the present critical state of affairs, I am unable to make my usual arrangements as regards hunting this season.'*

It was in agriculture, however, that the full impact of the War was felt. Just as the crops were ready for harvesting farms lost both men and horses to the military. Farmers were told to consider accepting unskilled volunteers, including women, to help with the

1   *Without knowing Mr Walkley* - Edith Olivier
2   *Wiltshire Times* - 29 August 1914
3   *Wiltshire Times* - 8 August 1914
4   *Devizes and Wiltshire Gazette* - 6 August 1914
5   *Western Daily Press* - 20 August 1914

harvest and prepare the land for the following years crops.

In the High Street, German manufactured items, such as tin plate toys and textiles, disappeared from the shop windows. Even the drug Aspirin, which had been developed by a German company, was rebranded and given the trade name of Helicon to satisfy British patriotism.[1]

Suddenly there were spies everywhere. Germans and Austrians, who for years had happily lived and traded in Britain were detained. An Austrian man who had spent many years working in Chippenham was arrested and interned in a camp in Newbury.[2] Innocent picnickers were arrested on the Downs near Devizes on suspicion of planning to sabotage the Marconi radio towers. At Chippenham station the authorities were alerted to a man taking particular interest in the railway bridges and the signalling infrastructure. He was later arrested at Bath, but after interview was released to continue his journey.[3]

Men Leave for War

BY THE END of August forty men from Saxby and Farmer had signed up for military service. The Directors of the Chippenham Cloth factory, Pocock's, reported a similar number of men had volunteered.

William Brewer, the foreman at the factory and a well-known local footballer,[4] was one of the Wiltshire Territorials who joined his regiment on Salisbury Plain to await orders to embark for France.

The Wiltshire Yeomanry received their orders to move to their war station and left the town on 12 August.[5] They marched through the High Street to the railway station, where trains were waiting to take them and their horses to Winchester to await further orders:[6]

> The C Squadron Wilts Yeomanry, which has been billeted at Chippenham since mobilisation, left last evening. The squadron consisted of 200 officers and men, which is at full strength, they had a hearty send off and the premises in the main thoroughfare were decorated with flags.

The Squadron was led by Major William Fleetwood Fuller, whose family home was Neston Park. His sister in law, Mabel Fuller, was the Commandant of the rapidly formed Melksham Voluntary Aid Detachment. Amongst the crowds were the ladies of the Chippenham VAD cheering as their friends and relations in the squadron marched out of Chippenham.

1 *Illustrated London News* - 3 October 1914
2 *Western Daily Press* – 24 October 1914
3 *Bath Chronicle* - 22 August 1914.
4 *The Great War Chippenham Soldiers* – Richard Broadhead
5 *The Royal Wiltshire Yeomanry* – J R I Platts
6 *Western Daily Press* - 13 August 1914

The Story of Chippenham's Red Cross Hospital

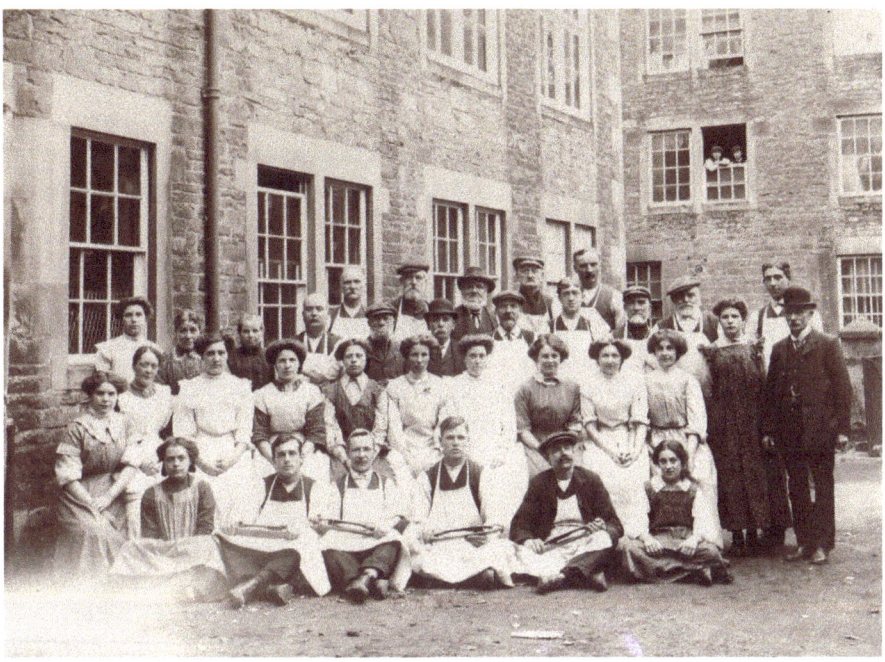

Cloth workers at Pocock's factory. Many of the young men signed up for military service in 1914. William Brewer is first right back row

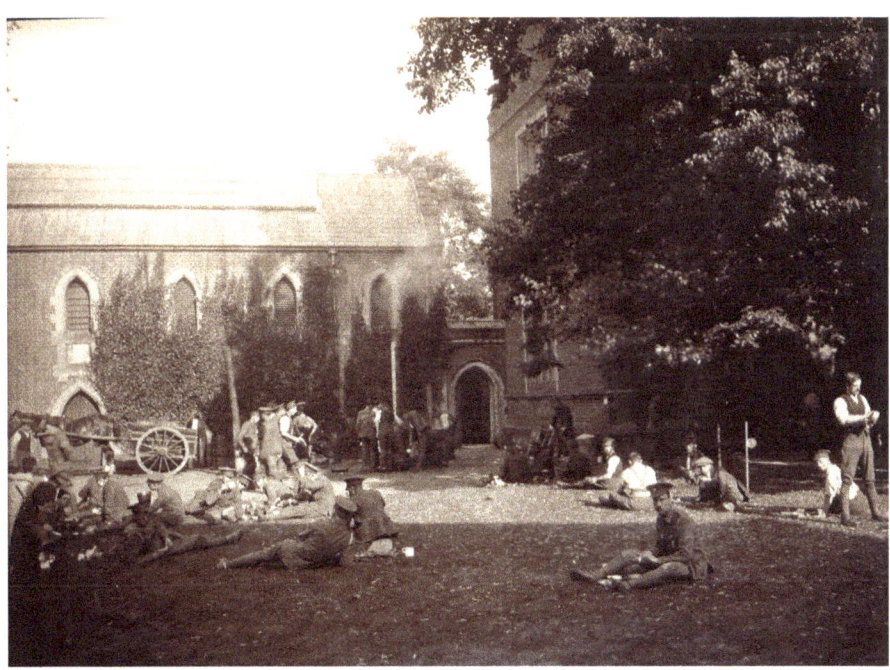

August 1914. Chippenham Squadron of the Wiltshire Yeomanry camped at Winchester College

By the third week of August the newspapers announced that the first men of the British Expeditionary Force (BEF) had landed in France. The public were able to read positive reports of action against the Germans,[1] but a few weeks later news filtered through of a number of setbacks suffered by the Allies. At the battle of Mons, outnumbered by the Germans, the BEF were forced to withdraw from their positions. In October the first battle at Ypres began and heavy casualties were reported. Then, in November, the North Wilts Herald[2] carried the headline that everybody in Wiltshire feared, '*The Wiltshire's Second Battalion meets with a reversal. Many reported killed*'.[3]

Chippenham, like every other town in the country, received its share of bad news. By the end of the year the toll of men lost from the area was well over twenty. Amongst them was William Brewer, who had left Pocock's cloth factory, and Lord Charles Mercer-Nairne, son of Lord and Lady Lansdowne.

VADs Mobilise

NOW THE COUNTRY was on a war footing the Red Cross organisation in Wiltshire mobilised.

In Chippenham Mrs Wilson, the Commandant, reacted immediately and gave the Borough Council notice that due to the declaration of war the Red Cross may need to requisition the Town and Neeld Halls for hospital service.

The Quartermaster of the Detachment, Mrs Ennis, prepared letters to be sent to all households in the town asking that they be ready to loan furniture and equipment.[4]

On 7 August, two days after the announcement that Britain was at war, a meeting took place in Corsham to report on Red Cross preparations in Chippenham Division.

Basil Hankey, of Stanton Manor near Chippenham, who had replaced Colonel Fletcher as Red Cross County Director, informed the Vice President, Lady Methuen, that Chippenham Division had been very active and could say that work was progressing well in preparations to receive the wounded.

He confirmed that three of the four detachments in the Division had plans in place to provide temporary hospital beds; Corsham were planning for 30 beds having gained agreement to use Corsham Town Hall; Chippenham anticipated fifty beds in their Town Hall and the recently formed Melksham, under Mrs Robert Fuller, were offering up to 70 beds. Mr Hankey said the beds would go a long way to meeting the 500 or 600 patients he expected would need to be accommodated in Wiltshire.

Two days later, on 9 August, an emergency meeting of the Wiltshire Red Cross County Committee was held at Trowbridge. The County Committee were responsible for

1 *Daily Mirror* - 27 August. The BEF bore the brunt of six attacks which were successfully repulsed.
2 *North Wilts Herald* - 13 November 1914.
3 The Wardrobe Museum Salisbury - The 2nd Battalion lost 76 men and 7 officers and 229 were wounded and many more taken prisoner.
4 *Devizes and Wiltshire Gazette* - 6 August 1914

The Story of Chippenham's Red Cross Hospital

updating the military authorities at Bristol on progress to secure accommodation. Basil Hankey was able to report that plans were underway throughout Wiltshire and over three hundred bed places had already been promised, with numbers continuing to increase. He went on to tell the Committee that every day more volunteers were coming forward to join the Red Cross and offer help when the hospitals were open.[1]

Similar meetings were taking place throughout the country and regular updates were sent to the Central Committee of the Red Cross, who were meeting daily to coordinate the immediate needs of the War Office. The Times of the 5 August:

> The British Red Cross Society held a council meeting yesterday at St. James's Palace. Another meeting will be held to-day. Meanwhile the society's final arrangements to meet immediate needs are being rapidly pushed forward.

The Central Committee issued a public appeal for donations of bedding, bandages and, for the men at the Front, warm clothing. There was also a national appeal for the loan of empty warehouses and other suitable buildings to be used as temporary auxiliary hospitals, should the need arise.[2]

The Red Cross Society and the Order of St John continued to work independently, but with the developing emergency the two organisations agreed it would be sensible to join together to avoid duplication and to ensure a consistent policy to Voluntary Aid. By October 1914 this joint effort was formalised when the Joint War Committee[3] was established. The two organisations acted in total unison throughout the War under the banner of the Red Cross. This meant that across the country detachments like Chippenham saw members from both organisations work side by side under one command.

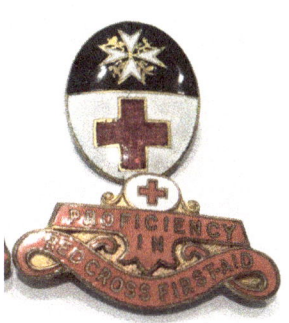

The Joint War and Proficiency badges belonging to Chippenham VAD Amy Bolton.

The VADs wore badges with emblems of both organisations showing the commitment to this joint working.

The order was also given that all Voluntary Aid Detachments were placed under the direct control of the War Office. The Red Cross would continue to take an administrative role but act on the direction of the Military Command. The British Nursing Journal of 15 August 1914 gave notice:

> War having been declared the Voluntary Aid Detachments have ceased to be under the orders of the British Red Cross Society and are now under the orders of the local military authorities with whom they are registered.

1   *Devizes and Wiltshire Gazette* - 13 August 1914
2   *The Times* - 5 August 1914
3   *The British Red Cross in Action* - Dame Beryl Oliver

Unity and Loyalty

The organisation of the Red Cross Society will be employed to assist any detachment mobilised by replenishing stores and drugs and in supplying hospital and general comforts.

In the case of Chippenham Division, the Second Southern Command at Bristol took command and orders were passed to the Red Cross Director, Basil Hankey.

Of the four detachments in Chippenham Division only Derry Hill had not offered plans for beds as they had been unable to secure premises. It was decided they would work with Chippenham Detachment and a joint meeting was held at the Institute in Derry Hill chaired by Lord Walter Hervey, husband of the Derry Hill Commandant.[1]

The Derry Hill Detachment proposed they share responsibility for the Hospital in Chippenham Town Hall. 50 beds had already been planned by Chippenham VAD and it was estimated, with Derry Hill's help, a further 15 beds could be made available. This was approved and the two Commandants, Mrs Wilson and Lady Walter Hervey, agreed to meet the Chippenham Council to formally requisition the Town Hall.

The Chairman raised the matter of equipment. Mrs Ennis, the Chippenham Quartermaster, had already written to residents in the town asking for their help in providing beds and bedding and furniture. It was decided to follow this letter up with house to house visits to ask for suitable items.

Lord Walter Hervey went on to say that there would be an unavoidable cost to buy medical equipment and establishing kitchen and sanitary facilities. He said the initial expense would have to be found locally from Red Cross funds and public subscription, however, he fully expected a refund from War Office funds once the wounded arrived.

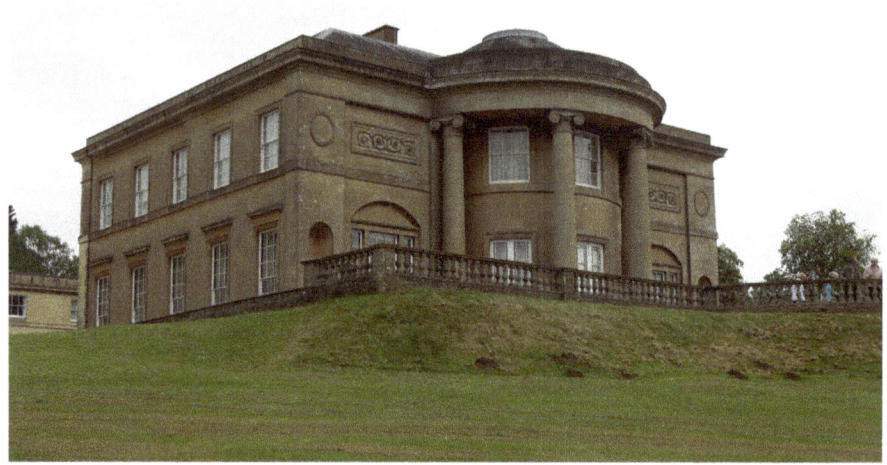

Bowden Park, the home of the Gladstone family, where a work group met to make hospital supplies

---

1   *Devizes and Wiltshire Gazette* - 13 August 1914

To meet this initial financial outlay it was decided a further leaflet should be distributed around the district seeking guarantees from the public towards the cost of setting up.

The next item on the agenda was the transport of patients. It was expected that they would arrive by train at Chippenham station and most would be stretcher cases. The shortage of male members in the Red Cross was as acute as ever and the detachments were unable to provide qualified ambulance orderlies. Nancy Briscoe, the wife of Dr William Briscoe, said she had been able to muster a squad of six trained St John Ambulance men from the police and railway to volunteer their services as stretcher bearers.

The meeting then turned its attention to the need for consumables: a constant supply of pyjamas, bandages and bedding was needed to satisfy the expected demand. It was agreed that these could easily be made by volunteers locally and groups of workers should be organised by the Red Cross Committee. Lady Walter Hervey, Lady Margaret Spicer of Spye Park, Mrs Gertrude Gladstone of Bowden Park and Florence Money-Kyrle of Whetham House all agreed to arrange work groups.

Mrs Gladstone and Lady Spicer made their homes available for ladies from the surrounding villages to meet to sew pyjamas and bedding and roll bandages.

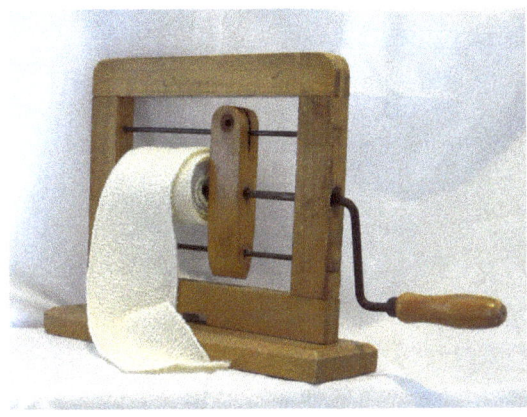

A bandage roller used by work groups

Florence Money-Kyrle arranged for the volunteers to meet in the village hall in Heddington. Her daughter, Joan, who helped organise the group, wrote in her diary[1] for 11 August:

> At 2.00 (p.m.) had a Workparty at Heddington and 30 mothers and girls attended. We got through a splendid amount of work. On the following day she wrote 'Did sewing etc. for hospitals and garments. On the twenty fourth she wrote 'Afternoon, we went up to Aylmer's and helped her cut out shirts and bed jackets and things for her Work party.

Meeting with Chippenham Council

On 11 August, as agreed at the Derry Hill meeting, Mrs Wilson, Lady Walter Hervey and Nancy Briscoe met Chippenham Council to explain the Red Cross plans for the Town Hall and the alterations needed.[2]

1   Wiltshire and Swindon Archive - 1720/720 *Diaries of Joan Money-Kyrle*
2   *Western Daily Press* - 12 August 1914

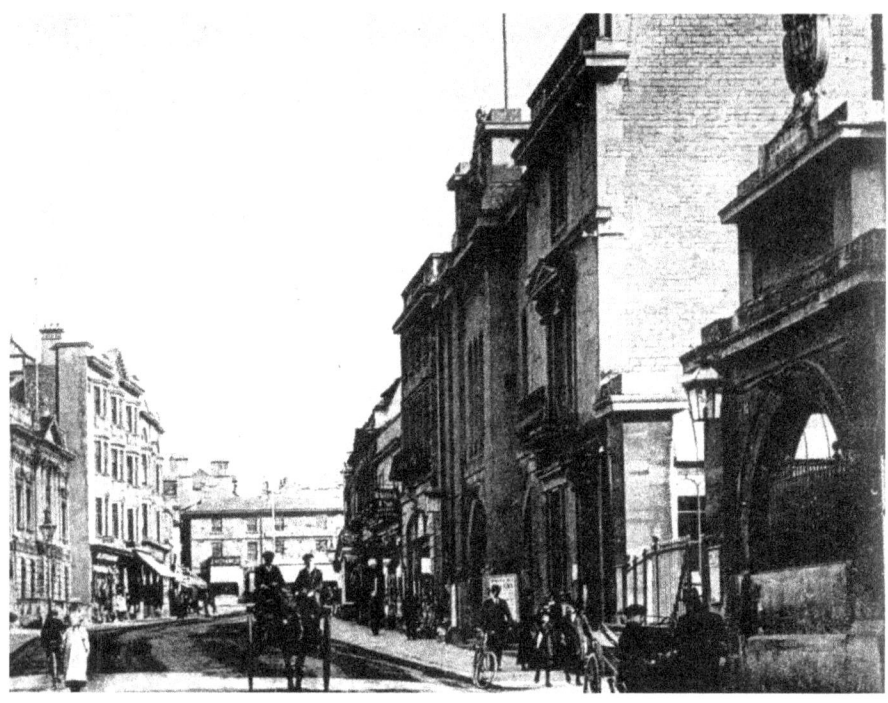

Chippenham Town Hall

The Town Hall was above the covered market and consisted of a large hall facing the High Street with ante rooms and stores to the rear of the building. The ladies explained to the Town Councillors that it was proposed the main hall would be converted to a ward with capacity for fifty beds and one of the smaller ante rooms would be fitted out to take a further 15 patients. The other adjoining room would be needed for cooking and as a mess room. To achieve this a number of structural alterations were needed to provide toilet facilities and install the kitchen.

They explained that after the alterations were complete the halls would be cleaned and decorated and the beds and medical equipment could then be installed. The employees of the cloth factory in the town had already offered their services to clean the wards.

The response from the Council was unenthusiastic. The Town Hall was regularly used for business and social occasions. Its loss would be detrimental to the town both as a venue and lack of revenue. The ladies representing the Red Cross detachments were told that the Council needed further information and the Town Clerk was instructed to deal directly with the Red Cross County Director.[1] Although the response appeared to be a delaying tactic organisations, such as the Lansdowne Lodge, who regularly met at the Town Hall were given notice to vacate on the assumption the rooms would to be handed over to the Red Cross

---

1   *Chippenham Council minute book 9*

The Story of Chippenham's Red Cross Hospital

Red Cross Training

First aid and nursing classes were rapidly established to address the sudden influx of volunteers who came forward. The Red Cross monthly journal for August 1914 said, '*There has been a great rush of women of all classes to join the various branches.*' In Wiltshire courses were arranged around the County. The medical staff at Devizes Asylum offered to train Red Cross volunteers with classes on Mondays and Fridays at 5.30pm for women and Mondays and Thursdays at 8pm for men, the cost being 2s 6d.

In Chippenham, the Drill Hall in Bath Road had been used for classes before the War but, with increasing numbers of candidates, two wooden huts behind the Technical School in Cocklebury Road were brought into use for Red Cross instruction and examinations.[1]

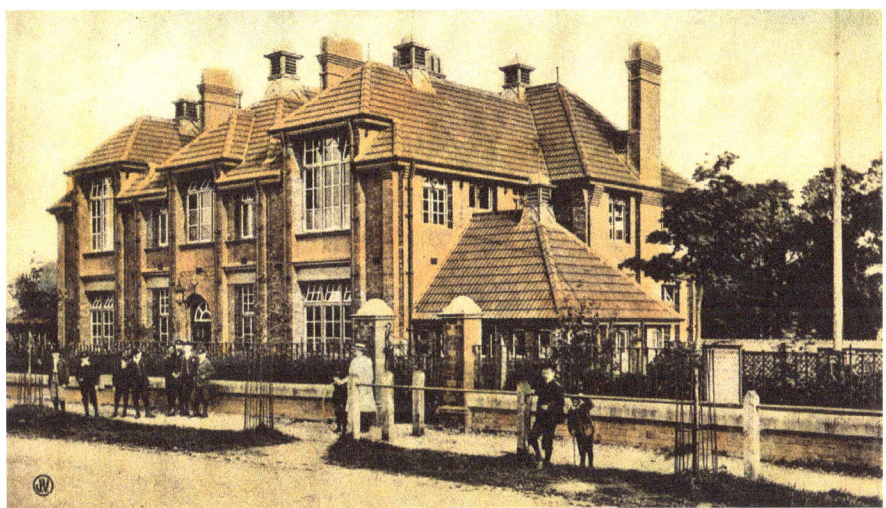

The Technical School Chippenham

For those living outside the towns classes were arranged in village halls. Joan Money-Kyrle wrote in her diary on the twelfth of August, '*Went to Red X practice meeting at Derry Hill and did bandaging etc.*' On the twenty second she wrote '*Afternoon, went to lecture at Lacock by Dr Taylor. Most interesting*'. Her diary confirms she regularly attended sessions at both Derry Hill and Lacock, where she also sat her exams.[2]

The First Wounded

When war was declared the Territorial Force General Hospital scheme was approved and in Bristol the recently opened King Edward VII Memorial

---

1   Chippenham Museum – Article from magazine *Education* 3 June 1960 and undated news cutting about Chippenham College extension.
2   Wiltshire and Swindon Archive - 1720/720 *Diaries of Joan Money-Kyrle*

Unity and Loyalty

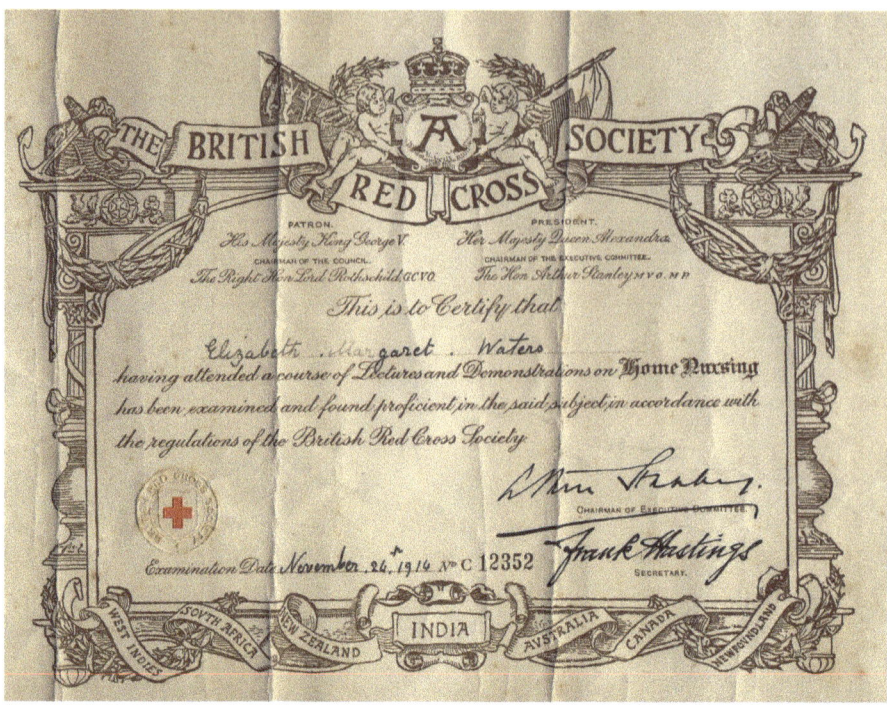

Home Nursing certificate awarded to Elizabeth Waters of Steinbrook Cottage Kington Langley in September 1914

Extension of the Bristol Royal Infirmary was handed over to the military. A further hospital, Southmead, was also allocated and these establishments become the Second Southern Military (or Base) Hospital.

Within days of the first engagement with the enemy wounded men arrived back at English ports. The first ambulance train, bringing men from Southampton, arrived at Bristol on 2 September.[1] The Bristol Voluntary Aid Detachments were ready to transfer the men to the city's military hospitals. With the allocation of beds at Southmead the Red Cross county organisations were told that there was no need to evacuate civilian patients from Bristol and therefore they need only prepare to receive convalescent wounded soldiers.

When the trains carrying the wounded arrived in Bristol the public lined the streets and cheered the men as they were conveyed to the hospitals. The newspapers were very positive telling how well prepared the organisation was and the men were recovering rapidly from their injuries. The Western Daily Press:

> GOOD NEWS FROM BRISTOL MILITARY HOSPITAL- It is pleasing to know that all the wounded soldiers from the front who are at the Second General Hospital are progressing very favourably. A large number have recovered from their wounds

---

1 *The Forgotten Front Bristol at War* – James Belsey

The Story of Chippenham's Red Cross Hospital

sufficiently to enable them to go to their regimental depots and almost every other day others are leaving.

A batch left yesterday and everything is in readiness for receiving more wounded from France, who may be sent to Bristol Military Hospital at any time.

The hospital trains that carried men from Southampton to Bristol passed through Trowbridge, the county town of Wiltshire. The Red Cross County Committee asked that trains stop at the town's station so that refreshments could be offered to the men by their members.[1] Red Cross workers from around the area attended the trains and it is quite likely some of the VADs from Chippenham Division offered their services.

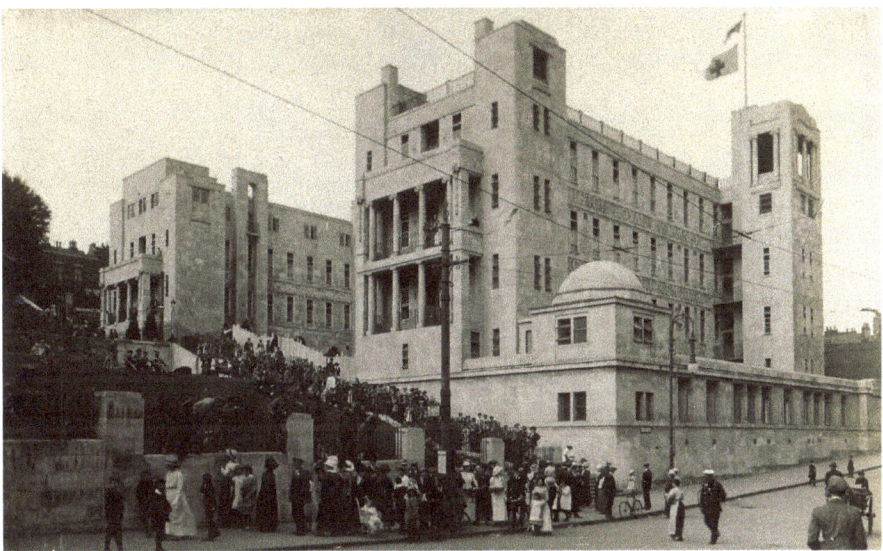

Bristol Royal Infirmary

As the first wounded arrived in Bristol the VADs in Chippenham Division were busy preparing wards for their convalescence. In Corsham, nineteen wounded men arrived from the King Edward VII wing of the Bristol Royal Infirmary on 26 October[2] and were taken to the Red Cross Hospital, which a few weeks earlier had been the Town Hall.

A few days later 32 men arrived in Melksham from Tidworth Military Hospital and were accommodated at the Conservative and Liberal Clubs, where the rooms had been converted to wards at the expense of the Melksham Commandant, Mrs Robert Fuller.[3]

The news in Chippenham was not so encouraging. The Council hadn't responded to Mrs Wilson's application to use the Town Hall. Instead the Town Clerk said he had

1   *Wiltshire Times*- 3 and 17 October 1914
2   *Wiltshire Times* - 31 October 1914
3   *Wiltshire Times* - 07 November 1914

heard directly from the War Office during September confirming they did not need to establish a hospital in Chippenham. The Council minutes: [1]

> The Town Clerk read a reply he had received from the War Office stating that there was no intention to use the Neeld Hall or Market Yard for the purposes of a Military Hospital.

No mention was made of the Town Hall in the minutes but this was clarified in November when the Halls Committee made the following statement:[2]

> The committee has considered the application of the Wiltshire Branch of the Red Cross for use of the Town Hall etc. as a Voluntary Aid hospital. They did not consider the premises suitable due to the smell and noise from the cattle market.

Auxiliary Home Hospital Department

During the first days of the War the Red Cross Central Committee appealed nationally for empty buildings to be used as temporary hospitals for convalescents. The response was far greater than expected and within a few weeks over 5000 buildings throughout the country had been offered. It fell to three retired Army Medical Officers to assess the suitability of each one and recommend them to the Auxiliary Home Hospital Department of the Joint War Committee.[3] With such numbers to consider the Department probably heeded Chippenham Council's opinion that the Town Hall was unsuitable and decided against using it.

The properties offered, as a result of the Red Cross appeal, included public buildings, country estates and private houses. Buildings were classified according to their appropriateness for convalescents. An 'A' Classification referred to buildings suitable as a Red Cross hospital, equipped and staffed to take stretcher cases. Any lower classification was simply a rest home for ambulatory convalescents who needed little or no medical treatment.[4] By November 1914 over 300 buildings throughout the country had been accepted by the Auxiliary Home Hospital Department providing 10,325 beds.[5]

Locally Basil Hankey saw the importance of properties of all classifications and said private houses and estates would be suitable for many convalescents.[6] Owners of country estates offered their houses as relaxed homes for recovering officers. The Bath

---

1 *Chippenham Council minute book 8*
2 *North Wilts Herald* - 20 November 1914
3 *The British Red Cross in Action* - Dame Beryl Oliver
4 *Wiltshire Family History Society magazine* —July 2003- Susan Mole, in an article about her grandmother Kate Hinton a staff nurse at Chippenham describes the classification from research with the Red Cross -.
5 British Red Cross report for week ending 4 November 1914 published in the newspapers.
6 *Devizes and Wiltshire Gazette* - 13 August 1914

Chronicle of 15 August reported on a number of grand houses in Wiltshire:

> Mr and Mrs E C Schomberg of Seend, have placed their residence, Seend House, at the disposal of the King Edward VII's Hospital for Officers as a convalescent home. Other Wiltshire residences kindly offered for similar purposes include Charlton Park (Lady Suffolk), Grittleton House (Sir Audley Neeld) and Mrs Garnett's residence at Chippenham.

Elsewhere boarding houses advertised in the Army and Navy Gazette, offering special terms to convalescing officers. Mrs Howard of Lowfield Heath, near Crawley in Sussex offered rest and quiet with good cooking and the added bonus of a nearby golf course.[1] There were even offers to convalesce on the French Riviera.[2] Near Chippenham the Rector of Yatton Keynell offered his home as a quiet retreat for the wounded.

These private arrangements were often not included in the thousands of offers being dealt with by the Auxiliary Home Hospital Department and soon the initial enthusiasm was overtaken by the need for greater organisation as it became increasingly difficult to account for recovering military personnel. The War Office anticipated that public eagerness could lead to chaos and instructed that the Red Cross should be solely responsible for coordinating all offers of help. By the third week of the War they had issued a memorandum:[3]

> The military authorities are most grateful for the generous offers of private houses to be used as temporary hospitals but the time has not arrived when definite assurance of the necessity of utilising these houses can be given. Funds should not be prematurely laid out on the preparation of these hospitals which might be more usefully expended in other directions.

The memorandum also made it quite clear that individual Voluntary Aid Detachments had no authority to take over any public or private building without the agreement of the Central Committee, suggesting that enthusiastic groups were establishing hospitals without approval.

'Mrs Garnett's residence at Chippenham,' mentioned in the Bath Chronicle on 15 August, was Greathouse in the village of Kington Langley, the Garnett family having moved to Wiltshire a few years earlier. They had extended and remodelled the property extensively, turning a farmhouse into what was described as a mansion large enough to warrant a number of indoor and outdoor servants. Charles Garnett was a barrister who practised in London and when he moved to Wiltshire he took an active role in local affairs, serving on the Chippenham Cottage Hospital Committee and as a governor of Chippenham Secondary School.

1   *Army and Navy Gazette* - 12 December 1914
2   *Wiltshire Times* - 31 October 1914
3   *Western Daily Press* - 22 August 1914

Unity and Loyalty

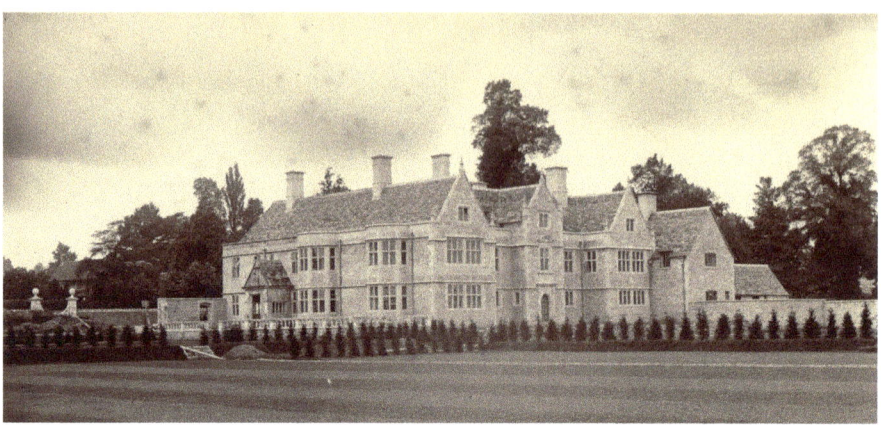

Greathouse Kington Langley

In the early days of the War Charles Garnett volunteered to go to the front and joined the Red Cross Headquarters in Ypres.[1] He drove his own ambulance to France and served for eight months on the front line, transporting wounded men to base hospitals and when he returned to Wiltshire his ambulance was loaned to the Red Cross locally.

There are no records of Greathouse being used as a convalescent hospital and it is unlikely it was classified by the Red Cross. An employee at Greathouse, however, recalled preparations that led to opening of a ward in the house.[2]

Elsie Fortune was born and grew up in Chippenham and by 1914 she was employed as Mrs Garnett's lady's maid. When Mrs Garnett set out to prepare her home for the arrival of convalescents Elsie was asked to help.

A complete floor of the property was cleared of the family's possessions and the staff were instructed to pack them away in the attic. Mrs Garnett decided this was also the opportunity to dispose of unwanted family possessions, which were put aside to be sold at a garden party, with proceeds going to the Red Cross.

Mrs Garnett was a member of the Chippenham Red Cross Divisional Committee. With this connection to the auxiliary hospitals and Mr Garnett's practical experience of ambulance work it is thought they regularly invited wounded men to Greathouse for a few days rest and to enjoy evenings of amusement and entertainment. Elsie recalled how the men enjoyed visits by musicians and comics or simply entertained themselves with board games.

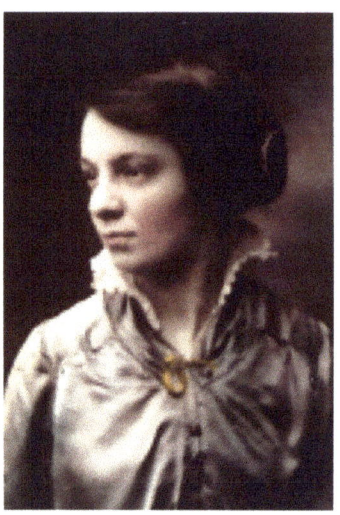

Elsie Fortune

1   *Wiltshire Times* - 20 September 1924, Charles Garnett's obituary.
2   Meeting with Bryant Vincent who recalled the reminiscence of his mother, Elsie Fortune

The Story of Chippenham's Red Cross Hospital

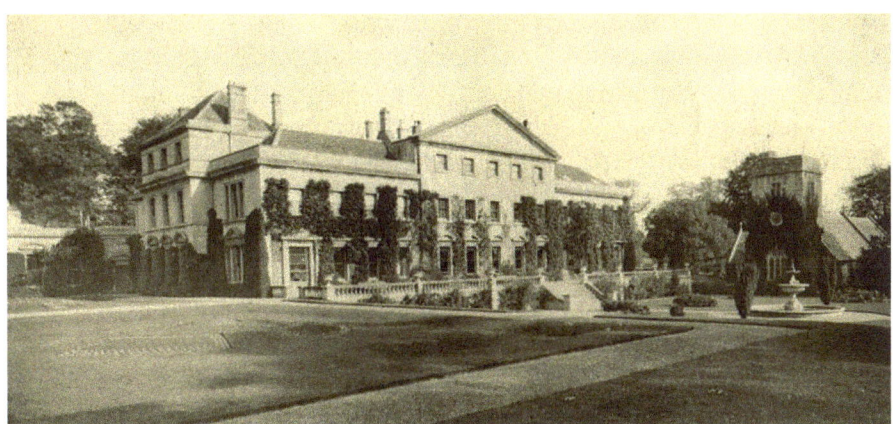

Draycot House

Another private property that was offered for convalescent men was Draycot House at Draycot Cerne, a few miles from Chippenham. Unlike Greathouse, Draycot House was listed and recognised by the Red Cross, but little is known about the staff or patients. Part of the house was set aside and fitted out as a ward by the tenant, Princess Hadzfeldt, who raised a Voluntary Aid Detachment with members coming from the villages of Christian Malford, Sutton Benger, Draycot Cerne and Seagry.[1] This Detachment was registered with the Red Cross as Wilts 38 and eventually came under the command of Chippenham Division. There is no further mention of Draycot until the summer of 1915 when it appears the property was closed and Princess Hadzfeldt had moved to Windsor.

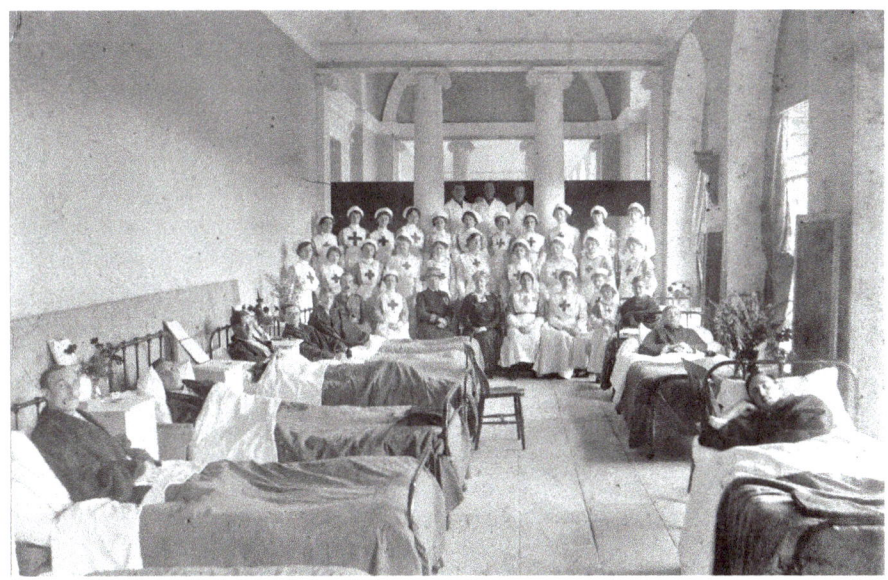

Patients and VADs at Bowood

1 *Devizes and Wiltshire Gazette* - 9 January 1916

The owner of Draycot House, Lord Cowley, had taken possession of the property and made plans to undertake extensive modernisation work.[1] At that time the Wilts 38 Detachment appears to have fallen dormant.

A number of other country estates in North Wiltshire opened as Red Cross hospitals. Lord and Lady Suffolk received the first wounded men at their home, Charlton House near Malmesbury, in November 1914. A few weeks earlier Lord and Lady Lansdowne opened Bowood House, near Chippenham, elsewhere in the county Wilton House and Longleat also received patients.

As a hospital was not required in Chippenham, some of the members of Derry Hill and Chippenham Detachments were allocated to Bowood House, while others joined the Red Cross Hospital in Corsham. The remaining VADs in Chippenham turned to providing care to Belgian refugees who were expected to arrive in the town at any moment.

Belgian Refugees

DURING THE NINETEENTH century Britain had committed to maintaining Belgium's independence and neutrality.[2] When Germany invaded Belgium on the 4 August, they violated this agreement and almost immediately there were horror stories of atrocities against civilians. In December 1914 the Daily Telegraph published King Albert's Book, a compendium of tributes in support of Belgium to raise money for the Belgian fund. The book described the horror in Belgium:

> Her beautiful country has been laid waste. Her harvests, which were ripe for the gathering, have been trodden into the earth. Her villages have been given up to the flames. Her cities have been made to resound with the screams of shell and the cries of slaughter.

To escape the German aggressor thousands of Belgian civilian refugees arrived in Britain. Towns and cities across the nation welcomed them with open arms and offers of help from the public poured in. The Red Cross and the Order of St John worked together and organised a refugee service for displaced people in Britain.[3] Two years later a committee under the Chairmanship of the Duke of Norfolk reviewed the welfare arrangements for the Belgians. The report described the first months of the War:[4]

> In the autumn of 1914, His Majesty's Government offered the hospitality of the British Nation to these victims of the war, and arrangements were made by the (Local

1 *Wiltshire Times* - 25 September 1915
2 The Treaty of London 1839
3 The British red Cross Society – Information sheet: *Our Refugee Service during the First World War*
4 Imperial War Museum – Article - *Women at War collection*. Report dated 8 September 1916.

The Story of Chippenham's Red Cross Hospital

Government) Board for their transport to this country and the provision of refuges in which they could reside pending their allocation to hospitality. Some 250,000 refugees have come to this country, and the great work of providing them with temporary homes was taken up with enthusiasm and liberality by the public themselves.

Numerous local committees were formed for the purpose of providing hospitality and caring for refugees, and many private individuals also gave them shelter and maintenance. The War Refugee Committee in London acted as a central organising body, and rendered most valuable service in the allocation of refugees to the hospitality which was so generously offered.

In Wiltshire the Local Government Board asked the County Branch of the Central War Relief Committee to appoint a number of district representatives to form refugee sub-committees. Lady Methuen, the Vice President for the Chippenham Division of the Red Cross, was appointed to lead the committee that included the towns of Corsham, Chippenham and Calne.[1]

The Mayor of Chippenham chaired a meeting in October to organise a local relief fund to help the refugees. Temporary accommodation and the loan of furniture were needed when the Belgians arrived in the town.[2]

Chippenham VADs were at the meeting and offered their services. Ethel Williams arranged for the Detachment to provide welcoming meals for the Belgian families. Elizabeth and Alice Collen, offered financial and practical help and, as they were also members of the Chippenham Red Cross sewing work group,[3] they were able to arrange for bedding and clothing to be made available.

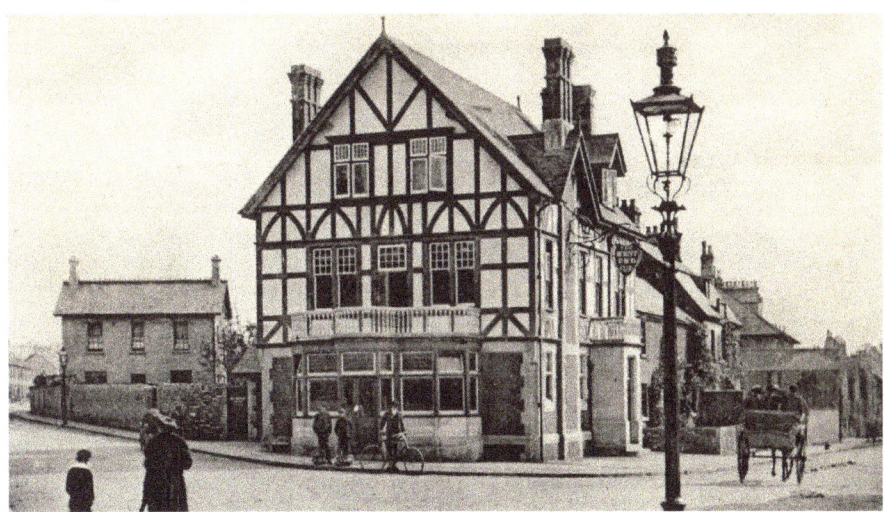

The old West End Club became temporary accommodation for Belgian refugees

1 *Wiltshire Times Letters to the Editor* – 26 September 1914
2 *Wiltshire Times* -31 October 1914
3 The British Red Cross Society - VAD index card record

Unity and Loyalty

Another VAD, Rachel Coward, the wife of Frederic Coward, the Manager of the Union of London and Smiths Bank on the Bridge in Chippenham, gave much of her time helping the refugees. Her husband was also involved with the refugees and was the treasurer of the Belgian Relief Fund in the town.[1]

To accommodate the Belgians in Chippenham the Bath Brewery Company provided the old West End Club at Landsend at no charge and Frederic Coward arranged for the Relief Fund to pay for any furnishings needed to make it ready to receive the first refugee. Doctor Wilson, the husband of the Chippenham VAD Commandant, provided £10 towards the running costs of the accommodation and the use of a small cottage he owned to house further refugees.

Joan Money-Kyrle, a member of Derry Hill Detachment and her mother Florence, who was on the committee of the Chippenham Red Cross Division, were responsible for finding additional accommodation for refugees. In her diary[2] Joan describes how she successfully negotiated accommodation for 11 Belgians in the village of Heddington, near Calne.

In Lacock, Matilda Talbot, who was in charge of cooking at Corsham VAD Hospital, arranged for a family of Belgians to occupy a house in the village[3] and organised donations of food to ensure they were well fed.

Elinor Davis, another member of the Chippenham VAD and a well-known singer in the town, arranged a concert to raise money for the refugees. The Western Daily Press:[4]

> A successful concert, organised by Mrs W. C. Davis, was given in the Neeld Hall on 'Wednesday evening on behalf the funds of the Belgian hostel, in which 20 refugees are accommodated and maintained by public subscriptions. Songs were admirably rendered by Miss D. Aylmore, Miss G. Beaven, Messrs T. H. Fogg, J. Pearn , F J. Troughton, H. Eldridge, and several of the refugees, one of whom sang the French British, and Belgian National Anthems. Mrs Davis's elocutionary powers were displayed in the recital of Harold Simpson's poem, 'Unconquerable.' The part-songs and choruses were successfully given by a choir of 50 voices, under the direction of Mr George Freeth, and the instrumental music was provided by Lady Muriel Coventry's orchestra. The programme concluded with a brilliant and patriotic spectacle, in which was represented the colonies coming to the help of the Motherland.

Some of the Belgians remained in Chippenham for the duration of the War. When they first arrived in 1914 it was decided that they should not take up work but by 1915 this rule was rescinded. In Chippenham Belgians were employed in a number of industries including Saxby and Farmer making munitions[5] and at least one young Belgian lady

---

1 *Wiltshire Times* 19 December 1914
2 Wiltshire and Swindon Archive - 1720/720 *Diaries of Joan Money-Kyrle*
3 *My life and Lacock Abbey* – Matilda Talbot
4 *Western Daily Press* - 4 December 1914
5 *Devizes and Wiltshire Gazette* - 3 February 1916. Charles Wellens worked at Saxby and

The Story of Chippenham's Red Cross Hospital

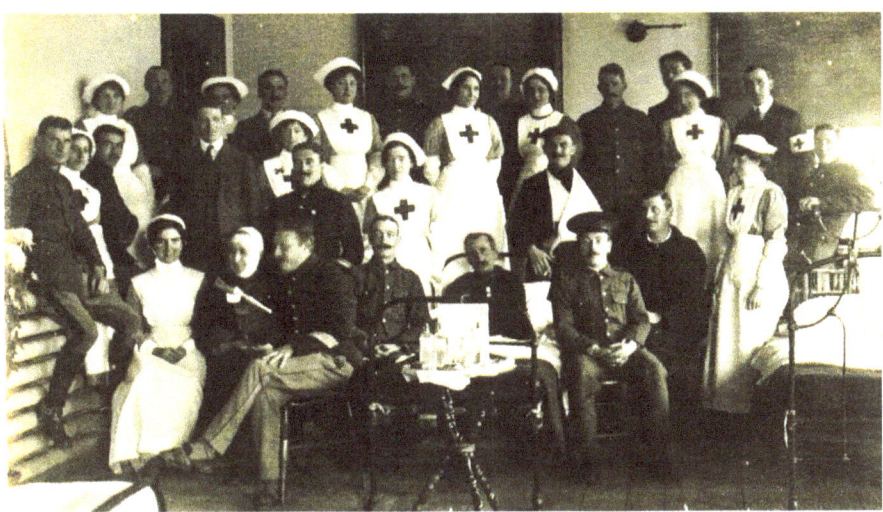

VADs and wounded at Corsham. Some of the men were Belgian soldiers.

joined the VADs in Chippenham. Some of the patients at Corsham were Belgian soldiers and were welcomed by their countrymen.[1]

Comforts for the Troops

THE GENERAL PUBLIC were looking for ways to help the soldiers at the Front. Newspapers published articles giving practical advice and called for the public to *'do what you can to cheer and encourage our soldiers. Gladly help any organisation for their comfort and welfare.'*

Nora Phillips of Kington Langley, the daughter of Chippenham's Town Clerk, F H Phillips, was one of many voices who suggested that ladies should group together to make warm clothing to send to the Front. In a letter to the London Times she wrote:[2]

> The women of the country should set to work immediately to provide large stores of boots, socks, flannel shirts, knitted cardigans, balaclava helmets, and tobacco packed in small cases, in order that a regular distribution to our troops may be maintained either through existing organisations or by means of a Women's Patriotic Fund.

Lady Neeld of Grittleton endorsed this in a letter on behalf of the North Wilts Needlework Guild, saying she hoped in the national crisis there would be a great increase in the number of items given to the Guild that would be of use to the men at the front.[3]

Farmer.
1. *A Life revealed. The Diaries of Herbert Spackman* – Ernest Hird. Spackman took in several Belgians as lodgers and also describes concerts for the Belgians and the patients.
2. *The Times* - 11 August 1914
3. *Wiltshire Times* - 22 August 1914.

Unity and Loyalty

She joined the Mayor at a meeting at the Town Hall Chippenham in September 1914 with the aim of organising groups to make 'comforts' for the troops. Twenty ladies came forward immediately prepared to provide their sewing services.[1]

In many of the villages around Chippenham 'comforts' groups were formed to make socks, balaclavas and blankets for the Tommies, some groups even sent cake and chocolate.

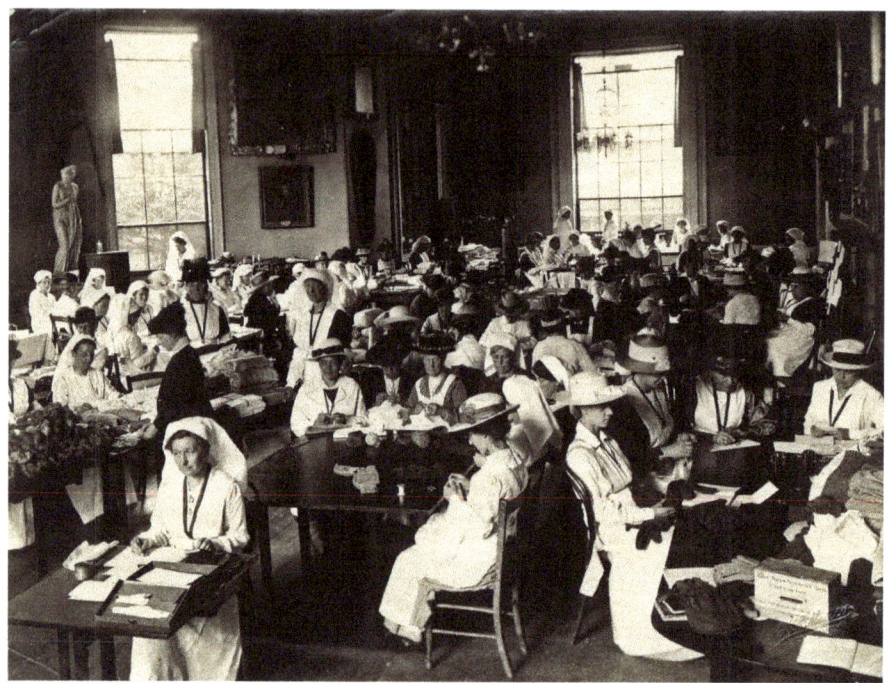

The Queen Mary Needlework Guild in Salisbury making comforts for the troops

In the village of Nettleton the wife of the vicar, Gladys Stafford Jones, formed a committee to raise money and make garments. By the beginning of October they had raised £13.15s and 150 articles had been made. Easton and Pickwick near Corsham sent 24 shirts and 24 pairs of socks during one week in September.

These groups of volunteers were keen to do as much as possible to help the war effort and sent off parcels of clothing to various organisations, including the War Office, in the hope they would reach the men at the Front. It soon became apparent that this uncoordinated approach led to confusion and waste. There was no control of quantity or quality or even the appropriateness of clothing. A comment made by one organiser was that silk pyjamas were of no use to men in the trenches. To bring some order to the donations the Red Cross were asked to coordinate contributions and issue standard patterns for blankets, socks, gloves and balaclavas. The sewing groups were instructed to send parcels to the Society's Central Committee at its Headquarters at Devonshire House in London.

1 *Western Daily Press* – 23 September 1914

The Story of Chippenham's Red Cross Hospital

The Western Daily Press published a letter from C R White, Vice-President of the Bristol Branch of the British Red Cross Society giving advice on the matter:

> We cannot too strongly urge upon all who are desirous of assisting this direction (sewing and knitting garments) that they should organise themselves under the British Red Cross Society, as not only will more effective work be done, but, in the distribution, the Society will exercise the necessary care in seeing that the fruits of their efforts are not frittered away by unorganised distribution.

The Red Cross Central Committee was soon overwhelmed with parcels and enquiries about making clothing for the troops and they turned to their County Branches for help.

Sewing and Knitting Work Parties

IN MANY COUNTIES, including Wiltshire, the Red Cross Divisions were asked to form Comforts Sections to take responsibility for organising donations and the distribution of the work from the sewing groups in their area.[1]

In Chippenham Division the section became known as the Chippenham Red Cross Divisional Needlework Association and was led by Lady Margaret Spicer with Gertrude Gladstone as secretary. They were both influential ladies in the county, able to guide the sewing and knitting groups to meet Red Cross standards. They also had experience of organising sewing groups following the Derry Hill meeting in August 1914, where they had taken responsibility for hospital supplies work groups.

Lady Spicer and Mrs Gladstone issued instructions to improve the organisation

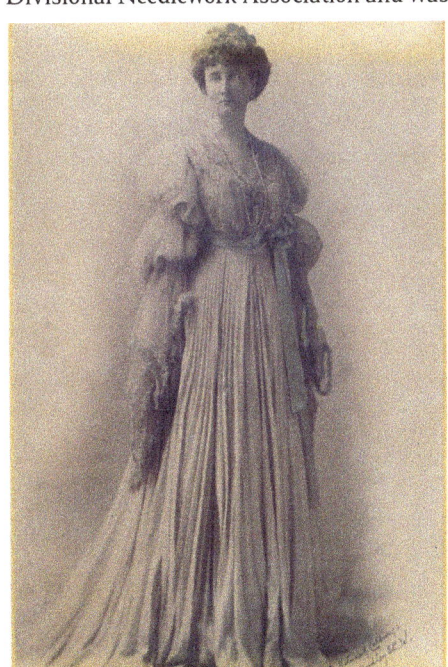

Lady Margaret Spicer led the Needlework Association. In 1915 she also became Vice President of Chippenham District

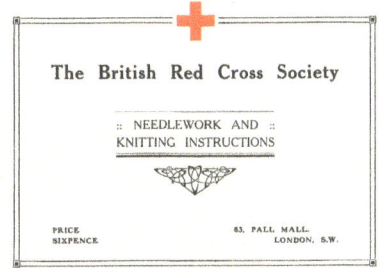

The Red Cross issued standard patterns to work parties

---

1   *The Story of British VAD work in the Great War* - Thekla Bowser

Unity and Loyalty

> **RED CROSS WORKERS!**
>
> You can considerably increase your output of work by using a
>
> # SINGER
>
> ## SEWING MACHINE
>
> Made in the huge Singer Factory at Clydebank, Scotland.
>
> **IF YOU POSSESS A HAND MACHINE**
> go to the nearest Singer Shop, or ask any Singer Salesman about having it fitted to a
>
> **COMBINATION HAND & TREADLE TABLE AND STAND**
>
> With it you can produce twice the work in half the time.
>
> For temporary use, Singer Sewing Machines can be rented by the week or month.
>
> SINGER SEWING MACHINE CO., LTD., 42, ST. PAUL'S CHURCHYARD, LONDON
>
> *Shops Everywhere.*
>
> RED ✚ workers can find them by the sign of the RED S

The Singer Sewing Machine Company offered Red Cross workers improvements to their machines

of the Needlework Association to ensure distribution of articles became more efficient. These instructions included that every sewing and knitting work group should register with the Red Cross and that their workers join the Red Cross Society.[1] This meant all the work groups, both those making hospital supplies and those making clothing for men at the front, would be under the control of the Red Cross and a coordinated approach could be achieved.

---

1 The British red Cross Society – Information sheet: *Volunteers during WW1*.

The Story of Chippenham's Red Cross Hospital

Some groups, such as the North Wilts Needlework Guild and the Chippenham St Paul's Church Women's Union, decided to remain independent but agreed to work alongside the Red Cross.

Once a group registered with the Red Cross, it became part of a national organisation of Work Parties. Each Work Party was given a unique four-digit number and formally placed under the command of a Division. The membership of Work Parties varied: some had less than 10 members, others over forty. They were organised under a Work Party Leader, who would be a prominent lady in the community, often the wife or daughter of the local vicar.

Amy Bolton, daughter of Allan Bolton, the Rector of Yatton Keynell, led a Red Cross sewing group in the village, while vicar's wife Annie Ramsbottom organised the work party in Lacock.

It was usual for the Work Party to meet as a group in a local hall but some ladies, through choice or necessity, would sew at home. Mary Deane, who was a member of Box Work Party, wrote in her diary how she often did Red Cross work alone at home.[1]

The members were responsible for the purchase of materials and equipment and relied on fund-raising events and door to door collections. Mrs Ramsbottom and the ladies of the Lacock Work Party arranged whist drives and dances. A particularly successful event at the Oddfellows Hall in 1916 raised the magnificent sum of £8 2s 3d.[2]

A report for Chippenham Division in March 1916[3] said that the sewing and knitting work had been taken up with great enthusiasm by ladies of all classes and some excellent results were achieved. Mrs Gladstone's group, who met at Bowden Park, had produced 1200 garments in less than a year.[4]

It is thought that during the War over 20 Work Parties were attached to Chippenham Division and organised by the Chippenham Red Cross Divisional Needlework Association. They worked throughout the War and some groups continued after the war making items for voluntary organisations such as St Dunstans who cared for blinded servicemen.

The following is a list of those work parties registered with the Red Cross and their leaders:[5]

Number	Work Party	Work Party Leader	
1404	Derry Hill	Lady Walter Hervey	Rumsey House, near Calne
1614	Grittleton	Hon Lady Neeld	Grittleton House
1625	Corsham	Hon. Mrs E Talbot	Hartham Park, near Corsham
1628	Bradenstoke	Miss E F Wiltshire	Bradenstoke
1672	Bowden Park	Mrs Gladstone	Bowden Park near Chippenham

1 *The Shadow of Mary Deane* – Patricia Whalley
2 *Wiltshire Times* - 5 February 1916
3 *Devizes and Wiltshire Gazette* – 23 March 1916 Annual report of Chippenham Division
4 *The Tatler* - 15 August 1917
5 The British Red Cross Society Archive

Unity and Loyalty

1686	Spye Park	Lady M Spicer	Spye Park near Chippenham
1701	Sutton Benger	Countess Cowley	Draycot House, Draycot
1702	Box	Mrs Stephen Langton	Sherbrooke, Box
1703	Slaughterford	Mrs Bolwell	Slaughterford
1725	Corsham	Mrs C H Williamson	Middlewick, Corsham
1731	Chippenham	Mrs Newton Heath	Market Place, Chippenham
1771	Lacock	Mrs Ramsbottom	Lacock Vicarage
1784	Corsham	Miss K L Goldney	Beechfield, Corsham
1786	Corsham	Lady Goldney	Monks Park, Corsham
1883	North Wraxall	Mrs B C Langley	North Wraxall Rectory
1893	Bowden Park	Mrs Gladstone	Bowden Park near Chippenham
1916	Yatton Keynell	Miss A Bolton	Yatton Keynell Rectory
1917	Colerne	Mrs Stephens	Colerne Rectory
4914	Chippenham	Hon Mrs Allfrey	Greenways, Chippenham
4933	Tytherton	Mrs W Collett	Barn Bridge, East Tytherton
5174	Lacock	Mrs John Taylor	Bowden Hill, Lacock
5679	Dauntsey	Mrs W Winwood	Idover House, Dauntsey

There was also sympathy for the plight of our allies and appeals to help them. In February 1915 a bale of blankets and shirts[1] was dispatched by Corsham Work Party as part of the Serbian Relief Fund. Serbia had been fighting the Austrian armies and suffered heavy casualties, both military and civilian. The Spectator magazine summed up why we should help:[2] *'Serbia is as much our ally as Russia, and as such is entitled, not merely to our esteem and sympathy, but also to assistance of a more practical kind.'*

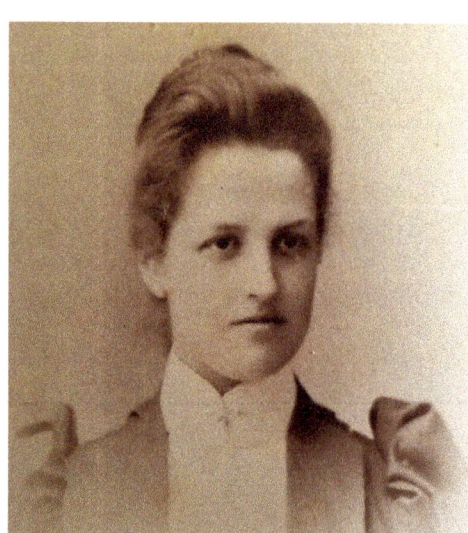

Florence Lane

Chippenham had two work parties, numbers 1731 and 4914. Little is known about 4914 as few records have survived but we know that 1731 had a membership of over forty ladies, led by the wife of draper Newton Heath, Helen Heath. Due to the size of the work party she shared the responsibility with Florence Lane. Florence was the daughter of a retired bank manager and lived in St Mary Street. She and her father had been keen supporters of the Red Cross, since the first meeting in the town in 1909.

1   *Gazette and Herald – From the Files* - 26 February 2015.
2   *The Spectator* - 26 September 1914

The Story of Chippenham's Red Cross Hospital

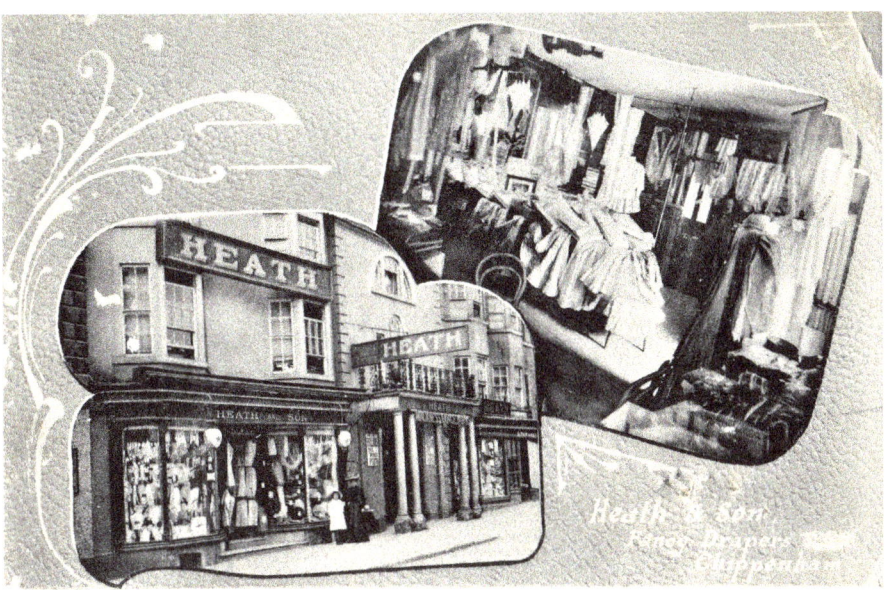

Business card for Heath and Son Fancy Drapers. The rooms above the shop were used as the Red Cross depot

To receive donations brought in by members of the public and items made by work parties the Red Cross introduced central depots where volunteers sorted and distributed bedding, pyjamas and bandages for the hospitals and clothing for the troops at the front. In the early days of the War a Wiltshire Red Cross depot was established in Calne[1] and another depot was opened at Wicker Hill in Trowbridge.

As the War continued more depots were needed and it was decided to open one in Chippenham. Helen Heath's husband owned the draper and outfitters shop in the Market Place and in 1916 he agreed that the rooms over his shop could be used as a Red Cross Depot where a group of ladies spent two or three days each week distributing donations.

---

1   Wiltshire and Swindon Archive - 1720/720 *Diaries of Joan Money-Kyrle*. Miss Money-Kyrle refers to the Calne Depot in her diary of 1914.

Chapter 6
1915

THE GERMANS BOMBARD English towns and cities. There are complaints that the production of munitions can't keep pace with the War in France and factories turn to armament production. Casualties are greater than anticipated and more hospitals are urgently needed. In November Chippenham VAD Hospital opens and the town celebrates Christmas with the wounded men.

New Year and German Raids

AS 1914 DREW to a close there was little sign of the anticipated victory, and the slogan 'Over by Christmas' took on a hollow ring.

The mayor, John Cole, gave his traditional New Year address to the town. He reflected on the previous months of war and spoke of the need for the town to maintain its spirit and do its duty:[1]

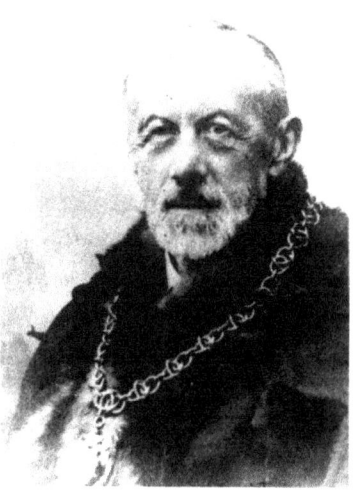

Mayor John Cole

> As this is the first meeting of the Council for the year it has been customary for the mayor to offer to the Council the greetings of the season. This year I think it will be the form of wishing that the end of 1915 may be happier than the beginning.
>
> The great nations of the earth are at war: duty has called this country to take part and I am sure we all trust that duty will sustain this nation until the work is accomplished.
>
> I had a very excellent motto sent to me by a friend this Christmas, it is this, 'He conquers who endures.' I convey it to my fellow townsmen: may the spirit of endurance and the spirit of determination sustain us to the end.
>
> And gentlemen may we abide patiently these days of sorrow and sacrifice and look forward to a brighter and happier time when our nation shall again possess quietness and peace.

Particularly heavy rainfall for much of January saw Chippenham suffer levels of flooding not seen for over ten years. The first day of the year also brought the grim news

---

1   *Chippenham Council minute book 9.*

The Story of Chippenham's Red Cross Hospital

that the battleship HMS Formidable had been sunk by a German submarine in the English Channel, with many lives lost. Mr and Mrs Day, of Parkfields, suffered many sleepless nights before they heard their son Alfred had survived the sinking, but lay injured in hospital.[1]

The War came to Britain when the ports of Scarborough, Hartlepool, and Whitby were shelled by the Germans in December 1914 with hundreds of civilian casualties. Joan Money-Kyrle wrote in her diary:[2] '*Rather disturbing news tonight Germans have been shelling Scarborough and Hartlepool several people killed.*'

On 19 January 1915 the Germans launched the first Zeppelin raids on the East Coast and by May 1915 London was the target. The public became increasingly nervous as the newspapers reported on these air raids.[3]

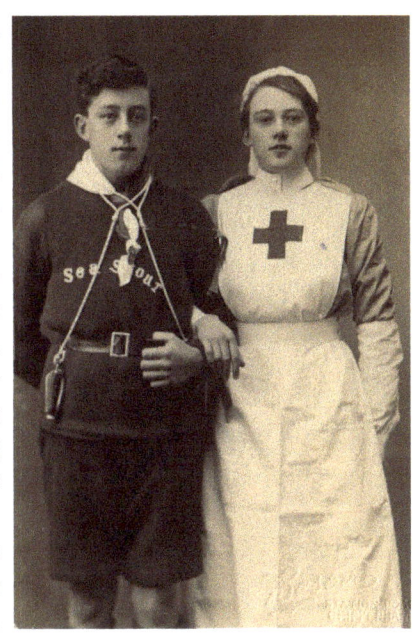

VAD Fanny Ferris and her brother Vivian. Scouts like Vivian were called upon for duty at the hospitals

Reflecting the escalation in the War the VAD hospitals in Chippenham Division, Bowood, Corsham and Melksham, were under increasing pressure to accept more patients.

VADs from Chippenham offered their help through the district. Mabel Tuck, Winifred King and Sarah Mackness joined Corsham, while Fanny Ferris and Norah Collen went to Bowood House, where Norah later became a staff nurse. In nearby Devizes the Central Wilts Division opened an Officers Hospital at Beltwood Dalling in January 1915.[4]

Chippenham Does its Duty

AT THE CHIPPENHAM Easter Vestry Meeting in April 1915 Rev Maxwell H. Smith, the vicar of the parish church, St Andrew's, gave his report for the year in which he described how the town had fared:

---

1   *Wiltshire Times* - 09 January 1915
2   Wiltshire and Swindon Archive - 1720/720 *Diaries of Joan Money-Kyrle* 16 December 1914
3   *All Quiet on the Home Front* - Richard Van Emden and Steve Humphries. The book describe how people felt demoralised and news reporting only led to greater anxiety.
4   *Gazette and Herald*– From the files - 17 January 2015. Beltwood Dalling was better known as Braeside

Unity and Loyalty

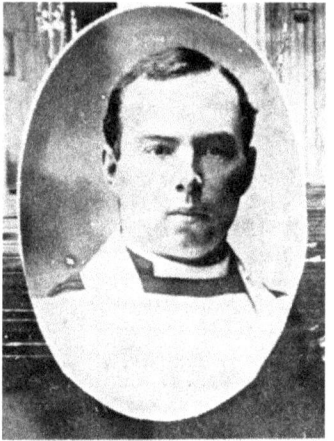

Rev Maxwell H Smith

The Year 1914-15 will ever be associated in the history of our parish with the war. We are engaged in a life and death struggle, our cause we believe to be a righteous one, and with the help of God we mean to fight until it has triumphed and until the menace of German militarism is no more.

In those dark days early in August, which now seem so far off, when the part Great Britain was to play hung, as it were, in the balance, the parishioners of Chippenham to a man stood loyal and true ready to endure hardships, prepared to make sacrifices and to support the Government in upholding the Empire's honour. The call to arms sounded and those amongst us of military age, as our roll of honour eloquently testifies, volunteered in their hundreds for service on behalf of King and country. To obtain a complete and accurate list of these is no easy matter, but I trust in course of time this may be secured and that in some form it may be placed in the church as a permanent memorial and record of willing service in the Empire's hour of need.

Our parish has contributed with its usual liberality to the various war funds which have been opened, and our parishioners have worked with enthusiasm upon the committees which have been formed to offer hospitality and sympathy to Belgian Refugees, to render assistance to the families of soldiers and sailors, and to relieve civil distress, whilst many have made themselves efficient members of the Red Cross Voluntary Aid Detachments. In these ways we have but done our duty: would that we could have done more!

For some months past one or two squadrons of the Royal Wilts Yeomanry have been billeted in our midst. I should be sorry to let this opportunity pass without saying a word of congratulation to the men for their exemplary behaviour at all times in the streets and in public places. They are shortly to go into camp at Bowood and when the time comes, we shall all be sorry to lose them, and they will take with them the heartiest good wishes of the parishioners of Chippenham.

Whenever soldiers are billeted in a town a difficulty invariably arises with the girls and young women of the place. The sight of a uniform appears to have a demoralising effect upon a certain class of young woman. It is a matter of regret that some few of our girls have had their heads turned and have behaved in the streets in an immodest way. It is to be hoped that the patriotic meeting for women and girls recently held will have been the means of bringing them to their senses and of teaching them self-respect, as well as respect for the Kings uniform.

The vicar recognised how the parish had helped the Belgians and applauded those who had joined the VADs.

The Story of Chippenham's Red Cross Hospital

The Shell Crisis

Now the certainty of a quick war was shattered official opinion indicated the likelihood of a protracted war, possibly a year or more, with both armies dug into trenches bombarding each other with heavy artillery. The amount of equipment this new industrial warfare demanded had never been anticipated and traditional shell and explosive production wasn't keeping pace with the rate of fire at the front.

Complaints of lack of munitions at the front were widely reported in the press. This rapidly escalated to a political scandal, known as the 'Shell Crisis', which resulted in a number of military and political resignations and the formation of a new coalition government led by H H Asquith, with David Lloyd George appointed as Minister of Munitions.

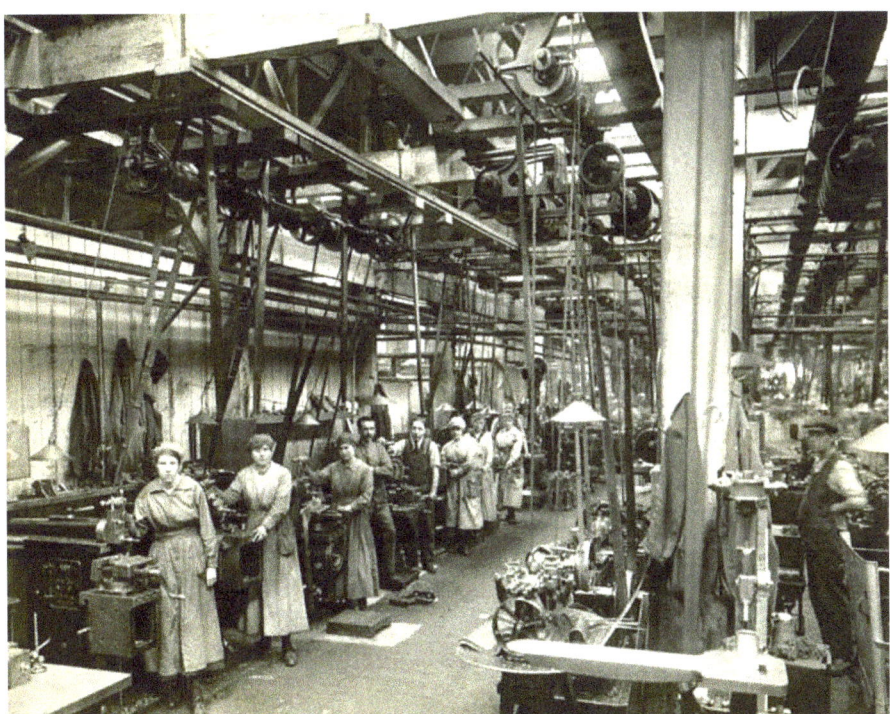

Munitionettes on shell production at Saxby and Farmer

To deal with the crisis Lloyd George introduced the Munitions of War Act in July 1915, which gave the newly created Ministry of Munitions power to direct factories to turn their production to armaments and restrict the freedom of workers to leave.

In Chippenham the railway signalling company of Saxby and Farmer was one of the businesses instructed to concentrate their efforts on shell production. Like many engineering companies it had lost a sizable portion of its workforce as they volunteered for war service. To meet the increased demand in production the company employed women on the factory production lines. Women turned to factory work throughout the country and were universally known as munitionettes proudly wearing the triangular 'On War Service' badge. What was not immediately appreciated, as women turned to work in factories, was a corresponding drop in numbers volunteering for the Red Cross.

Another Military Hospital in Bristol

In Bristol the Infirmary and Southmead Hospital were overflowing despite the civilian authorities allocating additional bed space. So many wounded were returning from the battles in Gallipoli and France that it was agreed by the War Office that a further military hospital should be opened.

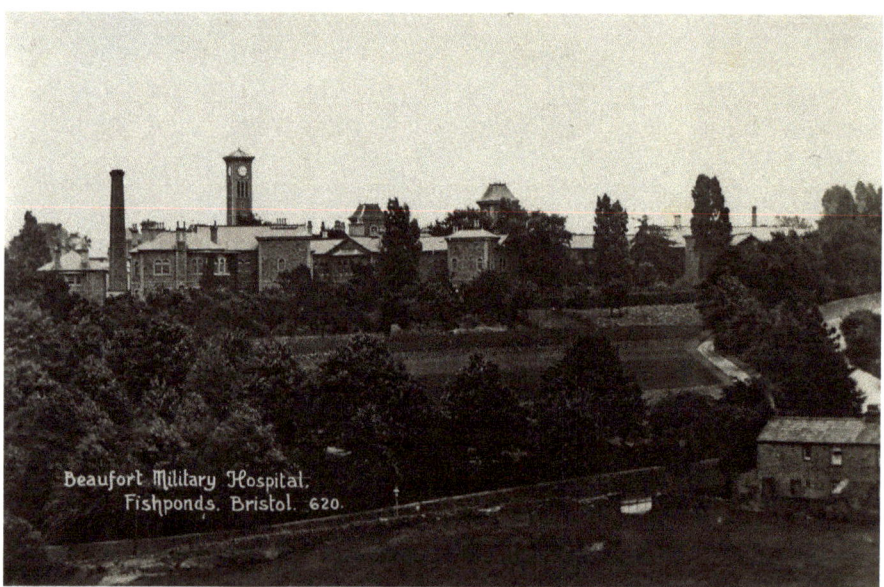

Beaufort Hospital Bristol

The Bristol Lunatic Asylum in Fishponds was identified as being suitable to receive wounded. The inmates were moved to other asylums around the country, although a number remained to help in the laundry and kitchens. It took three months to convert the building to provide full medical and surgical wards and two operating theatres. When it opened in May 1915 it was renamed Beaufort War Hospital and offered nearly one and a half thousand additional beds.

The knock-on effect for the Red Cross in Somerset, Gloucestershire and Wiltshire was that the VAD hospitals were constantly at full capacity and by the autumn of 1915 the Red Cross told the Military Command in Bristol no further beds could be allocated

The Story of Chippenham's Red Cross Hospital

in the area. Corsham VAD Hospital was described as reaching its utmost capacity.[1] The War Office realised that they had to ask the Red Cross to find additional suitable premises for convalescents.

The Chippenham VAD Hospital

THE WILTSHIRE COUNTY Director, Basil Hankey, received notification at the beginning of October 1915 that the War Office had agreed that Chippenham Town Hall was considered suitable and should therefore be requisitioned by the Red Cross as an additional VAD hospital in Wiltshire.[2]

Mr Hankey wrote immediately to Mrs Wilson, the Commandant of Chippenham:

> I have today heard from the Deputy Director Medical Services Southern Command, accepting the Town Hall for 40 patients. You will doubtless get to work at once and I will ask for your Detachment to be mobilised.

With the weight of the War Office behind him, Mr Hankey approached Chippenham Council to seek agreement that the Town Hall should be released to Mrs Wilson. With little debate this was agreed by the Halls Committee.[3]

Mr Hankey was told the first patients from Bristol were expected to arrive in Chippenham within a matter of weeks and so work to convert the Town Hall started immediately. The large hall was converted into the main ward to accommodate the majority of men. Two smaller adjoining rooms became side wards for those who needed additional care. A first-floor window at the rear of the building was enlarged and a doorway formed leading to a new passageway to link to the neighbouring Neeld Hall, where two upper dressing rooms were converted into a kitchen and bathroom.[4]

The new bathroom included the latest facilities. Fitted baths, hot and cold water and heated towel rails all served by a boiler under the stage of the Neeld Hall.[5]

It was agreed the stage of the Neeld Hall, when not needed for other purposes, could be used by the men as an area for recreation and

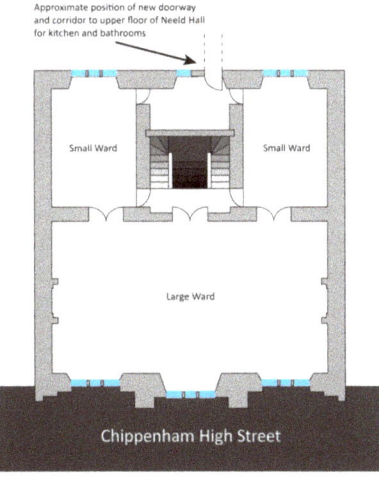

Sketch plan of Chippenham Town Hall showing the location of the wards

1   *Wiltshire Times* - 9 October 1915
2   *Wiltshire Times* – 16 October 1915. Basil Hankey's letter was dated 9 October
3   *Chippenham Council minute book 9*
4   Chippenham Museum - *Garlick Scrapbooks*
5   *Wiltshire Times* - 16 October 1915

reading. This became a favourite meeting place for patients and their visitors.

On the ground floor, in the covered market, a storeroom and additional rooms for the Commandant and Quartermaster were constructed.

The conversion work was carried out by the building company of Francis Hulbert, whose wife Emma was the Assistant Lady Superintendent.

Within a few weeks the alterations were complete and an army of volunteers from the town came to clean the rooms ready for the delivery of beds and equipment.

As soon as it was known the Town Hall was to be used as a hospital Evelyn Belcher, who had replaced Mrs Ennis as Quartermaster, asked the public for their help in donating money or loaning furniture and equipment. The response from the town was spontaneous. Within a week over £130[1] was received, including substantial amounts from Captain and Mrs Allfrey of Greenways House, Sir Audley Neeld of Grittleton and Mrs Garnett of Greathouse.

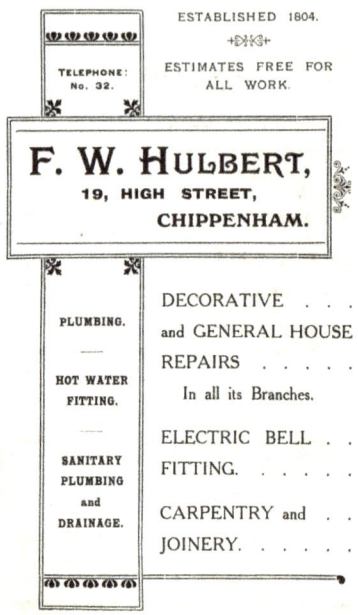

The building company of F.W. Hulbert carried out the conversion work at the Town Hall

People gave what they could afford from a few pence to a shilling or two, but all donations were gratefully received. The staff of Rowden Hill House, the home of the Whishaw family, clubbed together and raised five shillings.

Local organisations and businesses were generous. Edgar Neale, the Dispensing Chemist in the town, gave drugs and medical supplies and the brewers Slade and Sons donated bottles of aerated water for the patients. Beer was not offered, as wounded men were forbidden alcohol. Owner William Goold Slade and his wife Sara lived at Ferfoot, on the outskirts of Chippenham. In November 1916 Sara decided to join the VADs as a part time cook.[2]

Builders, Downing and Rudman and the Wilts Bacon Company provided their staff and vehicles to arrange collections of donated furniture, beds and kitchen equipment. Walter Ferris of Bosmere Farm in Tytherton, whose wife and daughter were both members of the Red Cross, volunteered along with Daniel Collen of the town mill and a group of Boy Scouts to collect smaller items. Another group of men, Messrs Richmond, Smallcombe, Hart, Tayler, Brock and Coleman were responsible for installing the furniture and setting up the equipment. The North Wilts Needlework Guild collected

1   Chippenham Museum - *Garlick Scrapbooks*
2   The British Red Cross Society - VAD index card record

The Story of Chippenham's Red Cross Hospital

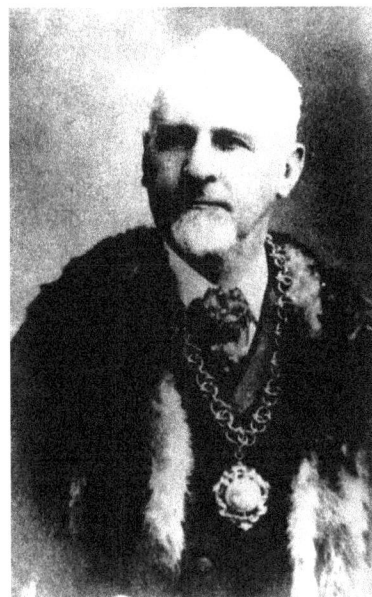
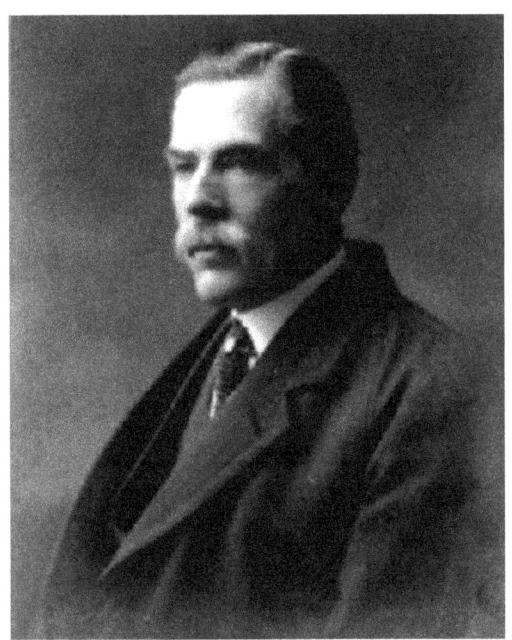

Daniel Collen organised the collection and delivery of furniture and equipment

Chemist Edgar Neale donated medical supplies

blankets, sheets and underwear to donate to the Hospital, while the St Paul's Church Women's Union made all the bedside locker curtains.[1]

The ladies of the Red Cross Divisional Needlework Association led by Mrs Gladstone and Lady Spicer co-ordinated the supply of bandages, bedding and pyjamas and detailed the Chippenham Work Party to maintain a constant supply of these items.

Cigarettes were one of the soldiers' greatest 'comforts' of the War. The Wiltshire Times told of a soldier corresponding with his parents in October 1914. He told them what he missed most was a smoke as tobacco was in short supply. The 'Smokes for the Troops' fund saw tobacco companies donate thousands of cigarettes for the men in the trenches, while Lord Kitchener opened a further fund to provide the wounded in hospital with tobacco and cigarettes. One company, Major Drapkin and Co, gave the Red Cross 100,000 cigarettes for wounded soldiers. When Chippenham opened James Whishaw, the father of the Assistant Commandant Phyllis Whishaw, gave a generous supply of cigarettes to be handed to the men on their arrival.

There was a great deal of public interest in the new VAD Hospital and at the end of October visitors were invited to admire the wards and their amenities. These visits were combined with a Red Cross flag day and the public were particularly generous with over £100 raised.[2] A few days later Colonel Bush, in charge of the Southern Command at Bristol, inspected the Hospital and Canon Maxwell Smith, conducted a service of dedication. It was decided to name the large ward Unity, the first part of the borough

1 Wiltshire and Swindon Archive 1488/42 *St Pauls Church Women's Union meeting minutes*
2 *North Wilts Herald* - 29 October 1915

Unity and Loyalty

motto, and the two smaller wards were named Evelyn and Geoffrey in memory of two sons of Mrs Wilson, who had recently lost their lives in action.

At the beginning of November the wards stood ready. They had been cleaned, blessed, inspected and the ladies of the Voluntary Aid Detachment were on standby.

Mrs Wilson received notification to expect ten wounded men from Southmead on 5 November, arriving at Chippenham station on the 4.34 train.

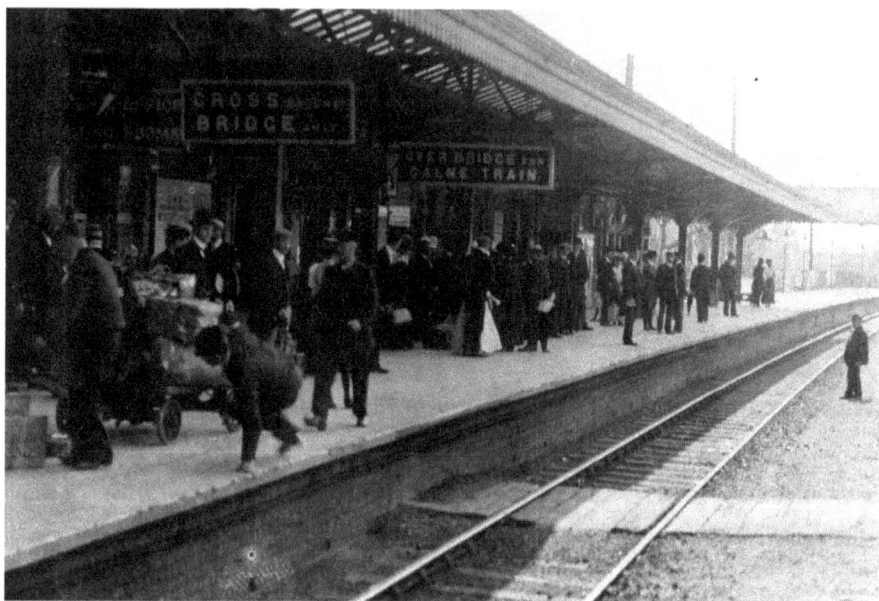

Chippenham Station

These men had spent weeks, even months in the Bristol hospitals and the transfer to Chippenham meant they could look forward to recuperating in a more homely and less formal environment. In 1919, when the wards closed a special mention was made that the Commandant, the nurses and the townspeople of Chippenham made every effort to brighten the soldiers' lives and made them feel thoroughly at home.[1]

This effort was particularly important to maintain morale, especially as many of the men were a long way from home and loved ones. The original hope that patients would be allocated to hospitals close to their homes had long been abandoned due to the considerable numbers involved.[2]

As the train arrived at the station a hastily formed Ambulance Section were waiting to welcome them. The orderlies on duty that afternoon were all Chippenham men; Frank Read, an engineer at Saxby and Farmer, Walter Archard[3], an ex-policeman and now a

1   Chippenham Museum - *Garlick Scrapbooks*.
2   *All Quiet on the Home Front* by Richard Van Emden and Steve Humphries. The idea that men would be allocated to hospitals close to home was soon forgotten
3   Walter died in 1916 but his son and wife continued their work with the Red Cross

The Story of Chippenham's Red Cross Hospital

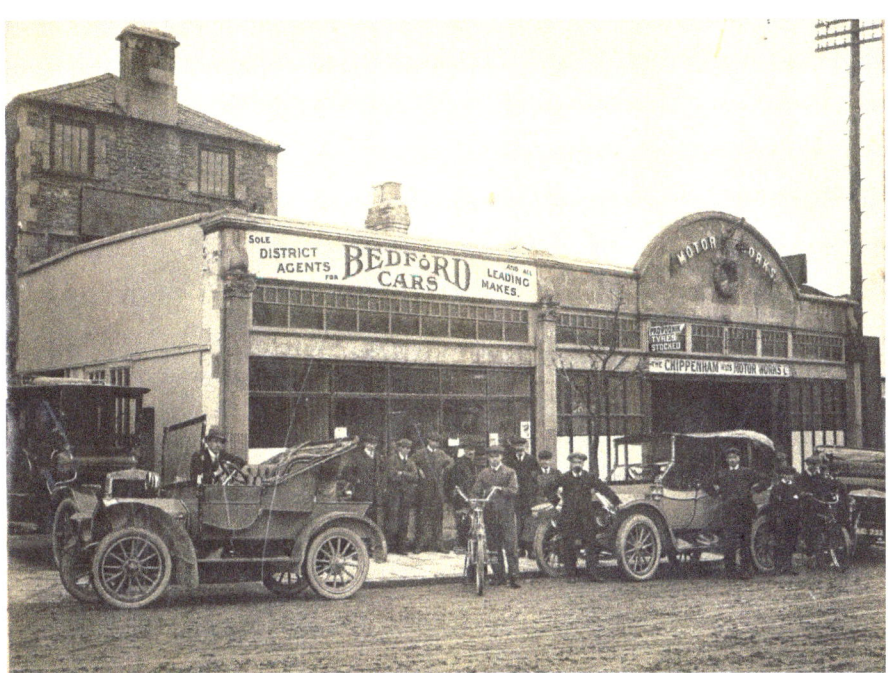

Chippenham Motor Works supplied vehicles to transport walking patients to the hospital

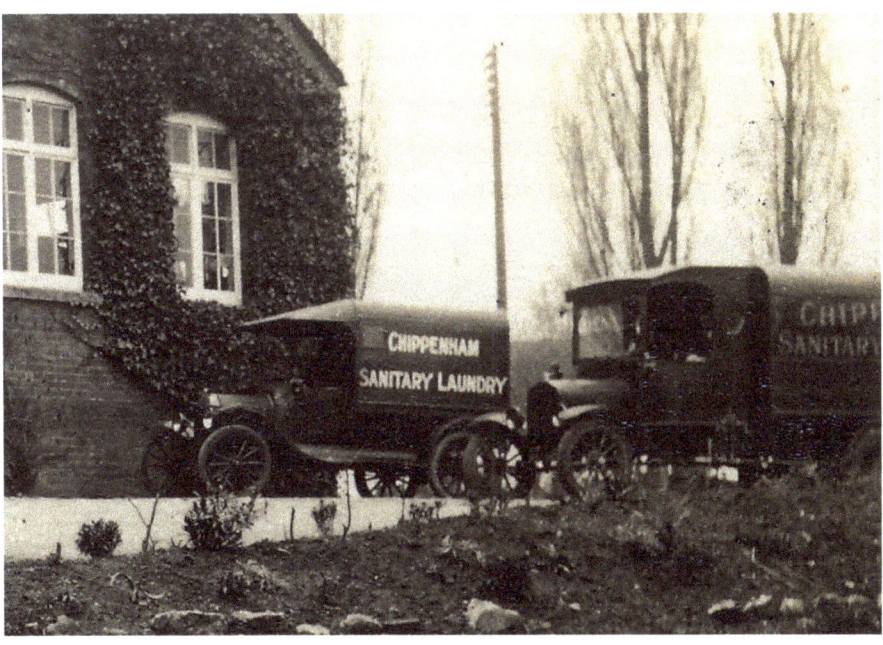

Vans of the Sanitary Laundry were brought into service as temporary ambulances for stretcher cases

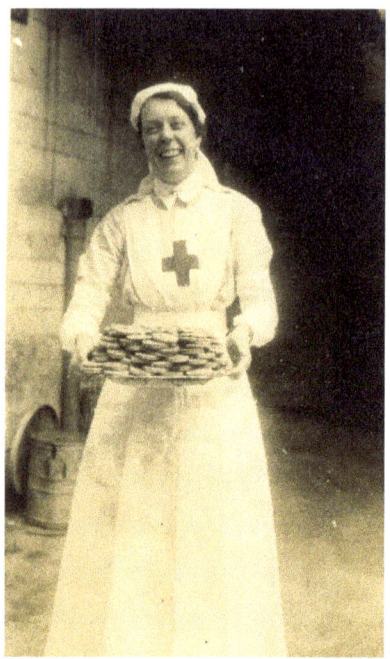

Ethel Williams with a tray of buns to cheer the patients

ticket collector at the railway station; and William King, an ironmonger working with in his father's business in New Road.

The fourth member of the section was Edwin Duck, a foreman porter at the station, who was also a leading member of the Great Western Railway Ambulance Section and had been awarded the gold medal for efficiency.[1] Within a few weeks of greeting the first patients at the station he learned that his own son George had been killed in Mesopotamia.[2]

Of the ten soldiers who arrived, nine were able to walk to the waiting cars lent by Mr Whishaw, Mr Barsted, the horse dealer in New Road, and William Burridge the owner of a motor garage, all of whom would go on to regularly supply vehicles for the use of wounded.

The stretcher patient was transferred to the Town Hall using a van borrowed from Chippenham Sanitary Laundry.

It was usual that crowds gathered when trains arrived with wounded and the men were cheered as they were transferred. The VADs would greet them, complete the necessary paperwork and make the men comfortable. The book Observations of an Orderly by L/Cpl Ward Muir describes the arrival of patients at a London hospital: a building that in peace time had been a school. Muir was a military orderly but many of his descriptions apply equally to a Red Cross hospital like Chippenham and give a sense of events as men arrived:

> The walking cases are the first to arrive, men who are either not ill enough, or not badly enough wounded, to need to be put on stretchers in ambulances, and are transferred from the station in motor-cars.

When the stretcher cases arrived:

> Four orderlies haul the stretcher from its shelf in the ambulance; two orderlies then take its handles and carry it indoors the stretcher is put on a wheeled trolley and he is taken straight away to his ward.

1   *Wiltshire Times* - 22 April 1944 - Obituary
2   *The Great War Chippenham Soldiers* – Richard Broadhead. George Edwin Duck died 22 November 1915 but his parents didn't receive the news until January 1916

The Story of Chippenham's Red Cross Hospital

He then tells that after initial reception, which included a welcome cup of cocoa, a cigarette and the inevitable paperwork, it was time for a hot bath. *'For the ritual of the bath must on no account be omitted.... The bath is thus a pleasure more than a necessity.*

The modern bathroom facilities at Chippenham must have been a firm favourite.

Walter Paddock, who had been a driver at the Angel Hotel in Chippenham until he enlisted in the Army, wrote about his experiences after being wounded at the front. He spent a month convalescing in Sevenoaks in Kent and described his arrival at the Red Cross Hospital, which was similar to Chippenham:[1]

> Had a bath, they dressed my wound and gave me a nice meal; then to bed. Oh, this bed was so cosy and comfortable after getting what rest I could lying in the trenches or on the ground, never taking my clothes or boots off. The sister brought me a cup of tea in the morning and said 'Breakfast at eight-thirty'. I asked if I could lay on for a little while as it was so comfortable; they agreed I could.

Every patient arriving would receive the customary packet of cigarettes and presents were given by members of the public. A man at Beaufort Hospital[2] summed it up in a letter:

> ... and one dear lady, thoughtful, motherly lady gave us luxury of luxuries! a nice pocket handkerchief each. And then there were the cigarettes. It all seemed so tender and homely it brought a little lump to my throat and made my eyes water.

The soldier went on to say: *'...before you could wink twice we were putting ourselves outside of tea and cake to our hearts content.'*

At Chippenham cakes and buns were immortalised by a wounded soldier when he penned a verse about Mrs Williams and her culinary skills saying *'Carefully mixing the dough and the plums, raising fine puddings and making nice buns'.*[3]

The Hospital Staff

A FULL COMPLEMENT OF VADs were present to welcome the first patients with additional help from the Scouts who were called upon to act as messengers and porters.

It is thought the following lady volunteers were on duty during the first days.

Commandant: Mrs Helena Wilson
Assistant Commandant: Miss Phyllis Whishaw
Lady Superintendent: Nurse Green

1   *A Country Boy* - W.J. Paddock
2   Glenside Museum Bristol Archive
3   Chippenham museum. CHIYH 2002-789 *Poem to Mrs Williams*.

Unity and Loyalty

Assistant Superintendent: Mrs Elizabeth Emma Hulbert
Quartermaster: Miss Evelyn Belcher
Assistant Quartermaster: Miss Dora Belcher

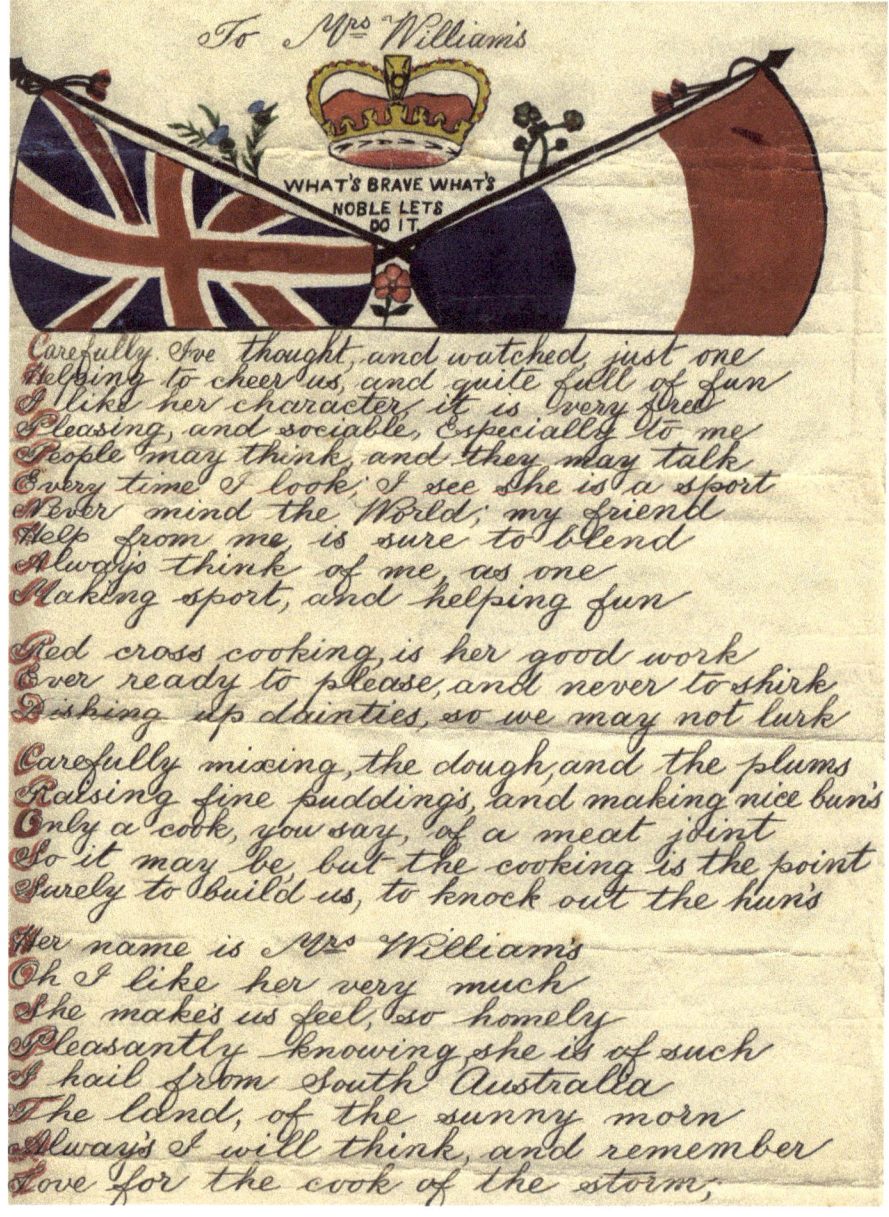

The poem presented to Ethel Williams praising her cooking composed by patient Joseph Dempsey

The Story of Chippenham's Red Cross Hospital

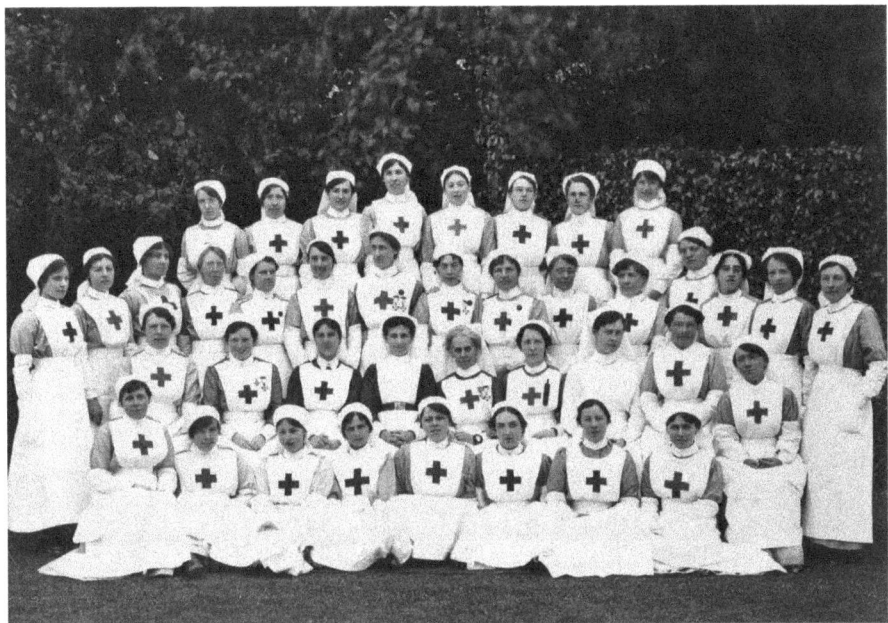

Chippenham Voluntary Aid Detachment, Wilts VAD 6. The photograph was taken soon after the Hospital opened

Nursing Staff:
    Miss Janet Awdry
    Mrs Alice Brett
    Miss Jessie Brinkworth
    Miss Norah Collen
    Mrs Rachael Coward
    Miss Fanny Ferris
    Miss Queenie Green
    Miss Louisa Grimshaw
    Mrs Ellen Hardiman
    Miss Dora Hart
    Mrs Kate Hinton

Cooking and Mess room:
    Mrs E Shipp
    Mrs Ethel Williams
    Mrs Beatrice Hetherington
    Mrs Pinfield
    Miss Kathleen Mackay
    Miss Spinke
    Miss Alice Munday
    Miss Amy Bolton
    Miss Norah Hetherington

Every VAD hospital was required to include a medically trained Lady Superintendent amongst its staff. In Chippenham this was Mary Green, who lived in Lowden Avenue. Miss Green was also the town's District Nurse and was, therefore, eminently qualified to take on the role. Her assistant, Elizabeth Hulbert, who had been a District Nurse before her marriage, took over as Lady Superintendent a year later and also took on duties as a Ward Sister.

For most of the Chippenham VADs this was their first taste of real hospital work. Eighteen months earlier they had practised bandaging in genteel surroundings and at the Trowbridge competition their compliant patients had text book injuries that were easily dealt with. Now they were going to be responsible for the care of soldiers, men, strangers, that had received real injuries and were suffering from sickness and disease.

Some of the Chippenham VADs who some months earlier had gone to Bowood and Corsham returned to Chippenham to share their experiences of Red Cross VAD hospitals.

Joan Money-Kyrle, who served at Bowood and later went to France, wrote in her diary[1] how she quickly came face to face with the reality of war. As part of her training she went to a Bristol hospital and helped with dressings and observed a number of operations and amputations.

The VADs soon proved themselves to be very capable dealing with finances and the logistics of feeding and cleaning on an industrial scale. They negotiated with the Council to place benches outside the Town Hall for the use of the wounded men. More seats were later placed nearby in Bath Road and on The Bridge.[2]

Avice Wilson recalled[3] how her grandmother, Ethel Williams, met with her friends many years after the War when they reminisced about life at the Hospital. She said it was clear they didn't always follow procedures: they just got on with the job and did what was best for the patients. She described her grandmother and her friends as *'very strong and efficient women.'*

A qualified night superintendent, Miss E Tomlin of the Middlesex Hospital, was employed during November 1915.[4] For the VADs shifts became a way of life. Joan Money-Kyrle wrote in her diary how her mother, also a VAD, took her turn for night duty at Corsham.[5]

The patients particularly appreciated the staff on night duty. This was a chance for a quiet chat and help with writing letters.

---

1 Wiltshire and Swindon Archive - 1720/720 *Diaries of Joan Money-Kyrle* 11 and 12 February 1915
2 *Chippenham Council minute book 9* - 7 August 1917. The council needed reminding by the VADs of the need to provide benches.
3 Meeting with Avice Wilson, author of a number of books about Wiltshire, at Chippenham Museum 25 September 2015.
4 *The British Nursing Journal* - 20 November 1915
5 Wiltshire and Swindon Archive - 1720/720 *Diaries of Joan Money-Kyrle* 13 March 1915

The Story of Chippenham's Red Cross Hospital

Nellie Farris recalled how the VADs always did a little extra:[1]

She did more than her share of the nursing. When she got a break she would sit by some helpless soldier and read his letters to him. She would often write their love letters and add little words of her own when the soldier seemed too weary to bother.

A soldier at Chippenham wrote a note to Ethel Brinkworth in her autograph album: *'To my night companion, with every good wish'*, probably referring to the fact that nurses often sat with soldiers during the early hours when the horrors of war brought on nightmares.[2]

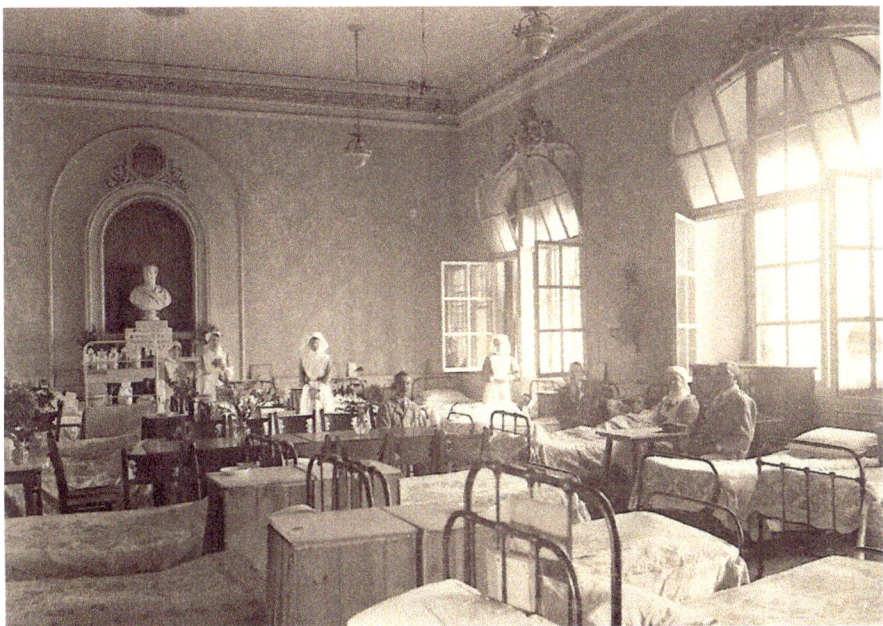

Unity Ward in the Town Hall where the first patients were accommodated

The First Patients

THERE IS NO record of the ten men who arrived at Chippenham on 5 November 1915, the newspaper simply said nine men had seen action in Gallipoli, and the tenth man was injured in Flanders, however with the help of the surviving autograph albums kept by the VADs it has been possible to identify some of those first ten men.

1   *The Downs and then Upps* – Nellie Farris
2   *All Quiet on the Home Front* - Richard Van Emden and Steve Humphries, describes men not sleeping for fear of nightmares.

Unity and Loyalty

Alexander Kinnear - Twenty year old Alexander Kinnear, a clerk in the Inland Revenue, had enlisted at Preston, in Lancashire, on 15 September 1914 joining the local regiment the Loyal North Lancs. He arrived in France in May 1915 and by June 1915 following action in the trenches he was diagnosed with a heart condition, known as soldier's heart, probably caused by stress and fatigue.[1] VAD Dora Hart, of Rooks Nest Farm at Pewsham, asked him to sign her album. He also drew a picture of a young lady, possibly Dora. Following treatment, he returned to his regiment and was finally discharged in 1920.

J E Parkinson - Sergeant Parkinson of the North Staffordshire Regiment also wrote in Dora Hart's album:[2]

Left England August 11th 1914. From Mons to Ypres.

Wounded at Ypres December 17th 1914. Left England for Dardanelles June 1915

Wounded at Suvla Bay August 1915

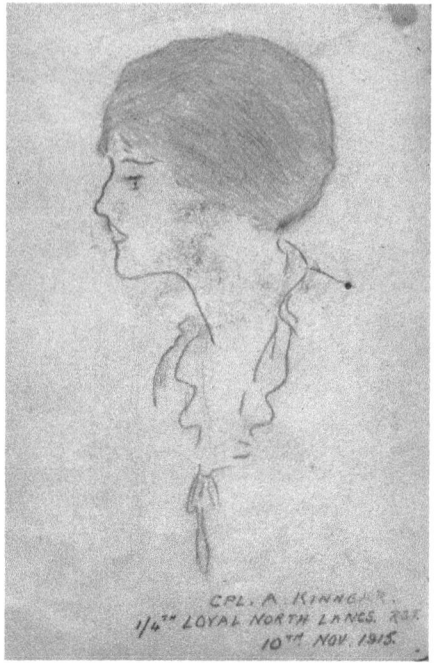

Picture drawn by patient Alexander Kinnear, possibly of VAD Dora Hart

G F Wheeler- Corporal Wheeler of 29th Signal Company gave a similar account of action in the Gallipoli campaign and returned to England suffering from sickness, probably Dysentery.

Joseph Dempsey - Amongst those first men to arrive at Chippenham was at least one Australian soldier, a novelty for the VADs, but as the War continued, they would meet many men from across the Empire.

Joseph Dempsey was a Londoner, born in Bromley in 1889. At the age of 20 he decided to try his luck in Australia where he found work as a driver. In May 1915 he responded to the call to defend his mother country and enlisted in the Australian Imperial Force. By late June he was at sea heading for Gallipoli.[3]

In Dora Hart's album he described what happened to him in Gallipoli: *'Wounded twice at Gallipoli and underwent an operation at Bristol through a blow from a Turk's rifle butt. I am now in Chippenham suffering from Rheumatism.'*

Having been wounded he was evacuated on 28 September on the Hospital Ship Grampian and arrived at Southmead on 11 October.

1   *Medical Diseases of the War* - Sir Arthur F. Hurst
2   The landings at Suvla Bay on the Gallipoli peninsular in August 1915 was a costly failure resulting in thousands of casualties.
3   Australian service records - J C Dempsey Regimental number 1685. 27 Battalion.

The Story of Chippenham's Red Cross Hospital

Lesley Arnold[1] a nurse at Southmead recalled, in an interview for the book All Quiet on the Home Front[2], how the men arrived:

> They shipped the soldiers straight to Southmead, up the River Avon, because they could take them straight off the boat and bring them into hospital.
>
> While the beds were got ready the men were laid on the hard, cold floor and we had to go around and take off their field ticket on which was written their name and injury. A lot of them were badly wounded, of course, moaning and screaming. We had to step over them, they were so close together, and lean down and cut this label off, after which they were gradually moved to the wards.
>
> Some of these men had come back from Gallipoli and they couldn't keep anything down, not a thing.

Joseph Dempsey's convalescence was slow and he remained at Chippenham for some months. By July 1916 he was fully recovered and re-joined his regiment in France. In February 1918 he was back in England when he married Hilda Hall from Cheltenham. He was treated for shell shock in 1919 and finally returned to Australia with his wife where he was discharged from the Army. According to his family Joseph suffered the disabling effects of shell shock for the rest of his life.

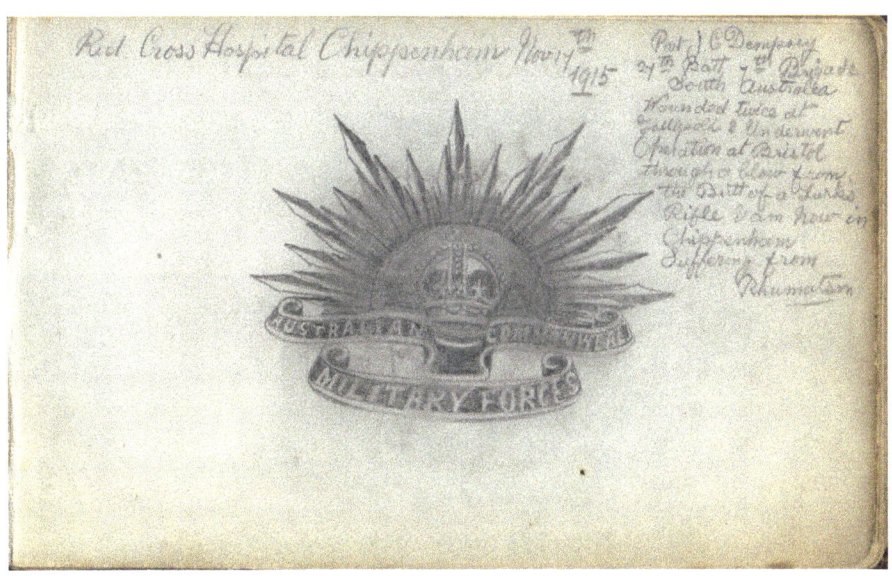

Joseph Dempsey told how he had been injured in Gallipoli

1 Lesley Arnold later became Lesley Leigh-Jones. She was the daughter of the vicar of Ebbesbourne Wake near Salisbury.
2 Extract from *All Quiet on the Home Front* - Richard Van Emden and Steve Humphries

Financing the Hospital

WHEN LORD WALTER Hervey spoke at the VAD Derry Hill mobilisation meeting, in August 1914, he said he anticipated the initial cost of setting up the hospitals for the War Office would be refunded to the Red Cross by the Government. This never materialised and the costs incurred by the Red Cross were met almost entirely by the generosity of local people and businesses.

Beryl Oliver wrote in the book 'The British Red Cross in Action' how the Red Cross financed the hospitals:

> The Auxiliary Hospitals themselves were placed under the direction of the County Director. Little difficulty was experienced in respect of funds, local subscriptions and collections of various kinds sufficed to meet current expenses while stores were ordered in bulk from headquarters. The War Office paid capitation grants in respect of occupied beds and as the war continued a small grant was sanctioned to meet the cost of unoccupied beds.

As wounded arrived a return was sent to the County Director each month to claim their capitation grant for the number of patient days. The War Office allowed three shillings per head per day to cover a patient's care.[1] It was often reported the War Office grant was barely sufficient for basic maintenance.

To provide additional comforts to supplement the grant the Red Cross relied on donations, both financial and practical, from the public. In Chippenham a hospital finance committee was established to oversee the accounting and collect donations. The following was placed in the newspaper at the beginning of 1916:[2]

> CHIPPENHAM RED CROSS HOSPITAL. A Finance Committee has now been formed:- Chairman Mr Chas. Garnett, Greathouse, Kington Langley; hon secretary, Miss Rich, Lowden Lodge; hon treasurer, Mr F Hake esq, Lloyds Bank.
> Donations are urgently wanted both for current expenses and to pay off the balance owing on the original outlay, and can be sent to either the Chairman, Secretary or Treasurer.

As soon as the Hospital opened fund raising events were organised in the town such as rummage sales, whist drives and dances. The Workers Union arranged a dance in the Neeld Hall in February 1916 that raised £10.[3]

The military units based in and around the town were keen to help. The Wiltshire Yeomanry, billeted in the town and at Bowood, also hosted whist drives and dances

---

1 British Red Cross Archive. Transcript of Chippenham annual accounts.
2 *Wiltshire Times* - 8 January 1916
3 *Wiltshire Times* - 11 March 1916

The Story of Chippenham's Red Cross Hospital

and the Motor Transport section of the Army Service Corps (ASC) arranged football matches in aid of the Red Cross.

Football

THE ASC WERE detailed to Chippenham during the summer of 1915 and more than 300 men were camped around the town, later billeted in the Temperance Hall and Skating Rink in Station Hill. Their drill ground and vehicle park was at the Folly in Bristol Road[1] and they soon used the open space to play football in their spare time.

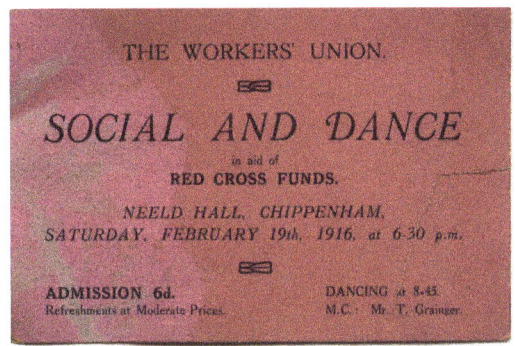

Ticket for a Workers Union Social and Dance in aid of the Red Cross

Members of the ASC were amongst the first to visit their wounded comrades and they soon got to know the staff and patients well.[2] The men shared a common interest in football and one of the topics of conversation was the unpopular decision by the Football League to adjourn its programme of matches for the duration of the War, as so many teams had lost players to the Services.[3]

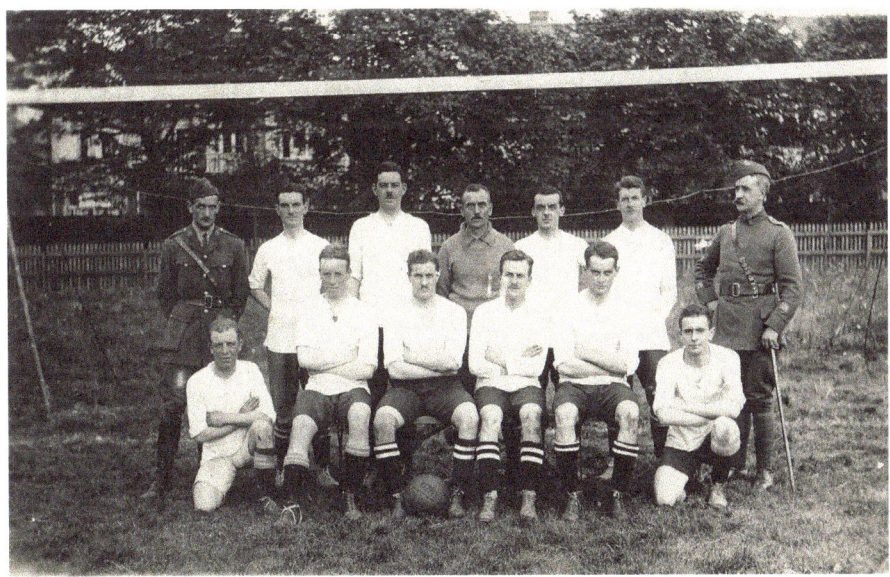

Thought to be the Wiltshire Yeomanry football team

1   *Chippenham Times* - 25 June 1915.
2   The VADs autograph albums include a number of entries from men of the ASC at the Skating Rink.
3   Imperial War Museum. Article – *9 facts about football in WW1*

Unity and Loyalty

In Chippenham the Rovers Football Club, The Rovers Wednesday Football Club and the Town Football Club had all been suspended. The football pitches lay idle with only occasional games by local juvenile amateur teams.[1]

The men of the ASC had organised a few informal inter-company matches at the Folly and the public had come to spectate. There was so much interest that the ASC challenged the residents of Chippenham to a match at the Chippenham Town ground.

On Saturday 20 November the team of Chippenham men lined up against 496th Company ASC. At full time the ASC had beaten Chippenham 7-2, but the defeat was taken in good humour. Patients were amongst the large crowd at the ground and organised a collection, raising over £4 for hospital funds.[2]

In December at the Technical School the Wiltshire Yeomanry team was defeated by the ASC from Lacock and once again the proceeds were donated to the Red Cross Hospital in Chippenham.[3] More matches followed throughout the winter.

Christmas 1915

By Christmas the number of patients in Chippenham had risen to 25 and those who were able had helped decorate the wards and put up the Christmas tree donated by well-wishers Mr and Mrs Leatham.

The people of Chippenham were keen to make Christmas day special for the men. Santa Claus made a special visit to the wards in the morning[4] and each man was given a present and cigarettes from the town and Mayor.

A short service was held at noon and the King's Message, which was published in Naval and Military Orders, was read to the men. In his message the King said:

> Another Christmas finds all the resources of the Empire still engaged in war, and I desire to convey on my own behalf, and on behalf of the Queen, a heartfelt Christmas greeting and our good wishes for the New Year to all who on sea and land are upholding the honour of the British name.
>
> In the officers and men of my Navy, on whom security of the Empire depends, I repose, in common with all my subjects, trust that is absolute.
>
> On the officers and men of armies, whether now in France, in the East, or in other fields, I rely with an equal faith, confident that their devotion, their valour, and their self-sacrifice will, under God's guidance, lead to victory and an honourable peace.
>
> There are many of their comrades now, alas, in hospital, and to these brave men also I desire, with the Queen, to express our deep gratitude and our earnest prayers for their recovery.
>
> Officers and men of the Navy and of the Army, another year is drawing to a close

---

1 *Wiltshire Times* - 04 September 1915
2 *Wiltshire Times* - 27 November 1915
3 *North Wilts Herald* - 3 December 1915
4 *Wiltshire Times* - 1 January 1916

The Story of Chippenham's Red Cross Hospital

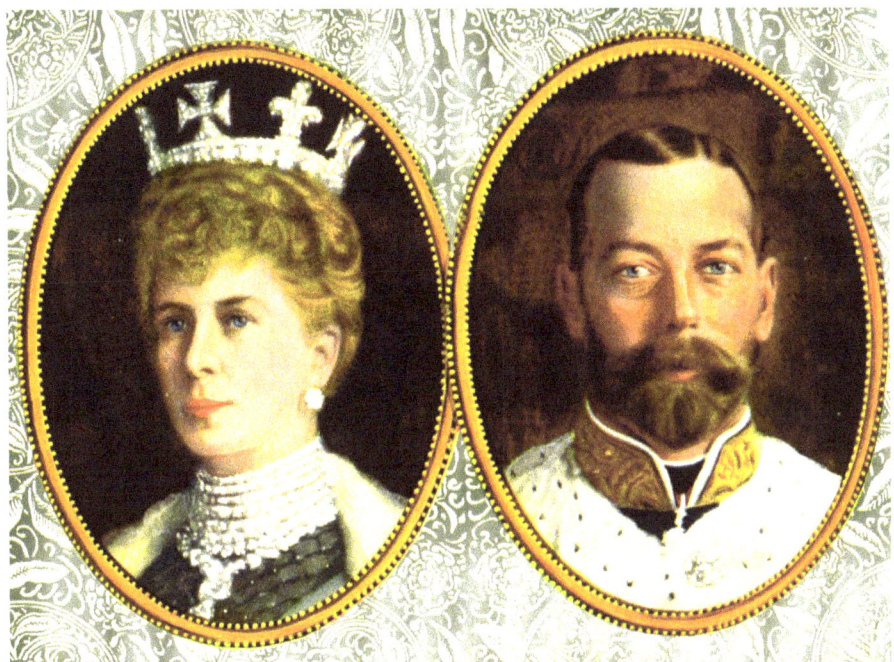

The King and Queen

it began in toil, bloodshed, and suffering, and I rejoice to know that the goal to which you are striving draws nearer into sight.

May God bless you and all your undertakings.

Christmas dinner followed, prepared under the direction of Mrs Williams and Mrs Shipp: traditional fare of turkey with all the trimmings followed by plum pudding. Joe Buckle officiated at the table and performed the carving duties assisted by Walter Hiscock and solicitor Edmund Awdry, whose daughter Unity was a VAD.

Later in the day more gifts were placed under the Christmas tree, visitors popped in to join the festivities and the day ended with singing and a whist drive.[1]

The men said they thoroughly enjoyed themselves and had the best time of their lives.

Two days later they were invited to the Picture Palace to enjoy a filmshow and later in the week they joined the men of the ASC in a programme of games and music in the Neeld Hall with a number of professional musical acts including Sisters Petite, a refined dancing and singing duo, who were well known around the country, and the singer Madame Dorria.

1 *Wiltshire Times* - 1 January 1916

Chapter 7
1916

THERE IS A shortage of VADs in the towns as women are attracted to other war work. Further detachments are recruited from the surrounding villages.

The battle of the Somme results in increased numbers of wounded and the Chippenham VAD Hospital is enlarged to deal with more patients. The VADs are asked to deal with increasingly serious cases.

The New Year

MAYOR ALDERMAN TOWNSEND addressed the Council at their first meeting of 1916. He wished them all as happy a new year as the present circumstances allowed and hoped that during his year of office peace would be proclaimed.[1]

The year opened with gales severe enough to uproot trees and cause structural damage. The Meteorological Office described January as stormy and abnormally mild caused by a deep depression travelling across the country.[2]

The morale of the country reflected the weather: the political problems that had tested the Government before the War had resurfaced. 1915 had seen increasing industrial action, shattering the Government's and the TUC's hope that all unions would observe an industrial truce for the duration of the War.[3] There had been intermittent strikes in the coal mines of South Wales and at the National Conference of the coal mining industry in January 1916 the Welsh miners were described as irresponsible when a strike was threatened.

The engineering industry was criticised for going on strike, in some cases for trivial reasons. Strikes were usually pay related, but one set of engineering workers went on strike in protest against a tax levied on ginger beer, a drink considered essential to their work. Another strike was prompted by the sacking of two munitionettes for wearing trousers outside the factory.[4] During 1916 the Munitions of War Act made strikes illegal in war industries and labour disputes went to compulsory tribunals, although in practice strikes continued throughout the War.[5]

1 *Chippenham Council minute book 9*
2 Metrological Office - *Monthly weather report*
3 *The History of the TUC 1868-1968*
4 The National Archive- MUN 2/27
5 www.parliament.uk – Living Heritage- *Parliament and the First World War. The Munitions of War*

The Irish Home Rule tinderbox was reignited on 1 August 1915 when Patrick Pearse, a Republican leader, gave a rousing speech at the funeral of Jeremiah O'Donovan Rossa, a prominent member of the Irish Republican Brotherhood, ending with, '*Ireland unfree shall never be at peace,*' a rallying call for Republicans which inflamed the simmering Irish problem and culminated in the 1916 Easter rising in Dublin.

The people of Chippenham were experiencing changes to the daily routine of the town. British Summer Time was introduced during 1916. This was not popular for the ordinary person in the street, but it was said it would allow businesses and farmers to take advantage of longer daylight hours and be more productive.

Air Raid Precautions were introduced throughout the country following the news of raids in London and the possibility of an attack by German aircraft was taken very seriously by the Council in Chippenham.[1] Public lighting was dimmed and windows covered with heavy curtains. Breaches of the regulations resulted in a hefty fine. Councillor Tuck was summoned by the magistrates for a breach of the Lighting Order when a doorway was left uncovered in the Neeld Hall.[2] It was even proposed that shops closed early in the winter to avoid the need to turn on lights.

The War was given as the reason to halt the annual visit of Bostock and Wombwell's popular travelling menagerie in February 1916. Their application to use the Market Place was refused on the grounds that cages and equipment may get in the way of the many large military vehicles now passing through the town.[3] By the beginning of 1916 it seemed the War was draining the town of popular recreation. The Angling Club abandoned its fishing competitions as so many members had left to join up. Even the popular musical societies in the town suspended their productions. Mr Parry of the Madrigal Society and Mr Burden of the Choral Society wrote a joint letter to the newspaper in January 1916:[4]

Air Raid notice issued by the Mayor in February 1916

> We should like to point out that both the above societies are still in existence but that in view of the strenuous and anxious times through which the nation is passing, coupled with the fact that so many men are on active service and the ladies on Red Cross work, it was thought desirable to suspend active work in the form of practices until the conclusion of hostilities.

1   *Chippenham Council minute book 9* - 14 February 1916
2   *Chippenham Council minute book 9* - 2 May 1916
3   *Chippenham Council minute book 9* - 1 February 1916
4   *Wiltshire Times* – 29 January 1916

It was further felt that at the present time the members available would be better engaged devoting their energies to various objects connected with war relief efforts and that it was therefore more fitting to postpone the resumption of rehearsals until a happier state of things prevailed.

News from the War was equally disheartening. The Western Front had reached stalemate. Both sides had dug in and the War had become one of attrition. In Gallipoli the disastrous offensive had finally come to an end when the last troops were evacuated during January 1916.

The initial enthusiasm to join up and fight the enemy had paled and in May 1916 the Government finally introduced the Military Services Act which brought in conscription to ensure a constant supply of recruits.

Women become War Workers

THE STRAINS OF war and the never-ending demand for men was taking its toll. Increasingly women were being called upon to fill the gaps at home and do men's work. The Great Western Railway in Chippenham engaged women to clean and maintain the trains and an offer was made by the Governors at the Technical school to train women in readiness to replace men in clerical and commercial positions.

In Bristol an increase in vandalism was blamed on the lack of numbers in the police force[1] and to fill the gaps women were recruited.

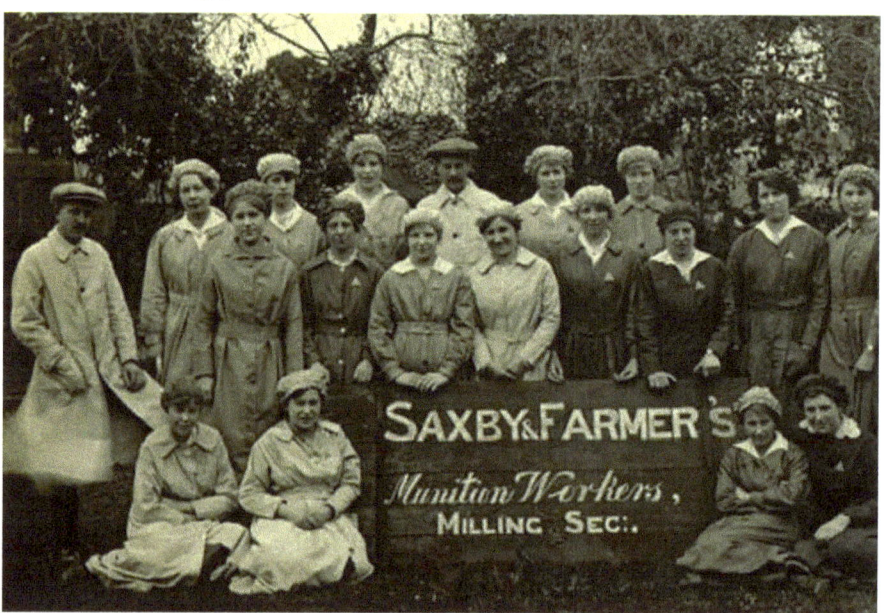

Saxby and Farmer Milling Section

1   *Western Daily Press* - 8 March 1916

The Story of Chippenham's Red Cross Hospital

The idea of engaging women in men's work was not popular. Even with the Munitions Act of 1915 there was opposition to employing women in shell and explosive production, even the threat of strike action, when unskilled women were employed.

In Chippenham, at the engineering works of Saxby and Farmer, there did not seem to be such hostility to women in the factory and it appears the munitonettes were accepted on the factory floor, although some people felt that allowing women to work alongside men in the workshops was 'faintly immoral'.[1]

Amongst the young women who joined Saxby and Farmer were Kathleen Granger, Elsie Brewer and Gladys Treweke. Gladys joined her father Ernest in the capstan lathe section along with Elsie while Kathleen joined the milling section.[2]

Shortage of VADs

WITH WOMEN TAKING on traditional male roles the task of recruiting VADs became more difficult, especially as those working in factories and on the railways were paid a wage. The Auxiliary hospitals had been established by the Red Cross under the Scheme for Voluntary Aid. The very name told that the work was unpaid and it was decided it should remain voluntary.

Some VADs applied for Special Service. This was work at military hospitals, either in Britain or overseas, that offered a small wage and expenses. To be considered for Special Service the recruit had to be a trained member of a Voluntary Aid Detachment and was required to sign up to 12 months service and undergo a rigorous selection interview.[3] In some cases she was also expected to be able to speak French. A number of VADs from Chippenham were interested in Special Service. Those selected included Amy Bolton, Ethel Brinkworth and Eva Hutton. Basil Hankey also received enquiries from members of the public who were interested in paid work with the Red Cross. He would reply to their questions suggesting they consider Special Service. Mary Bridges of Goatacre took Mr Hankey's advice and served at the Military Hospital on Salisbury Plain.

With the competition for women workers the Red Cross across the country were reporting significant shortages of VADs. In response the Chairman of the National Red Cross Executive Committee, Mr A Stanley wrote a letter to the newspapers calling for all women to consider joining the Red Cross as volunteers:

> A real and urgent necessity has arisen for more nurses, VAD nursing members (women) and VAD general service members in military and auxiliary hospitals at home........ We earnestly call upon these women to come forward and help us in this emergency.

For the first-time working-class women, who had never considered joining the

1   *Westinghouse Review* – October 1949. Article about women in the works.
2   *Westinghouse Review* – October 1951 and January 1955
3   Wiltshire and Swindon History Centre 3669/2/4 *Papers of Molly Bridges*. Special Service leaflet J VAD 11a

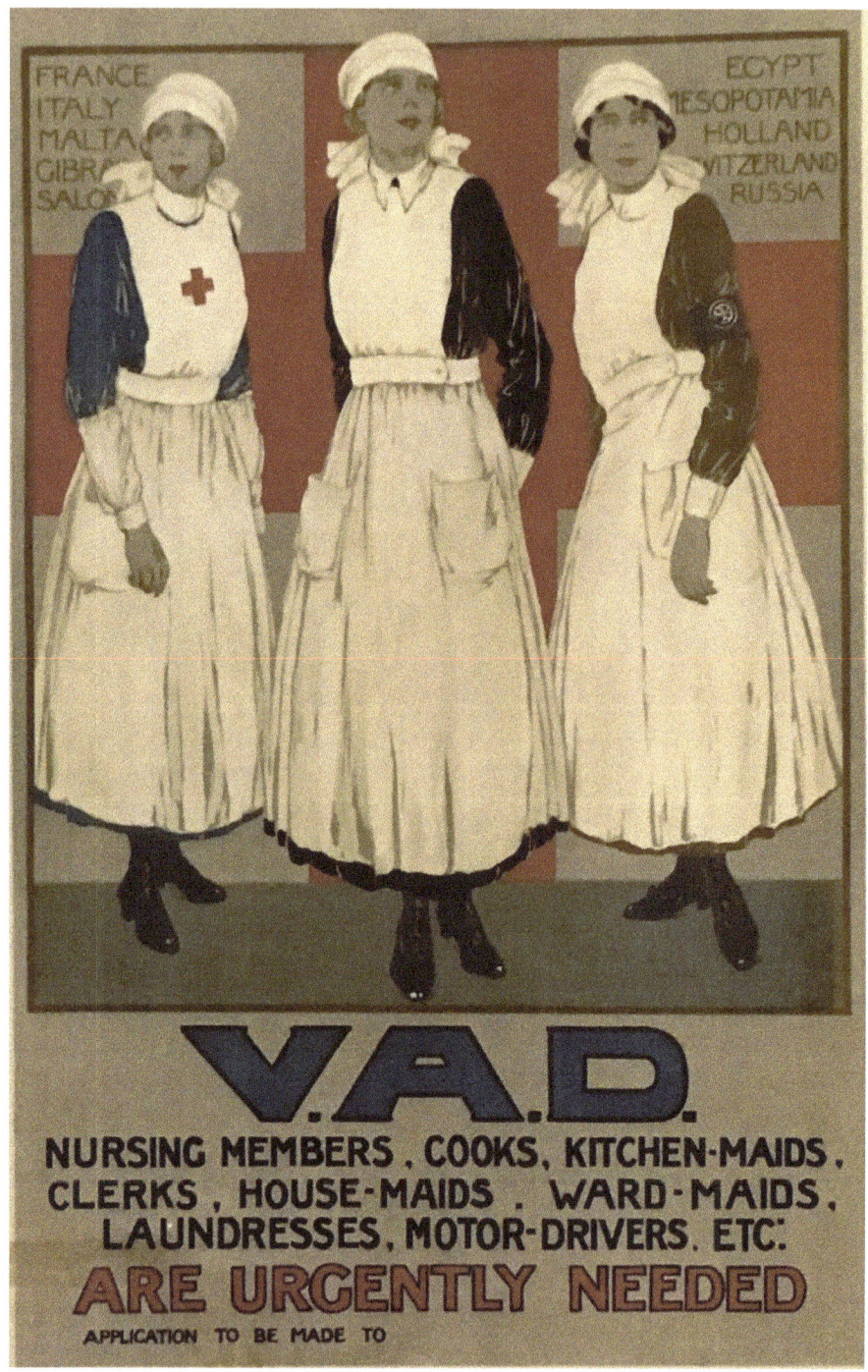

A VAD recruiting poster

The Story of Chippenham's Red Cross Hospital

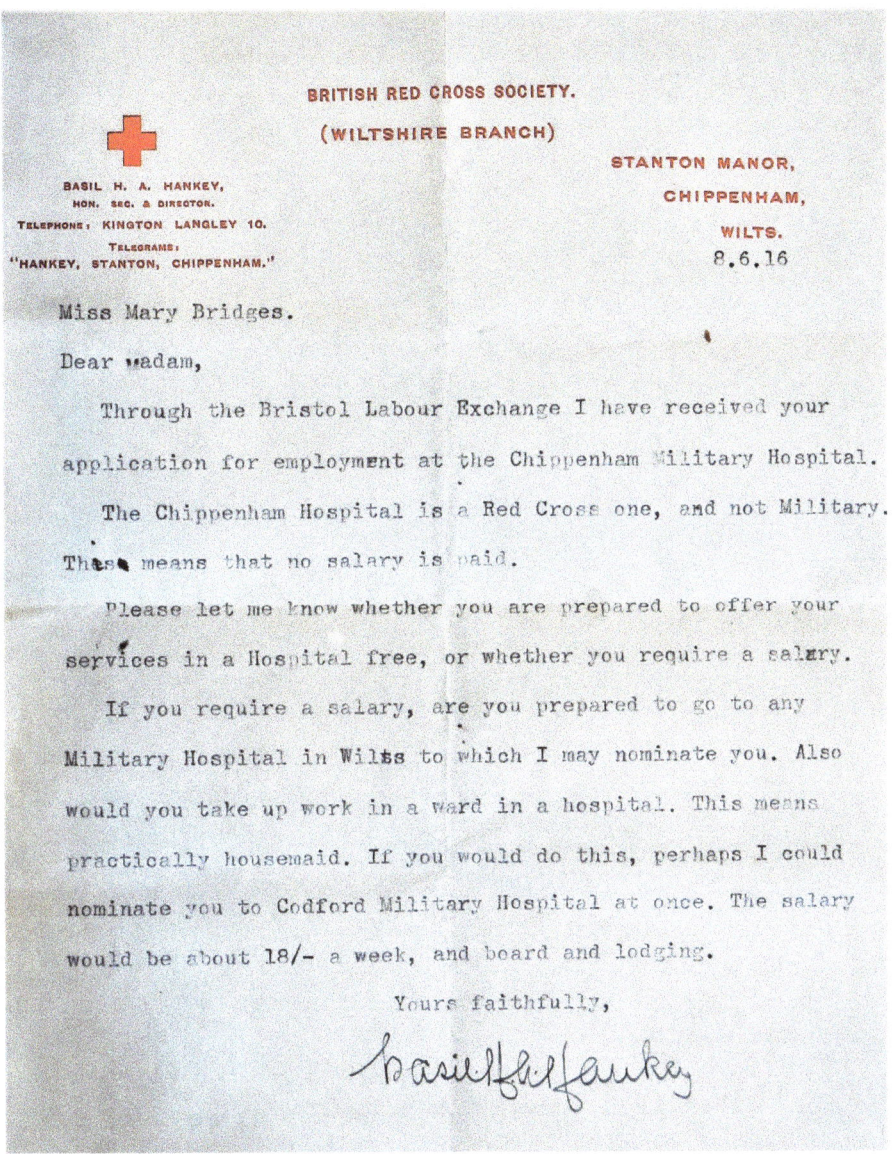

A letter from Basil Hankey explaining no salary is paid at Chippenham VAD Hospital

VADs, came forward. Having heard the urgency of the situation they offered a few hours each week: all they could spare as they had families and homes to look after.

In Chippenham Sarah Beaven volunteered every Sunday afternoon serving meals and washing up, she continued this work until the hospital closed in 1919. Sarah and her husband Frank, who worked at the condensed milk factory in Bath Road, lived in Park Lane and they were both very active members of the Salvation Army.[1]

1   *Wiltshire Times* - 4 February 1933 – Obituary

Unity and Loyalty

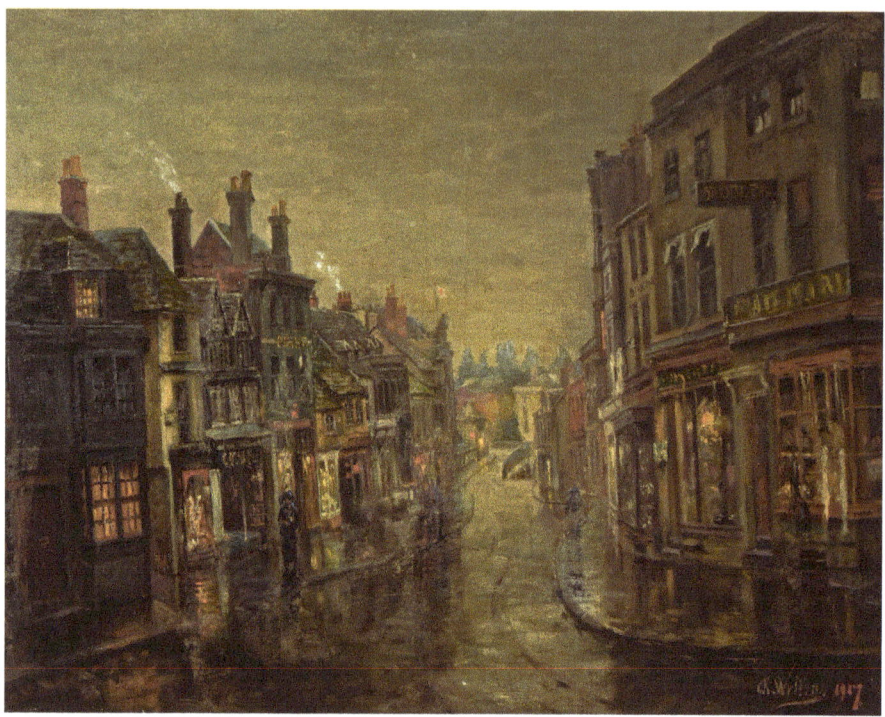

A painting of Chippenham High Street in 1917 by Belgian artist Charles Wellens

In May 1916 Florence Selman of Marshfield Road joined the staff in the kitchen. For seven hours each week she prepared vegetables. She also continued working until 1919.

Kate Bright lived in a small cottage in Emery Lane, which was almost opposite the Town Hall. She volunteered in January 1916 two hours a day cleaning the wards, but in December 1916 she received the dreaded news that her son, George, had been killed in action. She left in January 1917, seeing the wounded soldiers probably being a constant reminder of her son.

The plea for volunteers by the Red Cross also attracted unofficial helpers. These were people who wanted to support the hospitals without formally joining the Red Cross. Some simply visited and helped make afternoon tea. A number of munitionettes popped in to help and chat to the men. Hairdresser William Stephens, whose premises were in the Market Place,[1] called in regularly to shave and cut the hair of men who couldn't venture out. Charles Wellens, a Belgian Refugee, gave painting classes. He was a well-known artist in his home country and arranged drawing lessons for the men and VADs. Some of their work was included in an exhibition in St Paul's Church Hall, the proceeds from visitors and sale of paintings were donated to the Red Cross.

Children from the local schools collected mushrooms and blackberries from the fields and hedgerows and took them to the hospital kitchen. Mrs Williams' Blackberry

1   *Kelly's Directory* 1915

The Story of Chippenham's Red Cross Hospital

and Pear salad was a real treat for the men. Some children were volunteered by their parents to prepare huge baths of potatoes and carrots. In return they were rewarded with a cream tea at the home of Walter and Ada Hiscock in the Market Place. Their daughter Edith was a Brownie[1] leader and organised the children into work groups.[2]

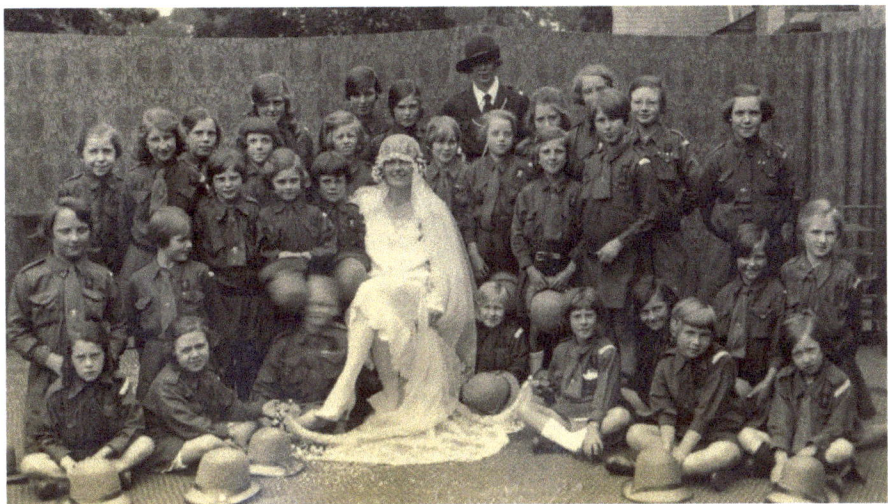

Edith Hiscock surrounded by her Brownie pack at her wedding in 1927. During the War she organised the children into work groups preparing vegetables

Colonel Sir Audley Neeld was a regular helper at the Hospital. His visits were eagerly awaited by the patients as his presence was said to be a real morale booster. He also arranged trips in his motor car for the men and VADs.

Additional Detachments

AT THE END of January 1916, the Hospital was at its capacity of 40. Although the extra help offered by well-wishers and part time volunteers was useful, it was clear Chippenham needed more trained VADs to provide constant care for the number of patients. The War Office rules dictated that an increase in staff meant raising further detachments.

Ladies from the surrounding villages came forward. In Biddestone and Box detachments were raised to supplement nearby Corsham Hospital, while in Chippenham it is thought a nursing unit of the Order of St John at Castle Combe increased the complement at the VAD Hospital.

In the villages of Christian Malford and Sutton Benger the Draycot House Voluntary Aid Detachment, Wilts 38, was reinstated and the members were first seen

1   First formed in 1914 Brownies were originally known as Rosebuds.
2   Recollection of Grace Hall, March 1992. From the albums of the Hiscock family courtesy Kate Tayler.

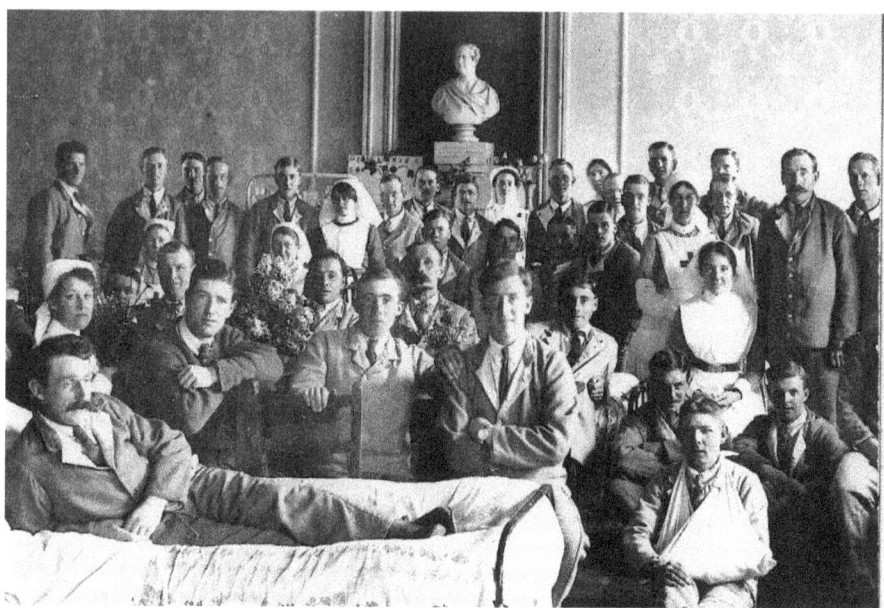
Unity Ward. By early 1916 the hospital was fully occupied

in full Red Cross uniform at a service of Intercession at Sutton Benger during January 1916.¹

A whist drive and auction took place at Paradise Farm in Christian Malford in March 1916 to raise money for the detachment and attract new volunteers to serve at Chippenham.² The sum of £13 6s 6d was raised which was used to buy equipment and help with the cost of training.

Katherine Harrison was appointed as temporary Commandant of the Detachment, which became known as Sutton VAD, Wilts 38.

Mrs Harrison and her Land Agent husband Henry lived at Park View in Sutton Benger. They were long standing supporters of the Red Cross and Katherine was instrumental in the opening of the Hospital at Draycot House while her husband joined a Red Cross unit that served in France.

Amongst the new volunteer members were local doctor's wife Ruth Barnes and farmer's wife Ethel Bodman. Others that joined were Katherine Bond, Alice Ellery, Grace Lavington and Ellen Cornish. Ellen Cornish had previously been a member of the Chippenham Detachment and in 1913 was one of the cooks at the Bowood Rally.

By the early summer of 1916 the VADs of Wilts 38 had completed their Home Nursing training and were working alongside their colleagues at Chippenham. The Detachment grew as more volunteers joined Wilts 38. One of the VADs, Georgina Sutton of Rookery Farm at Seagry, had valuable experience as she had returned from Special Service working in military hospitals in France.

1 *North Wilts Herald* - 9 January 1916
2 *Wiltshire Times* - 11 March 1916

The Story of Chippenham's Red Cross Hospital

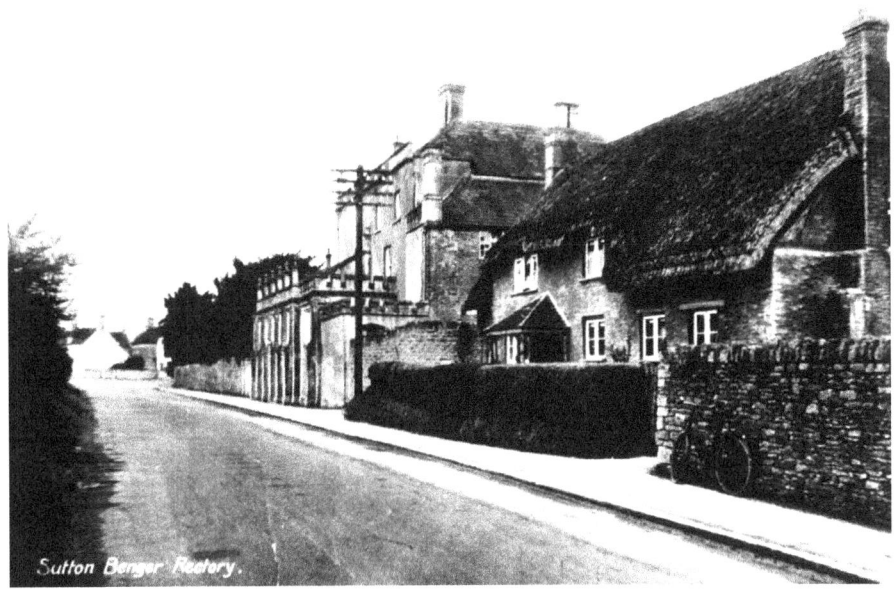

The village of Sutton Benger

As the VADS of Wilts 38 lived several miles from Chippenham, men from the villages were enlisted to drive them to attend their shifts.

One of these volunteer drivers was Bertie Sutton, who lived in Seagry. He was chauffeur to Lord Cowley[1] and regularly drove for the VADs. Despite this he received a notification that he was to be conscripted.

He appealed against this decision in November 1917 and Mr Carnley, the agent for Lord Cowley, spoke on his behalf at the tribunal. Mr Carnley told the tribunal the Red Cross Hospital in Chippenham was understaffed and if the nurses did not have transport it would be a serious matter. Despite this the tribunal dismissed the appeal suggesting the VADs could stay in lodgings in the town.[2]

It is not known if accommodation was provided in Chippenham, although there is a suggestion that Rowden House, the home of Mrs Cotes, was used as lodgings by some VADs.[3]

The Men's Detachment

IN JANUARY 1916 fifteen patients, some on stretchers, arrived at Chippenham Station from Bristol.[4] To greet them was Charles Garnett, of Greathouse, and a squad

1 Wiltshire Family History Society, *First World War Tribunals in Wiltshire* - Ivor Slocombe
2 *Wiltshire Times* – 24 November 1917
3 Chippenham Museum.- *Scrapbook of Ivy Gladstone*. A picture of Rowden House with a comment in 1919 saying goodbye Rowden
4 *North Wilts Herald* - 21 January 1916.

of ambulance orderlies. Mr Garnett brought his ambulance to convey the stretcher cases, while the walking cases were once again transported in private cars provided by volunteers in the town.

The need for ambulance orderlies and porters was critical and an appeal had been made to men in Chippenham to give up some of their spare time and come forward to join the Red Cross Ambulance Section.

Albert Maslen was an ideal candidate. He was a GWR locomotive driver and a long-standing member of the company's St John Ambulance branch.[1] He decided to join the Red Cross Ambulance Section in January 1916. A few days later he was at the Station with Mr Garnett to await the fifteen wounded men. Alongside Mr Garnett and Albert Maslen were a group of men from Saxby and Farmer; Arthur Stanley,[2] Lewis Jessop, William Bodman and Albert Tyler, who had all trained in first aid with the company.

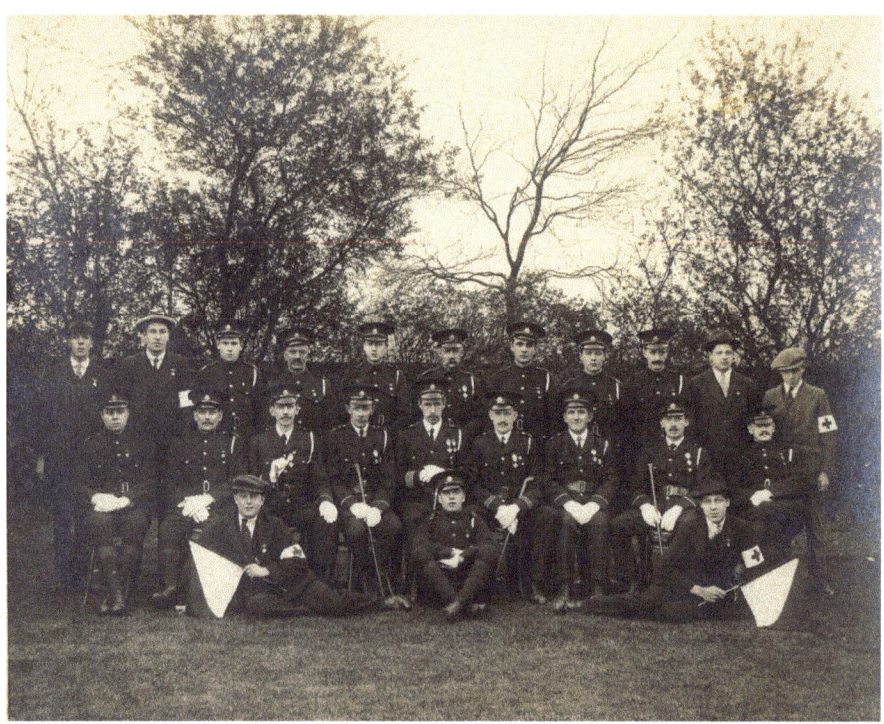

Members of Chippenham Ambulance Detachment, Wilts 13. Frank Read, the Commandant is centre middle row

At the Chippenham Red Cross Divisional meeting in March 1916 it was reported that the membership of the ambulance sections had improved. Corsham men's Detachment was at full strength with 47 members and at Chippenham, following the appeal for volunteers, enough men had come forward to form a section. As more men had

1   *Wiltshire Times* - 17 December 1921- Obituary
2   *Westinghouse Review 1950/51* Obituary. He was a long-standing member of the Red Cross

The Story of Chippenham's Red Cross Hospital

subsequently joined and were training it was hoped a full Detachment, numbering over 40 men, could soon be raised. The report of the meeting:[1]

> It is hoped a men's detachment will, be raised in Chippenham. They have already enough members to form a class for First Aid with Mr. F. D. Read as class, secretary. Doctor Laurence, of Chippenham, has given them their course of lectures, and if through scarcity of men they are unable to form a detachment; they will in any case be able to form one of the two sections.

By the summer of 1916 Chippenham had sufficient recruits. With many of the men already trained through their employment the War Office was happy to register the Detachment as Wilts 13 VAD under the leadership of Commandant Frank Read.

In March 1918 the Wilts 13 VAD held its first Annual General Meeting at the Technical School in Cocklebury Lane.[2] Chaired by Charles Garnett, the Honorary Commandant, the quartermaster Arthur Stanley, gave his report of the Detachment since its formation. He was able to tell the meeting that the volunteers had undertaken a great deal of training since 1916, including a course of lectures on Hygiene and Sanitation given by Dr Laurence. Twenty men passed the Home Nursing Examination, while others were awarded Red Cross Proficiency badges. In the early days of the Detachment most men did not have uniforms, but Mr Garnett, Mr Rogers and the Wiltshire Farmers gave donations to ensure the men were able to obtain them.

He went on to say they took regular duty at the hospitals, met the convoys of wounded at Chippenham Station and assisted at other locations, this included helping at Bath when full trains arrived with patients destined for the military hospitals.

The Somme

IN JUNE 1916 the Allied armies were preparing for a major push on the German lines. Days of heavy artillery bombardment on the German trenches preceded a massive infantry advance. This offensive, known as the Battle of the Somme, opened on 1 July and initial reports told of success for the Allies. This was the good news the public had been waiting for. The Daily Mirror announced that the situation was favourable to the Allies and 9500 German prisoners had been taken.

The Western Daily Press headlines on 6 July 1916, were equally positive:

GOOD BRITISH NEWS
SECURING IMPORTANT POINTS
FIGHTING AT CLOSE QUARTERS

The human cost of these initial successes was high and today the Somme is

---

1 *Wiltshire Times* - 25 March 1916
2 *Wiltshire Times* - 2 March 1918

Unity and Loyalty

considered one of the bloodiest battles of the War. By the end of the first day the British had suffered over 57,000 casualties and as the Germans launched a series of counter attacks thousands more were killed or injured. The battles continued throughout the summer and autumn. In September 1916 the War Office arranged to publish an account and showed film footage in the cinemas to convey to the public how well the Somme was going. As the weather deteriorated in November so the final push of the Somme offensive took place. By that time the numbers of casualties had escalated to levels never before imagined. It is estimated that total casualties were over a million, of which 420,000 were British.

Within days of the first battle the wounded began pouring back to Britain. Each day hospital ships offloaded their cargo into waiting trains and were despatched around the country. Bristol saw the first wounded from the Somme on 3 July. The train from Southampton arrived at Temple Meads station and 196 men were transferred to the Bristol Royal Infirmary and Southmead Hospital.[1] A further train arrived the same day with 90 men destined for Beaufort Hospital. Two days later a further one hundred men arrived[2] and over the weekend of the 8 and 9 July three fully laden trains arrived carrying 576 wounded, of which 350 were stretcher cases. As the trains continued to arrive the strain started to show on the men and women of the Bristol Detachments. It was said some volunteers didn't sleep for 48 hours as they cared for the men at the station and manned the endless convoys.

In Bath the same picture unfolded as trains[3] arrived with wounded destined for Combe Park, which had recently opened as a War Hospital. With some of the trains arriving carrying well over 200 wounded nearby Wiltshire Red Cross, including Chippenham Division, were called to help transport the patients.

As the fighting in France continued ever more patients arrived in Bristol and Bath and it became noticeable from the rail timetables that the hospital trains often arrived throughout the night: possibly a planned tactic to shield the public from the true scale of returning injured.[4] Even the VAD hospitals in Wiltshire saw trains arrive through the night. In Tisbury it was said of the trains arriving at the station, '...*it would not have done for any of their cargoes to have been seen in the cold light of day*'.[5]

The surge of injured arriving at Bristol had an immediate effect on the auxiliary hospitals with a massive demand for additional beds. In Chippenham Division, an extension to Corsham Hospital was opened during July 1916 at Monks Park,[6] the home of Sir John Goldney.

---

1   *The Forgotten Front Bristol at War* – James Belsey
2   *Western Daily Press* - 5 July 1916
3   *Bath Chronicle* - 8 July 1916. A train carrying 230 patients arrived on 6 July 1916.
4   *The Forgotten Front Bristol at War* – James Belsey. Belsey suggests the night timetable was intentional
5   *A Tisbury History* - Jill and Peter Drury
6   *Wiltshire Family History Society - January 1996* Article on Monks Park.

The Story of Chippenham's Red Cross Hospital

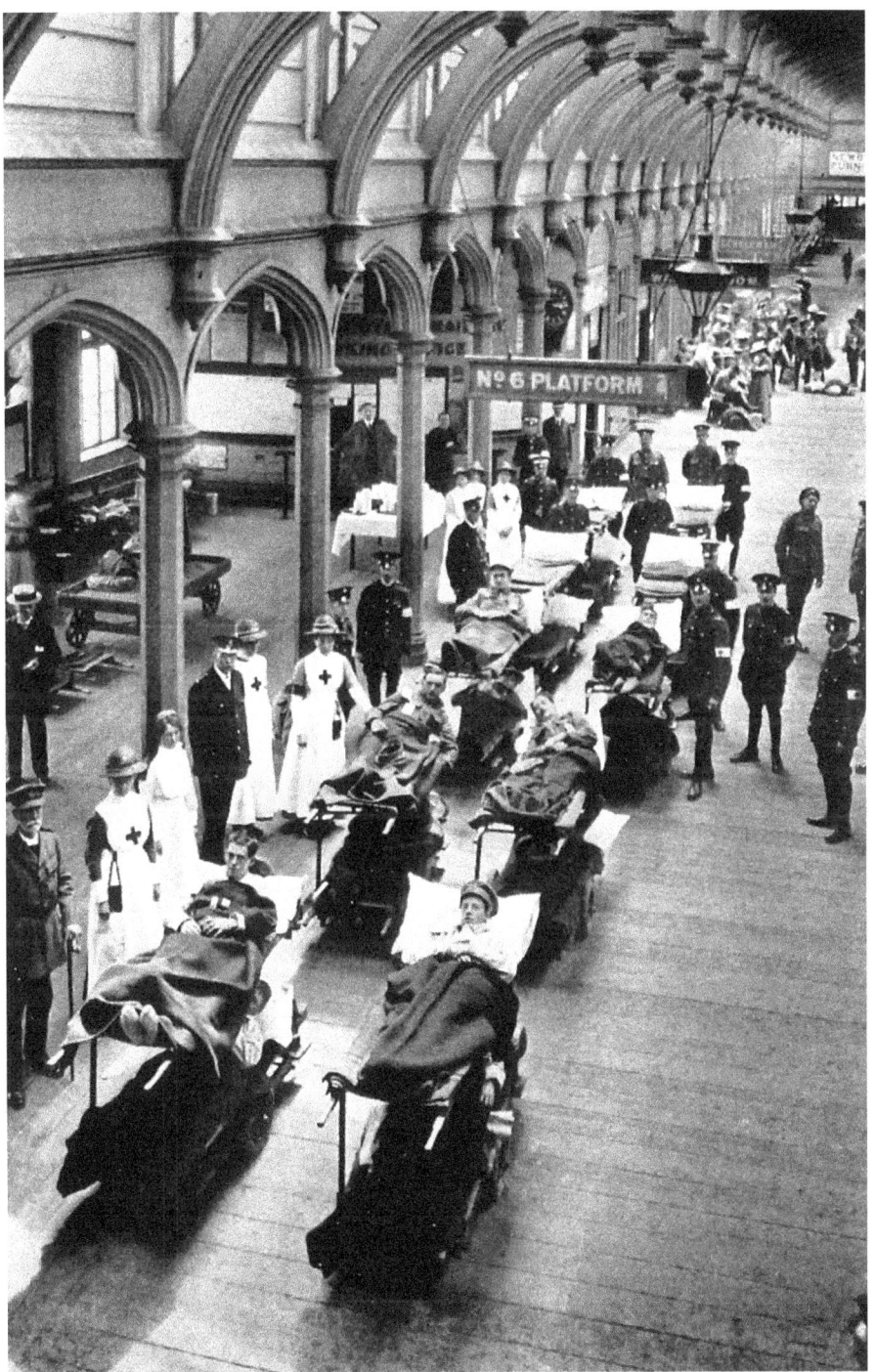

Wounded at Bristol Temple Meads Station

Unity and Loyalty

The Neeld Hall

A FEW EXTRA BEDS at Corsham were not enough to satisfy the flow of wounded to the Division. Basil Hankey wrote to Chippenham Council to explain the urgent need for more beds and asked for their agreement to release the Neeld Hall to the Red Cross as an extension to the Town Hall Hospital.

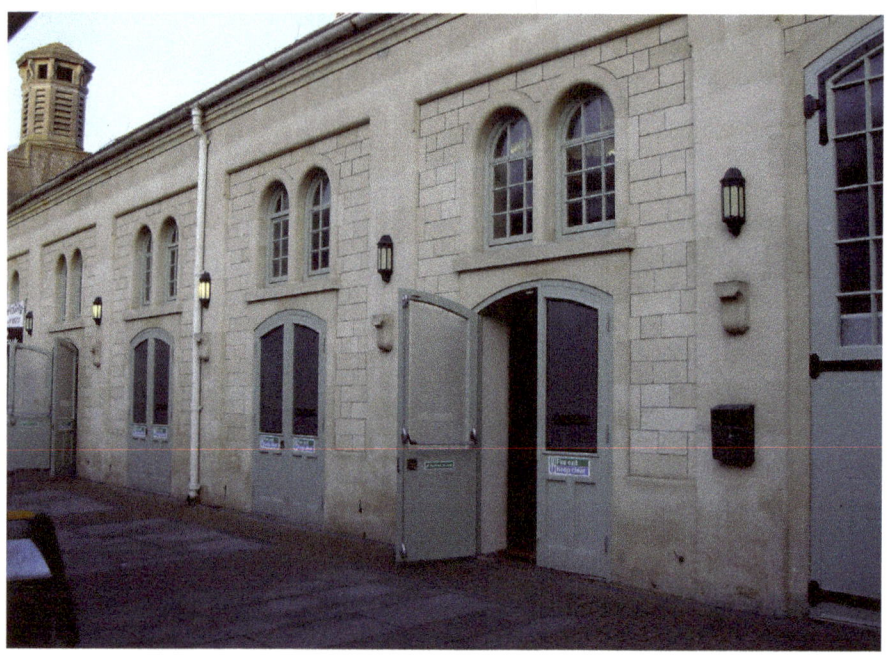

The Neeld today

The Council held a special meeting on 24 July 1916[1] to discuss Mr Hankey's letter, which had been endorsed by Colonel Bush, the commanding officer of the Bristol hospitals.

Councillor Mr Spinke, the owner of a printing works in the town, proposed that the application should be agreed. Samuel Spinke had a particular interest as his daughters Lilian, Mabel and Daisy were all serving as VADs.

The Council had reservations about the suitability of the Neeld Hall for wounded men. They would only give their approval on condition the Red Cross arranged a number of structural alterations, which included installing extra bathrooms and toilets, improving the drainage and erecting a panel partition in the hall to form a room at the opposite end to the stage, to allow the magistrates to continue to sit.[2]

They also pointed out that without the income they received from the Neeld Hall they would be out of pocket. Mr Hankey agreed, on behalf of the Red Cross, to apply to the War Office for a grant of £80 a year to compensate the Town Council for loss of income. He also

1 *Chippenham Council minute book 9*
2 *Chippenham Council minute book 9*

The Story of Chippenham's Red Cross Hospital

agreed to pay half the wages of the caretaker and a proportion of the rates and insurance. On these terms Mr Hankey's request that the Red Cross should use the hall was agreed.

The newspaper gave the following report following the Council's decision:[1]

> Owing to the large numbers of wounded soldiers now arriving daily at Bristol, Wilts 6 (Chippenham Detachment) have been asked to enlarge their Hospital.
>
> With the consent of the Mayor and Town Council part of the Neeld Hall is to be adapted for this purpose and will thus provide accommodation for 40 more patients.
>
> The Commandant asks for the co-operation of all friends in town and neighbourhood, that any who can lend or give any of the following articles should send a post card to the Quartermaster at the Red Cross Hospital, Chippenham not later than August 1st.

The newspaper also gave a lengthy list of items urgently needed for the new extension, including beds, mattresses and bedding, wheelchairs, kitchen equipment, knives and forks, clothing such as dressing gowns and slippers, and supplies of brandy, for medicinal purposes only.

As expected, the donations flowed in and within two weeks the Neeld Hall was fully equipped. The Commandant expressed her thanks in the newspapers and listed those who had donated to the new ward:[2]

> Amongst those who have so kindly equipped the Loyalty Ward are the following: - Miss Rooke, Mrs Elliott, Mrs R B Wood, Rev Bolton (Yatton Keynell), Miss Williams, Mr and Mrs John (Lea), Sutton VAD, Mrs Dickson, Miss Dickson, Mrs Ralph Pearce, Mrs Garnett, Mrs Taylor, Mrs Westoby, Mrs Post, Mrs Mackness, Mrs Chesterton, Mrs Hamlyn, Mrs Minty, Mrs Louis Brown, Miss Grainger, Mrs Stevenson, Mr Stevens, Miss Ashe (Market Place), the Misses Butler, Mrs Humphries senior, Mrs Allfrey, Mr Bergstrom, Miss Limbrick, Mr Fletcher, Countess Cowley, Mrs Singer, Mrs F E Wheeler, Miss Belcher, Mrs Llewellyn, Mrs Woods, Miss Farris, Major Cotes, Mrs Terrell, Mrs Britton, Mrs Bull, Mrs Lysley, Mrs Gladstone, Mrs Willie Lysley, Derry Hill VAD, Mrs Frank Spicer, Mrs and Miss Greenman, Mrs Patterson, Mr Dunford, Mrs Bryant, (Sutton Benger) Miss Bond, Miss Cornish, Lady Helme, Mrs Walters, Mrs Forgan, Mrs Sleight, Mrs Scott, Mrs E Hankey, Mr and Mrs Panel, Mr Mattingly, Mrs Bailey, Mrs Stewart, Mr Hull and others.

Such was the enthusiasm to support the hospital extension that within a matter of days 12 more men had volunteered for ambulance work with Wilts 13 VAD, and in December 1916 they were amongst nineteen men who were presented with their final examination certificates at the training room at the Technical School.[3]

1 *Wiltshire Times* – 29 July 1916
2 *Devizes and Wiltshire Gazette* – 10 August 1916
3 *Wiltshire Times* - 23 December 1916

Unity and Loyalty

It was decided to call the Neeld Hall ward Loyalty. With the large ward in the Town Hall already named Unity the joint names made up the Borough motto, Unity and Loyalty.

Many of the minor alterations required by the Council were carried out at no cost to the Red Cross by volunteers in the town.

The new drainage and toilets were installed by Mr Hulbert at a cost of £52 8s 6d, other structural work amounted to £51 17s 10d. These essential works depleted the Red Cross financial reserves however and an appeal for financial help resulted in the Wiltshire Farmers donating the sum of £240.[1]

On the 9 August the ward was ready for inspection. It was decorated with vases of sweet peas and on the front of the stage was a colourful collection of geraniums in pots lent by Mr Spinke, who a few weeks earlier at the Town Council meeting had championed the application from the Red Cross. In the evening the opening ceremony took place in the presence of the Mayor, Mr Townsend. A short dedication service was conducted by Canon Maxwell-Gumbleton[2] and Lady Margaret Spicer, the Vice President of the District, declared the ward open.

In his speech the Mayor thanked all those who had helped and reflected on how much was given voluntarily in aid of the Hospital to which he said:[3] *'It showed that those who could not go to the front and fight were ready to do their bit at home'*.

The Western Daily Press described the new ward:[4]

> The admirable work done by the Commandant (Mrs Wilson) and her staff has been highly appreciated by the Commanding Officer of the Southern Division, and at his request provision has been made for an additional 40 patients. This has been done by utilising the Neeld Hall, which is situated at the rear of subsidiary hospital in the Town Hall, and has been readily placed at the disposal of the hospital authorities by the Town Council.

With the addition of the new ward Chippenham Hospital could now treat 80 patients and within two weeks of opening 75 men were recuperating.[5] By the end of August it was at full capacity and, despite doubling the number of beds, the War Office asked the Red Cross to consider providing even more.

The news from the Front was grim. Despite the British employing a new weapon, the tank, in just one week in September 1916 the Allies suffered nearly 30,000 casualties, including the death of Raymond Asquith, the son of the British Prime Minister Herbert Asquith. The flow of wounded into the Bristol hospitals was never-ending and beds were continuously occupied. Men were being patched up by the surgeons at Bristol and rapidly transferred to the auxiliary hospitals.

1. Wiltshire and Swindon History Archive 1769/56 *VAD Hospital report 1 November 1916*
2. Maxwell H Smith adopted the surname Maxwell-Gumbleton in 1916
3. *Wiltshire Times* – 12 August 1916
4. *Western Daily Press* – 11 August 1916
5. *Devizes and Wiltshire Gazette* – 24 August 1916

The Story of Chippenham's Red Cross Hospital

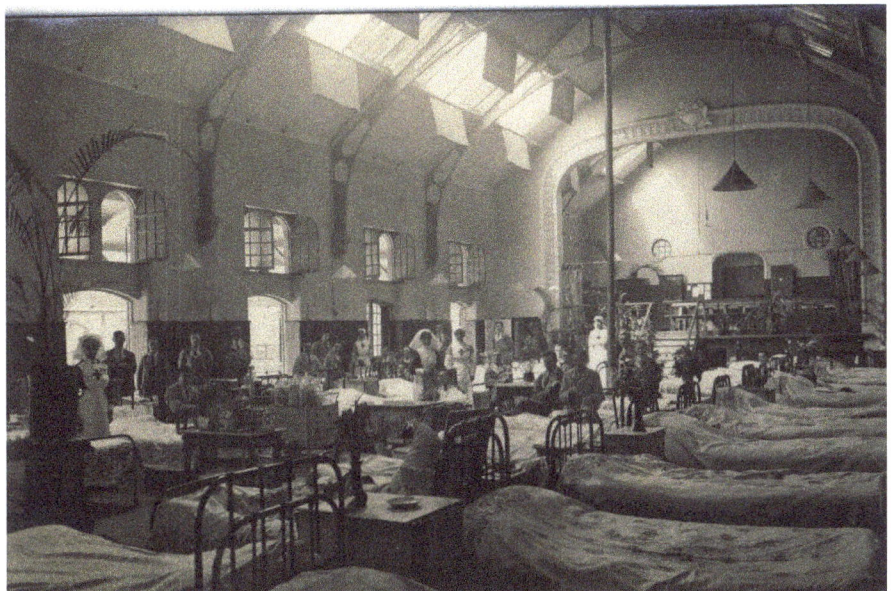

The Neeld Hall became Loyalty Ward

Basil Hankey wrote again to the Council in September 1916 to ask if they would consider releasing the remaining part of the Neeld Hall, the adjacent Corn Exchange and Store to the Red Cross.

The Town Council agreed to Mr Hankey's application on condition the Red Cross pay an extra £8 a year to cover loss of income and make alternative provision to accommodate the corn merchants for their market.[1] The Clerk to the Magistrates also agreed to release the space in the Neeld Hall on condition they could transfer their sittings to the Literary Institute in the Jubilee Building in the Market Place.

A temporary building was erected by the Red Cross in the Market Yard to house the Corn Merchants,[2] further building work took place in the Neeld Hall and the Corn Exchange was converted to a large kitchen. The stage in the Neeld Hall became the dining area and the recently erected partition in the hall was demolished. By the end of October the Hospital was at its increased capacity of 100 wounded men. There were reports that when the battles were at their heaviest the numbers being treated in Chippenham often went up to 106, with beds being squeezed into every space.

Cleaning and Laundry

THE TASK OF keeping the Hospital clean was a constant challenge. William Edwards was employed as caretaker and arranged for a team of cleaners, including Kate Bright, Emmie Finn, Elsie Hamlin, Alice Isaacs and Frances Jefferys to visit every

---

1 *Chippenham Council minute book 9*
2 Wiltshire and Swindon History Archive 1769/56 *VAD Hospital report 1 November 1916*

Unity and Loyalty

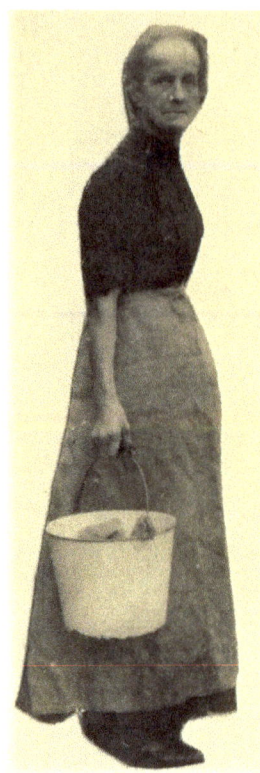

One of the domestic staff, essential to the maintenance of the Hospital

day. Cleanliness was so important that authorisation was given to pay some of the cleaners a wage to retain their services.

In 1917 Mrs Wilson gained further approval to extend the employment of staff into the kitchen as full time help was needed. An advert was placed in the local paper in March 1917:[1] *'WANTED. Strong steady kitchenmaid for Red Cross Hospital Chippenham. Apply personally after 11 o'clock to the Commandant.'*

Ada Merchant of London Road Chippenham started work at the end of March 1917 at a wage of 8s a week.

Laundry was an even greater challenge. Traditionally hospitals, such as Beaufort in Bristol, had their own large laundry to deal with the vast amounts of soiled bedding and clothing, but when Chippenham Town Hall was converted there was no such facility in the building.

Dora Belcher, the Assistant Quartermaster, was in overall charge of clothing and linen supplies and maintained a high standard of cleanliness. In 1919 she was commended by the Commandant for the *'The faultless manner in which the patients were turned out, which reflected credit on her department.'*

She probably looked to Chippenham Sanitary Laundry in Bath Road but also relied heavily on volunteers to keep costs down.

Lila Farries was the Quartermaster's Orderly and it was her job to gather the soiled linen and despatch it for cleaning. Ladies around the town would take in laundry and the senior girls at local schools helped with washing and mending.[2] Fanny Davis, who lived in Wood Lane and went to Westmead School was ten years old when the Hospital opened. She recalled how she and other girls did mending for the soldiers, darning socks that had such big holes their hands went straight through. She also said they made the sheets last longer by 'sides to middle.' She decided to do mending instead of art, as she disliked drawing and thought mending was far more helpful.[3]

As the Hospital increased in size and the amount of laundry reached industrial proportions another group of volunteers came forward to help. In the autumn of 1916, in the villages around Stanton St Quintin, a group of ladies organised by Maria Gardner, of Lower Stanton, formed a work party that took in much of Chippenham's laundry.

The Red Cross wrote about Mrs Gardner at the end of the War: *'She sorted,*

1   *Wiltshire Times* - 17 March 1917
2   *Wiltshire Within Living Memory* – Wiltshire Federation of Women's Institutes.
3   Betty Bird – Recollections from her mother Fanny Davis

The Story of Chippenham's Red Cross Hospital

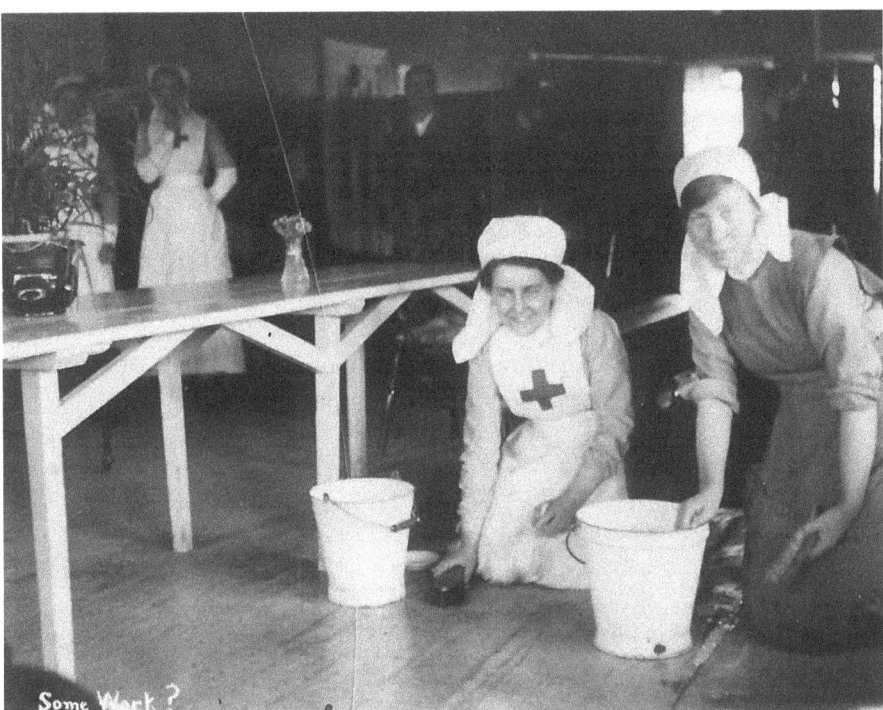

Cleaning the wards was a daily routine

distributed, collected and re-packed the washing done in Stanton for Chippenham VAD Hospital. she washed 24 articles weekly and made no charge whatever'.[1]

A routine was established. Maria Gardner's husband, Henry, travelled to Chippenham twice a week in his pony and cart to collect and return laundry. The soiled bedding and clothing was allocated to each volunteer and delivered by Henry.

Henry Gardner had lost a leg several years earlier, probably in an agricultural accident, and hadn't been able to work. He was dependent on poor relief, but he felt this work was his contribution to helping win the War.

The laundry workers were registered with the Red Cross as a Detachment known as Wilts 56[2]. Those who have been identified as belonging to the work party are listed below:[3]

Mrs Emma Allsop, of Lower Stanton. She washed 7 pairs socks and 12 other articles each week. She was 71 years old and a widow. Her son Albert was killed in action in 1917.

Mrs Sarah Bowsher, of Chippenham Road, Lower Stanton. She washed 18 Garments weekly. She was 77 years old and a widow.

Mrs Bessie Broom of Stanton St. Quintin. She washed 12 pairs socks weekly. Aged 39 she was married to Thomas, a cowman and had six children.

1   The British Red Cross Society - VAD index card record
2   The laundry workers may have been allocated to this Detachment for administration purposes
3   Ages given are at 1916

Unity and Loyalty

Mrs *Mabel Cottrell* aged 32, of Lower Stanton. She washed 18 garments weekly. Her husband William was an agricultural labourer.

Mrs *Harriet Couzens* aged 40, of Avils Cottages, Lower Stanton, washed towels weekly. Wife of a cowman she had four sons.

Mrs *Ellen Cripps* aged 51, wife of William Cripps, a Shepherd of Upper Stanton. Ellen washed six pairs of socks a week.

Mrs *Emma Fry* of Lower Stanton, aged 51 and wife of Omar, a cowman. She washed 12 shirts a week. It is quite likely her fourteen year old daughter Lilly helped with the laundry.

Mrs *Maria Gardner* of Lower Stanton, aged 46 was the organiser of the work party and washed 24 articles every week.

Mrs *Elizabeth Gillman* of Chippenham Road, Lower Stanton. Aged 67, she washed six pairs of socks a week, but was forced to give it up due to poor health.

Mrs *Nellie Miles*, aged 29, wife of Harry Miles, a farm labourer. Lived in Lower Stanton and washed 18 articles per week.

Mrs *Rhoda Millard* of Malmesbury Road, Lower Stanton washed 18 garments a week. It is thought that her husband William, known as Charles, volunteered as a full time orderly at the Military Hospital at Netley near Southampton.

Mrs *Kate Morse* aged 36 of Lower Stanton, wife of Charles, a shepherd, she washed 18 garments a week.

Mrs *Mary Savin* aged 49, wife of Tom, a gardener at Stanton Manor[1]- the home of Basil Hankey. In the 1911 census Mary Savin was described as a laundress working on her own account. Mary and her laundry may have been the inspiration for the work party.

Mrs *Edith Smith* aged 28, of Chippenham Road, Lower Stanton. Washed 12 articles for the Hospital each week. It is thought Edith was the daughter of Mary Savin.

Mrs *Annie Thomas* aged 60, of Avils Cottages, Lower Stanton. Washed 12 towels a week. Wife of Isaac Thomas a farmworker.

Mrs *Ellen Wallace* aged 71, of Lower Stanton. The Red Cross said about Mrs Wallace: *she is very old and infirm. She washes 2 pairs of socks weekly for the Hospital in Chippenham.*[2]

Mrs *Jenny Wallace* aged 29, of Lower Stanton. Washed 12 articles a week. Her husband, William, enlisted in the Artillery in November 1915. He was wounded in July 1917 and discharged from the Army in August 1918 with a disability pension. He died in 1923, it is thought his injury contributed to his death.

Miss *Sarah West* of Glede Farm Lower Stanton. Helped sorting and distributing washing.

Mrs *Fanny Whale* aged 49, of Lower Stanton. Washed 24 articles a week.

Mrs *Sarah Wheeler* aged 62, of Stanton St. Quintin. Washed 12 articles a week.

Serious Cases at Chippenham

BY THE LATE summer of 1916 there were so many wounded that beds at the Bristol military hospitals were constantly at a premium. Patients were released to the Red

---

1   *1911 census*
2   The British Red Cross Society - VAD index card record.

The Story of Chippenham's Red Cross Hospital

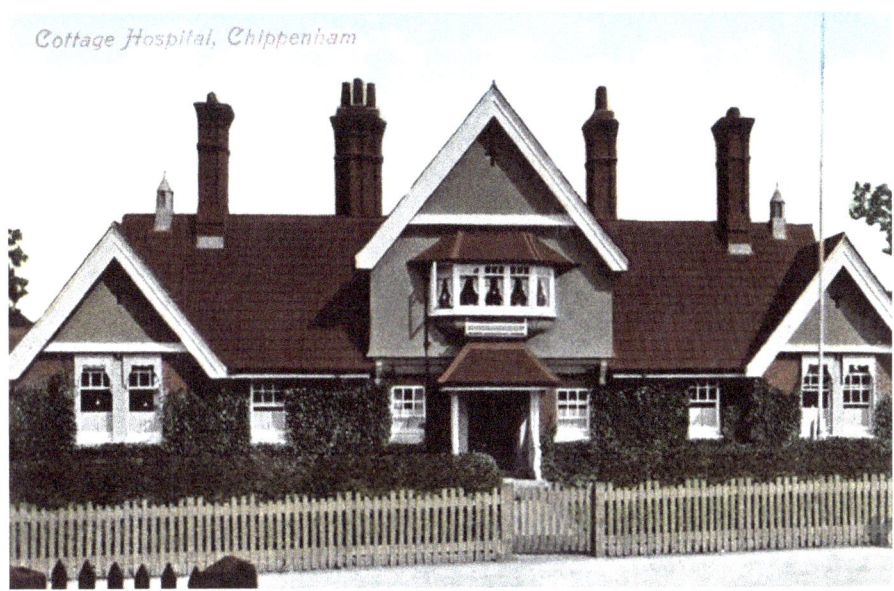

The Cottage Hospital

Cross auxiliary hospitals whilst still seriously ill. Some arrived at Chippenham in such a perilous condition that, despite being classed as convalescent, it was clear they needed a great deal of medical treatment in some cases even surgery.

This was a real test for the Chippenham VADs, whose training was limited to home nursing, first aid and general nursing care. The VADs had no option but to deal with the continuous flow of men regardless of their condition. Those who needed further surgery were taken to the Cottage Hospital where Doctor Wilson and his colleagues made use of the operating theatre.[1] Once the operation was completed the men of Wilts 13 returned the patient to the Red Cross Hospital and the VADs quickly learned to provide intensive post-operative medical care. By the end of the War over 200 operations had been carried out on wounded men at Chippenham Cottage Hospital and they were all cared for at the VAD Hospital.[2]

The VADs at Chippenham coped admirably under the leadership of the medically trained Lady Superintendent and doctors. In November 1916 Margaret Spicer, the Vice President of Chippenham division, wrote how well they had performed:[3]

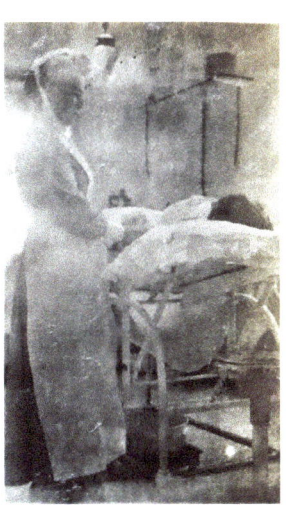

A wounded man in the operating theatre at the Cottage Hospital

1 Wiltshire and Swindon History Archive 1769/56 *VAD Hospital report 1 November 1916*
2 Chippenham Museum - *Garlick Scrapbooks*.
3 Wiltshire and Swindon History Archive 1769/56 *VAD Hospital report 1 November 1916*

Unity and Loyalty

The Hospital is much indebted to the Medical staff, Commandants, Quartermasters, Lady Superintendent, and Staff for their untiring devotion to duty; the numerous letters from men who have been discharged show their appreciation of the kindness received.

Grateful thanks are due to the large Number of residents both in Chippenham and the surrounding districts for their personal service and gifts of many necessities and comforts.

Hospitals Specialise

BY 1915 IT was recognised by the medical authorities that the system of sending wounded men to a general military hospital was not very efficient. A general hospital could not deal with such a variety of complex injuries suffered on the battlefield, especially when the numbers of returning wounded was so great. To deal with this and improve levels of treatment some hospitals were designated as specialist units treating particular types of injury.

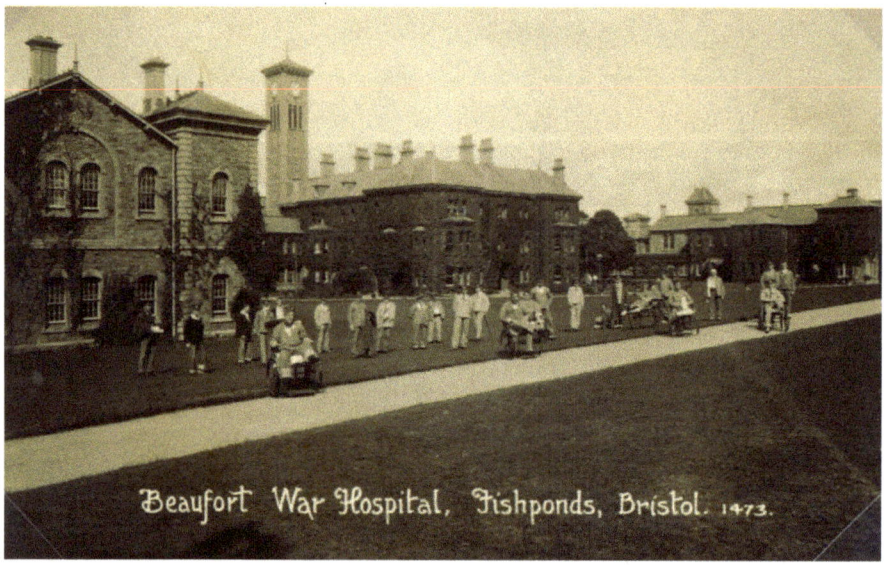

Orthopaedic patients at Beaufort Hospital in Bristol

The Queen's Hospital at Frognal House in Sidcup was dedicated to the treatment of facial injuries and went on to pioneer plastic surgery, while in Brighton the Pavilion Hospital opened in 1916 and treated and rehabilitated 6000 amputee soldiers. Louisa Grimshaw of Langley Burrell, one of the VADs at Chippenham, transferred to the Pavilion Hospital during 1916 and received a salary of £20 a year. Her work with the limbless was recognised in 1919 when she was presented with the Royal Red Cross second class.[1]

1   *London Gazette* - 31 July 1919.

The Story of Chippenham's Red Cross Hospital

In Bristol the Beaufort War Hospital was re classified as the Orthopaedic Centre for the Southwest,[1] treating bone and muscle injury caused by bullets and shrapnel. This took place at the beginning of January 1917 and the administration for Beaufort moved to the Fourth Southern Hospital Command at Devonport.[2]

With this change to specialism at Beaufort several VAD hospitals were nominated to receive Beaufort patients and specialise in convalescent orthopaedic treatment. The hospitals selected were:

Bruce Cole (Packer's Pavillion, Greenbank, Bristol), 120 beds;
The Pavilion, Calne, 45 beds;
Red Cross Hospital, Chippenham, 100 beds;
Oakland at Clevedon, 120 beds;
Relief Hospital, Longleat, 100 beds;
Standish Hospital, Stonehouse, 120 beds;
The Manor, Tockington, 20 beds;
Gourney Court, West Harptree 45 beds;
Ashcombe House, Weston-super-Mare, 166 beds.

Consequently, from the beginning of 1917, Chippenham concentrated on treating orthopaedic injuries although they also still received general cases of disease and illness from local military units.

The changes in command did not affect the day to day running of Chippenham Division, which remained under the administration of the Wiltshire Branch of the Red Cross. The Wiltshire Gazette in December 1916 reported:[3]

The Chippenham Red Cross Hospital is being transferred on January 1st (1917) from the Second Southern General Hospital to the Beaufort War Hospital. It is not expected that it will make any radical difference in the working and the staff hope they may still be kept busy as long as the war continues.

As a result of the impending change the flow of patients from the hospitals of the Second Southern Hospital Command, Southmead and Bristol Infirmary reduced in the weeks leading up to Christmas 1916. Over the holiday period there were only 63 men resident in Chippenham and the VADs took the opportunity to clean and decorate two of the wards. Most of the men were moved into Loyalty Ward: the recently converted Neeld Hall. Those needing most care were moved to one of the smaller wards, Geoffrey.

Unity and Evelyn Ward were stripped and fully cleaned. The Men's Detachment organised the cleaning duties, under the command of Frank Read. Many of them were

1   Glenside Museum Bristol Archive
2   *Bristol and the Great War 1914 to 1919* - Edited by George F. Stone and Charles Wells
3   *Devizes and Wiltshire Gazette* - 12 December 1916

employees of Saxby and Farmer and gave up their well-earned holiday from munition making to complete the work.[1]

Christmas 1916

COMPARED TO 1915, the Christmas festivities in December 1916 were a more energetic affair. On Christmas day the King's Christmas message included a special word for the sick and wounded:

> At this Christmastide the Queen and I are thinking more than ever of the sick and wounded among my sailors and soldiers. From our hearts we wish them strength to bear their suffering, speedy restoration to health, a peaceful Christmas and many happier years to come.

The people of Chippenham had taken the patients to heart and wanted to make Christmas one the men would remember. The North Wilts Herald described how they enjoyed the festivities: [2]

> The Loyalty ward was decorated with flags and pennants and lanterns lent by Col. Neeld and Geoffrey ward with flags lent by Mrs Dickson. The finishing touches, being the addition of evergreen on Saturday evening by the men's Detachment.
> On Christmas morning each man received a parcel containing fruit sweets and two presents. Dinner was at 12.45 and a very jolly party sat down. For those in bed who were well enough to be able to join in, eating the good things provided.
> The tables looked very pretty with crackers of every hue, dishes of fruit and nuts and flowers. Several gentlemen, including the mayor (Walter Hiscock) helped to carve the bird. After dinner a Christmas message was read from the King and this was loyally received and the National Anthem sung.
> After tea a Whist drive was organised and was much enjoyed by the men, members of staff and the men's Detachment, the prizes were given by the following. The Commandant (Mrs Wilson), the Mayoress (Mrs Hiscock) Mrs Newman, Mr Prior Mills, Mr Ludlow Tayler, Miss Hulbert and Mrs Williams.
> At 8 o'clock light refreshments were partaken of followed by games and 'Sir Roger de Coverley' the evening concluded with Auld Lang Syne and 'The King'.

On Boxing day, the wounded men were invited out to tea as guests of the Army Service Corps (ASC) who performed a revue for the patients and their friends The Wiltshire Times:[3]

---

1 *Devizes and Wiltshire Gazette* - 12 December 1916
2 *North Wilts Herald* - 29 December 1916
3 *Wiltshire Times* - 28 December 1916

The Story of Chippenham's Red Cross Hospital

Boxing Day, the wounded soldiers and their friends at the Hospital listened to an enjoyable entertainment given by the 733 Company M.T. A.S.C. Chippenham. They are a talented party and have trained their various gifts to a high state of efficiency so that that they would be welcome on any concert platform. A musical man was heard to say that if he had to join up and could get into such a company as that it would go a great way to reconcile him to the rigors of army discipline, especially under such an officer as Lieutenant Pine. Lieutenant Parkinson proposed a vote of thanks to the Company, and this was heartily accorded and replied to by Lieutenant Pine.

A few days later, as an additional treat, the ASC unit in the town arranged for a number of military ambulances to take men from the local hospitals to the theatre in Bath where they enjoyed the pantomime Sinbad the Sailor.[1]

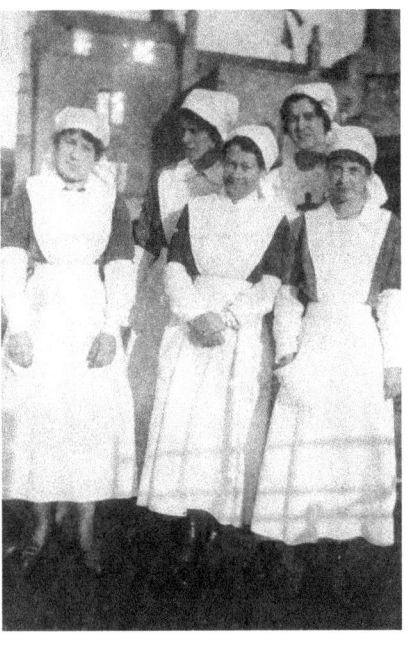

The cooks having prepared Christmas dinner

1 *Wiltshire Times* - 13 January 1917.

Chapter 8
1917

THE SHORTAGE OF VADs continues. The first patient dies in the wards of Chippenham Hospital.

German submarines inflict heavy losses on British shipping and rationing is introduced.

A Cold January

AT THE START of the year the men in the trenches in France were suffering the effects of the winter weather. The early part of 1917 was particularly cold resulting in many cases of frostbite.[1] The ground was frozen solid, and the snow and storms meant military action was limited to artillery bombardment and the occasional attack. The press even reported how little fighting had taken place. As spring arrived and the weather improved the British launched a major offensive in April 1917 known as the Battle of Arras.

In the Middle East fighting continued against the Ottoman Empire and Baghdad was finally taken by the British forces in March 1917. William Bodman, a member of the Chippenham Ambulance Detachment, received the news that his brother George had been killed, in January, during a battle leading up to the taking of Baghdad.[2]

There was growing unrest in Russia that escalated as the Bolsheviks organised demonstrations against the government. In March 1917 Tsar Nicholas II abdicated and a few months later Russia was in the grip of a revolution.

1917 started with a new Prime Minister. In December 1916 Asquith had stepped down and Lloyd George accepted an invitation to form a new coalition government.

Chippenham's Mayor, Councillor Walter Hiscock, opened the year giving the usual Mayoral New Year greeting:[3]

> Allow me to wish you all a much happier year than the one which is past. May 1917 be a year of victory and may permanent peace be established throughout the whole world before the year closes.

Chippenham, like the trenches in France, suffered a particularly cold spell during

---

1 Imperial War Museum. Article - *Voices of the First World War: Winter 1916*
2 *The Great War Chippenham Soldiers* – Richard Broadhead.
3 *Wiltshire Times* - 6 January 1917

The Story of Chippenham's Red Cross Hospital

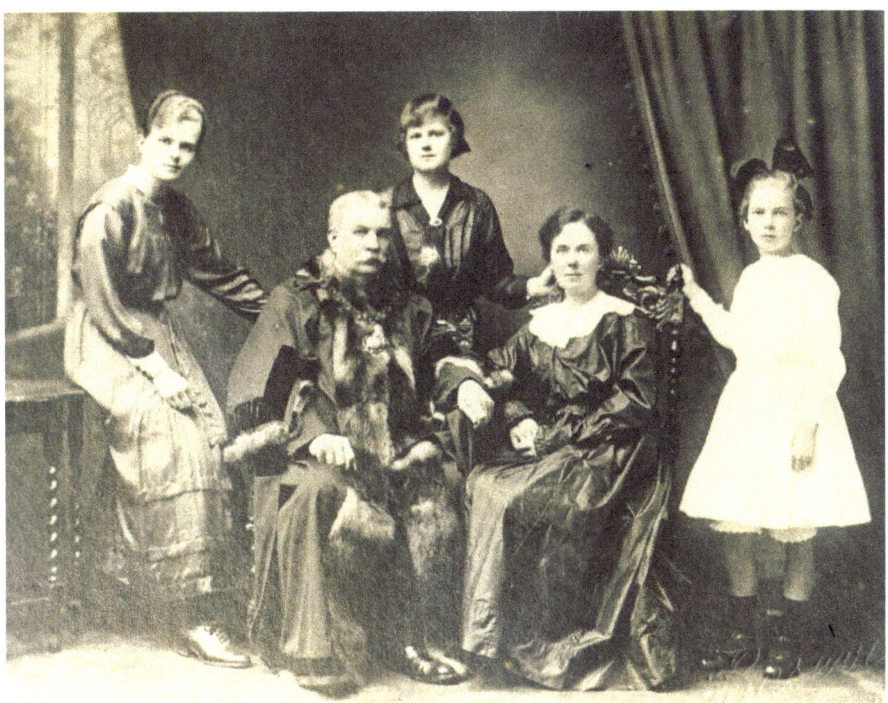

Mayor Walter Hiscock with his wife, Ada, and their daughters. The whole family volunteered at the VAD Hospital

January[1] and heavy snow had fallen in the town. In the Neeld Hall the heating system was insufficient to keep Loyalty Ward warm and Mrs Wilson approached the Council to provide extra heating, which they agreed and installed an additional two anthracite stoves.[2]

Mrs Ethel Bodman of Christian Malford, one of the cooks at the Hospital, with her friend Mrs Cooke of Foxham had arranged a collection in the villages before Christmas to buy turkeys for the men's Christmas dinner. Joe Buckle was able to supply good sized birds at a reasonable price, such a good price that a substantial amount of money was left over. The ladies used the money to buy ten shillings worth of sausages as a New Year treat for the patients.[3]

On New Year's Day members of the Chippenham Angling Club visited the Hospital and presented Mrs Wilson with a cheque for £5 to purchase a bed and bedding. This was money they had collected instead of holding their annual dinner, abandoned because most of their members were away on active service. Mrs Wilson thanked the Club and said donations of this type were always very welcome and if other organisations in the town were interested in doing the same it would be a great help.[4]

1   Metrological Office - *Monthly weather report*
2   *Wiltshire Times* - 6 January 1917 and *Chippenham Town Minute book 9*.
3   *Wiltshire Times* - 20 January 1917
4   *Wiltshire Times* - 6 January 1917

Unity and Loyalty

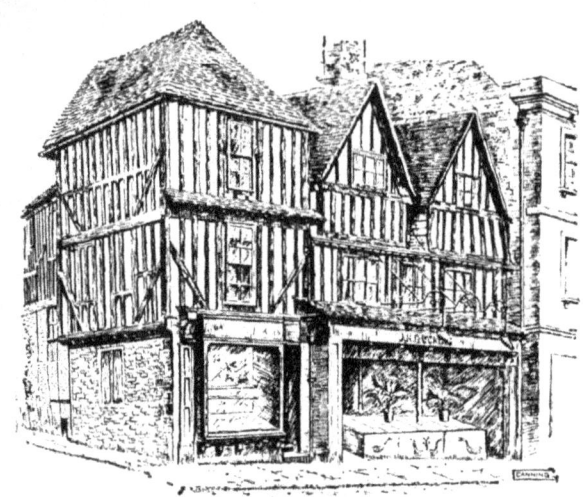

17, 18 High Street, Chippenham.

A Corner of Old England at Chippenham.

Advertising card for Joe Buckle's shop in Chippenham. Joe Buckle supplied poultry and cheese to the hospital

The men of the Ambulance Detachment had an ideal opportunity to test their skills when a special exercise was arranged in January 1917. For a few days nearby Box railway tunnel was closed for maintenance, meaning that trains between Chippenham and Bath were diverted along other routes. Box saw no rail traffic during the maintenance period and gave the chance to use the station as the centre for ambulance training. A number of carriages were pulled into the station and the men were able to practise de-training wounded soldiers.[1]

Orthopaedic Patients

THE NEW COMMAND structure under the Fourth Southern Hospital Command was implemented on the first of January and the freshly cleaned and decorated wards at Chippenham were ready to receive men classified as orthopaedic cases from Beaufort Hospital. Within two weeks the first men arrived, amongst them Private Bullion who had been badly injured with shrapnel and gunshot wounds to his legs.

David Bullion, a labourer from Forfar in Scotland, enlisted in September 1914. He reported to the recruiting office in Dundee and declared he was 19, when in reality he was only 16½. The recruiting officer turned a blind eye and he was assigned to 72 Brigade Royal Field Artillery as a Driver, arriving in France on 9 July 1915.

72 Brigade, Royal Field Artillery was part of Kitchener's Second New Army and David Bullion's first engagement with the enemy was at the Battle of Loos in September 1915. The Brigade then took part in the battles of the Somme and, during heavy fighting

[1] *Gazette and Herald - From the files - 26 January 2017*

The Story of Chippenham's Red Cross Hospital

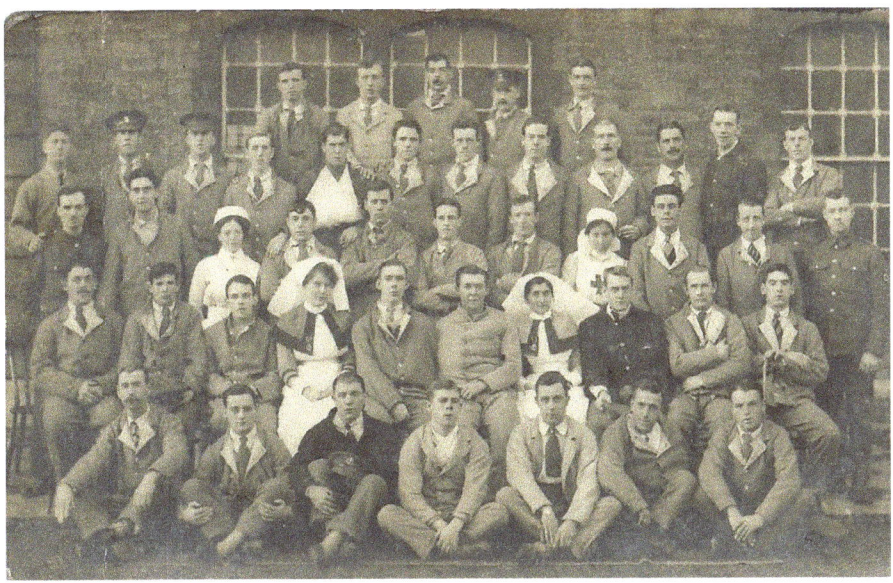

A Group of patients and nurses at Beaufort Hospital in December 1916. David Bullion is second row, first right, seated, with a walking stick

on 12 October 1916, Private Bullion was seriously wounded. He was evacuated to the military hospital at Rouen and then returned to Britain, arriving at Beaufort War Hospital on 17 October, where his treatment included a number of operations to his legs. He spent nearly three months at Beaufort and on 13 January 1917 he was sufficiently recovered to transfer to Chippenham. By the beginning of May he was confirmed as fit enough to return to his unit and he saw further action in France and Germany. He was released from his army service in March 1920 and returned to his home in Scotland. A year later he decided to emigrate and start a new life in Canada.[1]

The Wiltshire Red Cross reports for 1917 showed that a convalescent man remained in Chippenham for an average of seven weeks.[2] David Bullion's convalescence of over three months was not unusual however. Many orthopaedic injuries were complicated and required lengthy periods of treatment as muscles and bone healed and limbs were manipulated to bring them back into use.[3]

Massage treatment was introduced at Chippenham. This was an innovative treatment that proved successful in improving physical impairments caused by injuries to soft tissue and muscle. In Corsham accommodation was rented where men from

1   Chippenham Civic Society – *Buttercross Bulletin - August 2017*. The story of Gladys and David.
2   The British Red Cross Society archive RCB/2/14/2. *Wiltshire report 1917*. Men from the locally based regiments suffering from short term illness were also treated.
3   The National Archive Blog - There was a revolution in the treatment of orthopaedic cases during the War. Colonel Robert Jones an Army Surgeon wrote *Notes on Military Orthopaedics in 1916*, where he said, these types of wound need patience and time.

Unity and Loyalty

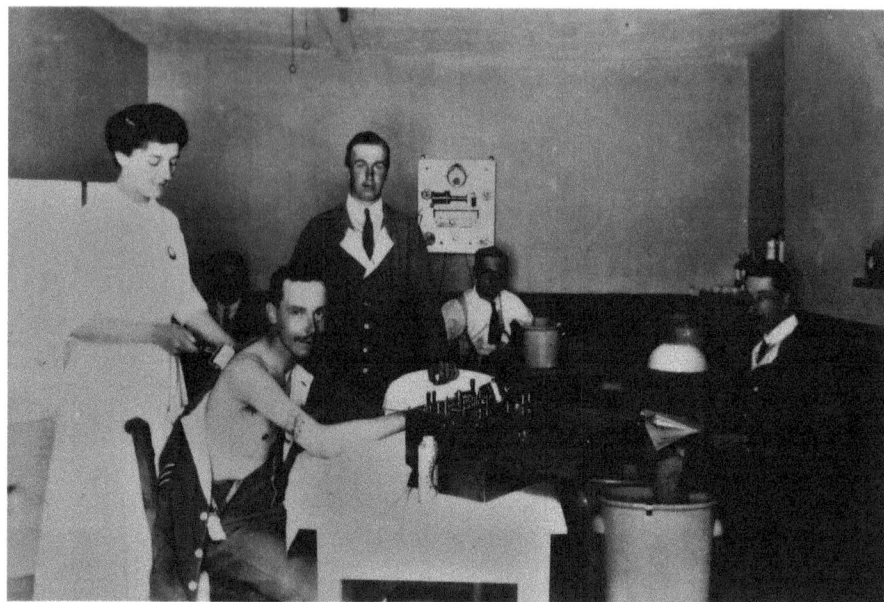

Men receiving massage treatment. There were treatment rooms in Chippenham and Corsham

Chippenham[1] and Corsham were treated with electric massage sessions.[2] Patients were also sent to the Royal Mineral Water Hospital in Bath for periods of treatment.

Amy Mack, an Australian newspaper reporter, visited Bath in 1916 and interviewed wounded men at the Mineral Hospital for the Sydney Morning Herald[3]. She told how even the depressing surroundings of the building could not dampen the spirit of the Australians she met:

> For surely in all England there is no dingier, duller hospital than that great square building. Outside the grim solid stone front is dark with age, but with none of that warm mellowing which comes to some stone buildings. Within the bare rooms, with their bare, benches and bare tables and tightly closed windows, make as dismal and unsuitable a setting as one could imagine for sick men. Yet even the dreariness of the rooms coupled with the depressing effect of the hot baths has not taken all the spirit from those Australian soldiers who are doing a cure there.

She went on to say that men stayed in Bath for no more than three or four weeks and those she met were looking forward to returning to the VAD hospitals. One man described how well he was looked after at Bowood: '*They were as simple and kind to us*

---

1 Corsham Civic Society Article. *WW1 Hospital, Corsham Town Hall 1914-1918* tells how the Town Council expressed concern that men came for treatment from Chippenham when there was an outbreak of measles in that town.
2 *The Corsham Commemorates project, Above and Beyond* - Corsham Town Council.
3 *The Sydney Morning Herald* - 22 March 1916

The Story of Chippenham's Red Cross Hospital

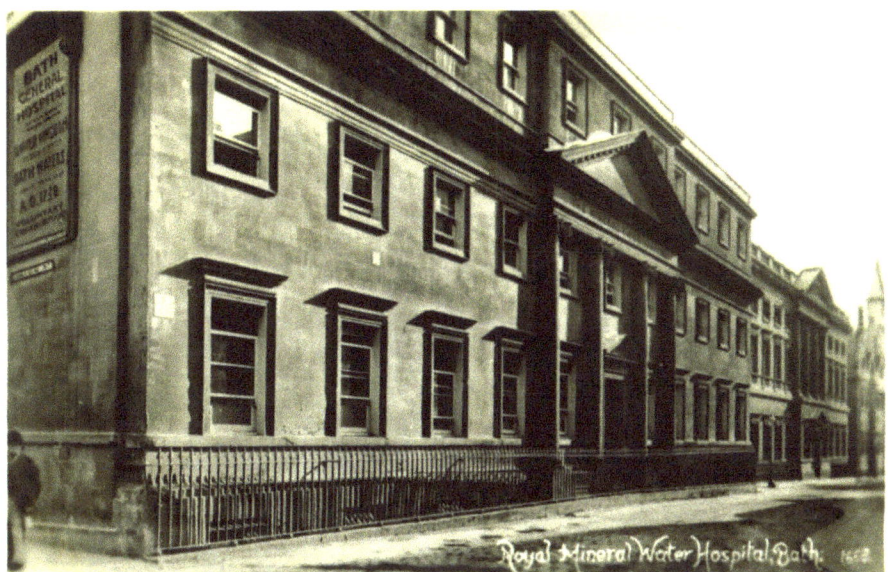

Royal Mineral Water Hospital Bath

as if they had known us always. Sometimes when I was ill in bed Lady Lansdowne used to come and sit beside me and talk.'

Bad News at Chippenham VAD Hospital

THE DAY AFTER David Bullion arrived at Chippenham a cloud fell over the Hospital. Doctor and Mrs Wilson received the distressing news that their last surviving son had died of wounds on 11 January in Mesopotamia.[1]

Herbert Raymond Wilson was the eldest of the Wilson's three sons, the two younger sons Geoffrey and Evelyn, after whom the two small wards at Chippenham were named, had both been killed in France during 1915.

Despite the dreadful news Mrs Wilson maintained her position. At the end of the War she was paid many compliments for her selfless service and her ability to maintain a happy hospital despite suffering such great personal loss.

A month later there was more bad news. Since the Hospital's opening, the Chippenham VADs had seen every patient recover with many being able to return to their regiments. This record was broken when Private Raymond Stubbert died.

Raymond Stubbert had travelled from his home in Nova Scotia in Canada to enlist in England. He joined the Army Service Corps and was part of the 829 Company ASC, the Motor Transport Section, based in Chippenham and billeted in the skating rink on Station Hill. A few weeks after he arrived in Chippenham he contracted pneumonia and was admitted to the Hospital in a very serious condition. Despite the attention of Doctor

---

1   *Western Daily Press* - 15 January 1917.

Unity and Loyalty

Laurence and the VADs his condition deteriorated and he died in Evelyn ward on 14 February 1917.

When the death of Private Stubbert was announced the whole town went into mourning. In the short time he was stationed in the town he had made many friends and a request was made that his funeral should be with full military honours and representatives from the town would be in attendance.

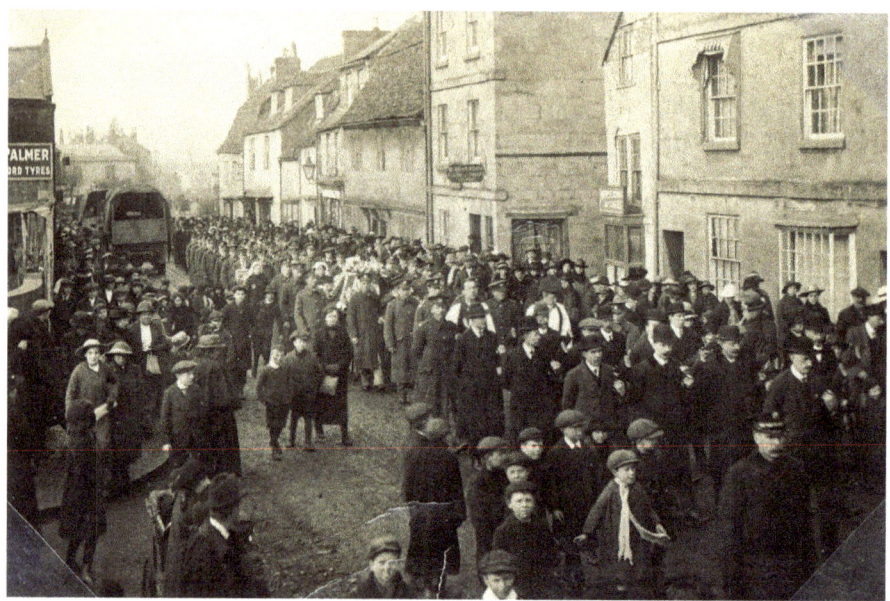

Funeral of Raymond Stubbert. VADs and wounded men can be seen behind the coffin

The funeral took place on the Saturday afternoon following his death. The shops in the town put up their shutters as a mark of respect. The coffin, draped with the union flag, was carried out of the Hospital and placed on a bier accompanied by a guard of honour made up of patients. The cortege was led through the High Street by the Mayor accompanied by the Superintendent of Police. The Wiltshire Volunteers paraded alongside the coffin with arms reversed. The Salvation Army band, officers of the Fire Brigade, men from the Army Service Corps, patients, nurses and cooks from the Hospital and many private individuals followed the coffin. The funeral service took place in St Andrew's church and the procession continued to the Cemetery in London Road, where three volleys were fired over the grave and the Last Post was sounded.

Amongst the many wreaths were several from the Hospital with the following messages: [1]

> Sympathy from the Officers of Wilts VI VAD.
> With deep regret from the Lady Superintendent, Nurses and the Men's

---

1   Chippenham Museum - *Garlick Scrapbooks*

The Story of Chippenham's Red Cross Hospital

Detachment, Red Cross Hospital.

In remembrance and regret from Sisters Reed, Vicborn, Davis, Houlston and Miller.

With sincere sympathy from the Cooks of the Red Cross Hospital.

A headstone was erected at public expense, but this was later replaced by the Commonwealth War Graves Commission.

Ten months later the Hospital suffered its second death. Private William Ellerton, of the 12th Battalion West Yorkshire Regiment, was seriously wounded in action.[1] He was treated for his injuries at the military hospital in Bristol and was then admitted to Chippenham. He never recovered and succumbed to his wounds on 30 December 1917. His family arranged his burial at Linthorpe Cemetery in his home town of Middlesbrough.

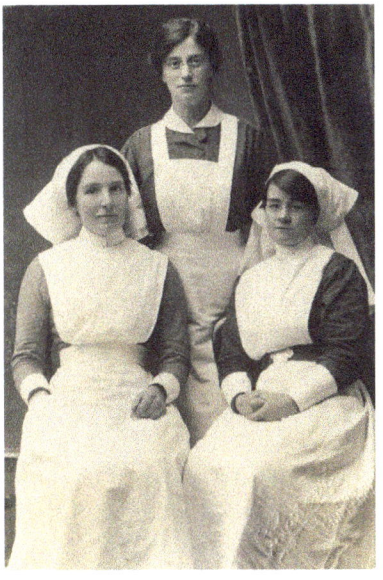

Ethel Vicborn, sitting on the right, joined with the sisters at the hospital to send a floral tribute

It is testament to the skill and care given by the VADs at Chippenham that no further patients died.

In 1918 the patients again formed a guard of honour at the funeral of a local hero. Richard Neate grew up in Castle Combe and later moved to Chippenham. In 1913, aged 17, he joined the Royal Marines. He volunteered for the attack on Zeebrugge harbour in April 1918 and was one of the heroes who died in action. Unusually his body was returned to his family, who lived in Wood Lane in Chippenham.

Four men from the Hospital accompanied the coffin in Chippenham from the station to Richard Neate's mothers house in Wood Lane and two days later, on 30 April, six men from the hospital, under the command of a Sergeant Wilson, acted as bearers, carrying the coffin to the Parish Church where the funeral service took place. The coffin was then taken to Castle Combe for burial.[2]

Rationing

IN JANUARY 1917 the German navy commenced a policy of unrestricted submarine warfare. This meant they would sink on sight any vessels, including those from neutral countries, bringing food and materials to Britain. The German's intention was that food shortages would bring Britain to its knees.

1   *Soldiers Died in the Great War, 1914-1919* published in 1921 by His Majesty's Stationery Office confirms died of wounds.
2   *Wiltshire Times* – 4 May 1918

Unity and Loyalty

A voluntary rationing scheme was introduced in February, with the aim of reducing the consumption of food in short supply and avoiding waste when cooking. Limits were set for the three staples of the daily diet: bread, meat and sugar.

The Government gave the Agricultural Committees more powers to increase food production in an effort to make the country self-sufficient. Tractors were imported from the USA and Canada to manage agriculture as efficiently as possible and where there were labour shortages the Army provided skilled drivers. In Wiltshire Mr William Burridge, one of the organisers of transport for patients in Chippenham, was appointed the District Supervisor of the scheme to distribute tractors to farmers in the county.

The Agricultural Committee also had the power to turn land over to agriculture. The Town Council in Chippenham agreed that more land should be given over to food production[1] and sites in Wood Lane, Marshfield Road and smaller plots in the town were designated as allotments with men, women and schoolchildren volunteering to tend them.

A Government leaflet for voluntary rationing

The voluntary rationing scheme was not as successful as hoped and in June the Local Government Board gave local authorities the power to enforce orders made by the Food Controller restricting the use of a number of foods. In August the Chippenham Surveyor identified a number of violations of the sugar order and notice was given that any future breaches of the order would result in prosecution.

Mr Kennedy Jones, the Director General of Food Economy, wrote in April 1917 to the Chairman of the Central Joint VAD Committee, Arthur Stanley, saying that apart from those on invalid foods he would expect wounded men in hospitals to conform to voluntary rationing. As a result at some VAD hospitals, particularly in urban areas, the patients raised grievances that food was in short supply and not well prepared.

By January 1918 the food situation had reached such critical levels that the Government introduced strict rationing. Rationing orders were introduced by the

---

1   *Chippenham Council minute book 9*

The Story of Chippenham's Red Cross Hospital

Ministry of Food for sugar meat, butter, cheese and lard. The penalties for misuse were severe.

At Chippenham there is no record of complaints at the VAD Hospital about the lack of food. Mrs Williams and Mrs Shipp, who were in charge of the kitchen, were well known for their culinary skills and to augment the rations the public regularly contributed food.

From the Hospital's opening donations of vegetables, fruit, salad eggs and poultry were given and continued, often with weekly deliveries. When voluntary, and later compulsory, rationing was introduced gifts from the public did not falter. Food supply in Chippenham appeared to remain plentiful. Produce was grown in gardens and allotments supplementing rationed foods. Tips on suggested recipes were published in the monthly journal of the Red Cross using foods that were not on the ration list.

During a typical week in April 1918,[1] at a time that saw compulsory rationing of sugar, meat butter and cheese, the following food was donated at Chippenham to supplement the hospital allowances:

Eggs, given by Langley Burrell, Kington Langley, East and West Tytherton, Foxham, Christian Malford, Mrs Freegard (Bencroft), Mrs Dickson, Mrs E Buckland (Kington St Michael) and Mrs Parry. A total of 15 dozen eggs.

Rhubarb, given by Mrs Hardiman, Mrs Miles (Sutton) and Mrs Wallace (Stanton),

Potatoes, one sack given by Mr Freegard

Greens, given by Miss Bishop (Kington St Michael), Mrs Garnett, Mr Swan (Castle Combe) Miss Gorst, Captain Leatham, Mr Freegard (Bencroft) and Colonel Neeld.

Flowers, given by Miss Joan Lysley, Mrs G A H White and Mrs Brotherhood.

In Kington St Michael the Congregational Chapel gave a donation of 10s 8d towards buying food.

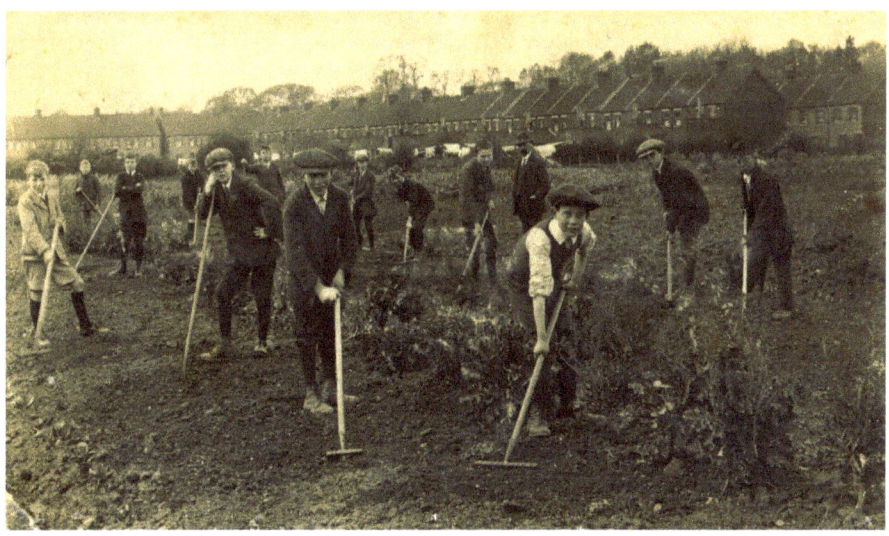

Schoolchildren working on allotments in Chippenham

1   Chippenham Museum - *Garlick Scrapbooks*.

Unity and Loyalty

Many of the donations were seasonal. Later in the year, as well as the staples of vegetables and eggs, donations included eight hares and eight pheasants from the tenants of Lucknam Estate: game was not subject to rationing. Mr Hankey supplied sacks of apples in the autumn from his orchard.

Often there would be cakes and jams: a certain amount of sugar was allowed for jam making. The local schools, Lowden and Westmead, would donate vegetables from the school allotment. The children had always helped gather fruit from the hedgerows and started collecting nettles for what became Mrs Williams's well-known nettle soup.

In 1919 when the Hospital finally closed Mrs Wilson reflected on the constant supply of donations saying that contributions came from every level: '*Many poor people in villages contributed one egg a week and these humble contributions have been as much appreciated as the larger supplies which came from the leading residents in the district*'.

When she thanked Mr Swan of Castle Combe, who from the opening to the closing of the Hospital never missed a week bringing a supply of vegetables, he replied by saying '*All I have done is a thank offering for having my boy return from the fighting in Mesopotamia without a scratch*'.[1]

America

WHEN THE GERMANS started their unrestricted sinking of ships in January 1917 there was no distinction between British and American vessels. As US merchant ships were sunk and American lives were lost the pressure on America to join the War against Germany grew and on 6 April 1917 America declared war against Germany.

In Chippenham the town showed its support for the Americans when on the 4 July the American flag was flown to mark American Independence Day. The local contingent of Volunteers, under the command of Captain Mills and accompanied by a band, marched up the High Street to the Town Hall, occupied by the Hospital, where the Stars and Stripes was raised. The patients and VADs formed up with the Mayor and Town Councillors to salute the flag.[2]

Review of the Year

AS 1917 CLOSED Chippenham Hospital was fully occupied. Mrs Wilson said that during the year Chippenham Detachment had worked well and the help of Sutton Detachment had been a great asset in dealing with such a heavy workload

The Vice President, Lady Margaret Spicer, in her review of 1917 reflected how busy the hospitals in the whole Division had been and published the number of patients, and more importantly, the patient nights (beds occupied) at each hospital.[3] At Chippenham the figures showed that on average 95 beds were occupied every night.

1 Chippenham Museum - *Garlick Scrapbooks*. Article the closing of the Red Cross Hospital
2 *Wiltshire Times* – 7 July 1917
3 Chippenham Museum. *Ivy Gladstone Scrapbook*.

The Story of Chippenham's Red Cross Hospital

	Patients treated during the year	Patient nights
Chippenham	712	34,680
Corsham	284	24,122
Melksham	1034	29,323

She went on to say as the ladies of Sutton Detachment travelled some distance to attend for duty in Chippenham a nurse's restroom was being built and would be opened by early January 1918. At the same time a corridor was to be constructed between the Neeld Hall and Market yard below the Town Hall to give easier access between all the wards, and the offices and stores on the ground floor.

Christmas

CHRISTMAS PROVIDED NO rest for the members of the Red Cross. The ladies of the VAD were fully occupied on Christmas Day when 100 patients celebrated in the Neeld Hall. The festivities equalled the previous year and the wounded men were given a Christmas to remember.

The men of the Ambulance Detachment remained on duty over Christmas to help with wheelchairs and carrying stretchers so all patients could join in the Christmas meal. They remained on standby with their ambulance should patients need to be transferred. On New Year's Eve, with colleagues from Corsham, they attended Devizes when an unexpected train arrived at the station in the town.

Members of the public were as generous as ever. At the Christmas poultry sale held by the local auctioneers Tilley, Parry and Culverwell a cockerel was given by Mrs Jones of Swinley Farm, Sutton Benger. After hectic bidding £3. 5s was raised for the Hospital Christmas fund.[1]

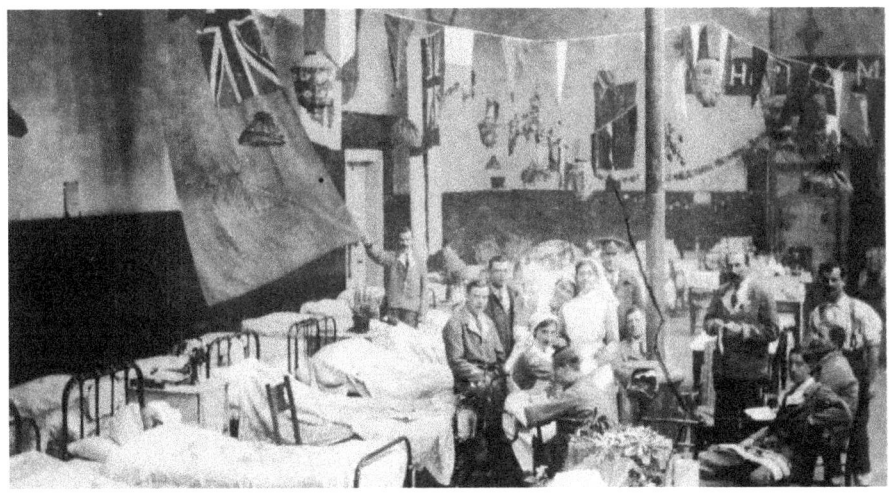

Loyalty Ward Christmas 1917

1   *Wiltshire Times* – 29 December 1917

Chapter 9
1918

THE VAD HOSPITALS continue to report serious staff shortages. The Ministry of Pensions is established and civilian hospitals are asked to treat disabled men. News from the front is encouraging and peace is in sight.

Optimistic News

THERE WAS SOME cautious optimism at the beginning of 1918 as the allies were beginning to score successes. America had joined the War against Germany the previous April and the first US troops had arrived in France in June 1917, by the spring of 1918 fully trained American men were arriving on the Western Front in large numbers.[1] They took a major role against the Germans at the battle of Cantigny in May 1918 which accompanied the news that the tank was showing continued successes on the battlefield. Further successes boosted morale throughout the country.

The Mayor of Chippenham joined in this optimism with his New Year message:[2] *'the hope that one of the sources of happiness which the New Year had in store was an end to the war.'*

The King made a proclamation that the first Sunday of the New Year, the Feast of the Epiphany, would be a Day of Prayer and Thanksgiving, giving a rousing message to the public:[3]

> This victory will only be gained if we steadfastly remember the responsibility which rests upon us, and in a spirit of reverent obedience ask the blessing of Almighty God upon our endeavours. With hearts grateful for the Divine guidance which has led us so far towards our goal, let us seek to be enlightened in our understanding and fortified in our courage in facing the sacrifices we may yet have to make before our work is done.

All denominations throughout the Empire observed the day of prayer and, as a mark of respect, licensed premises throughout the country remained closed for the day.

The Mayor and Corporation of Chippenham led the congregation at St Andrew's Church in praying for victory and peace. The VADs attended the Primitive Methodist

---

1 Imperial War Museum. Article - *Voices of the First World War: Arrival of the American troops*
2 *Wiltshire Times* – 5 January 1918
3 *Illustrated London News* - 12 January 1918

The Story of Chippenham's Red Cross Hospital

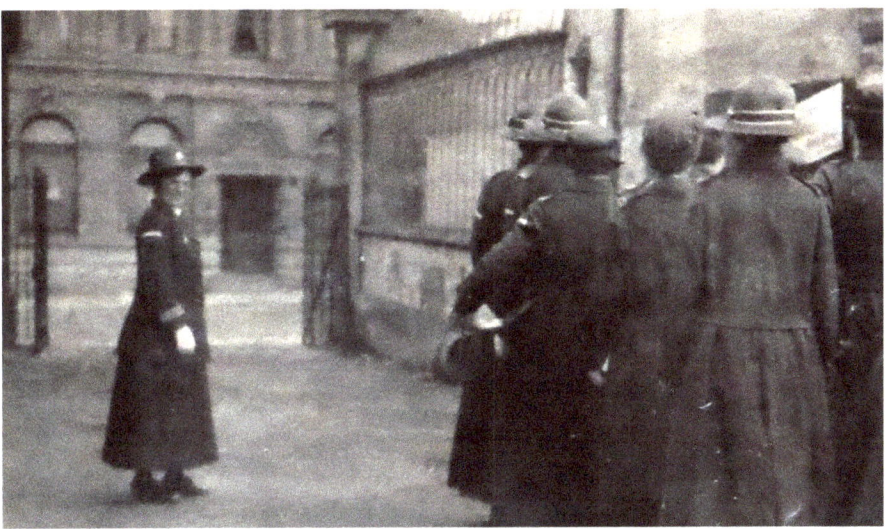

Chippenham VADs head for church parade

Church in the Causeway, where the retiring collection was in aid of the Red Cross Hospital.

Following the Church services a united gathering was held at St Paul's Parish Hall and the Mayor gave a hopeful message ending his speech:[1] *'...they (the people of the town) should all hope for a happy and speedy issue from this terrible conflict'.*

In January 1918 the weather was so bad, with torrential rain and snow, that the newly opened restroom was used as temporary accommodation for those VADs who were

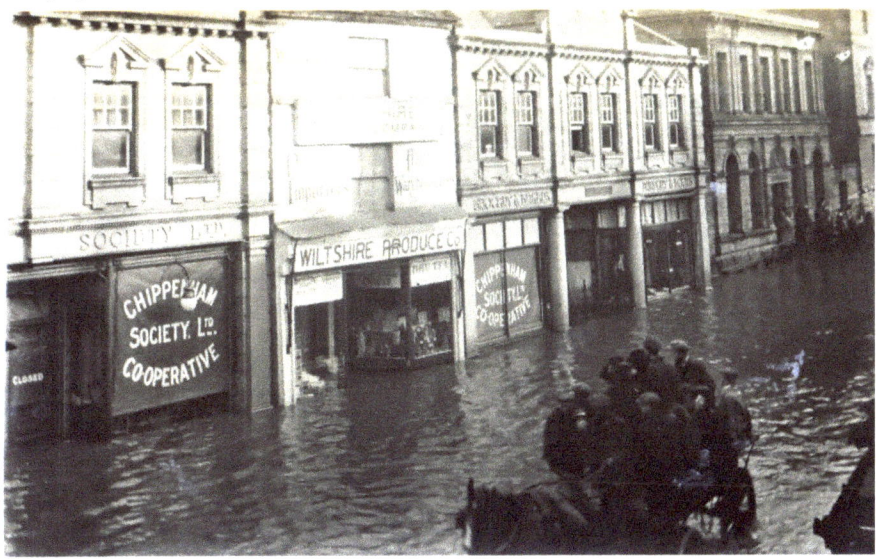

The flooded High Street in January 1918

1   *Wiltshire Times* -12 January 1918.

Unity and Loyalty

unable to get home. The river in Chippenham broke its banks, flooding the High Street and Bath Road, and the Town Bridge was under water. The Hospital escaped flooding but the VADs had difficulties getting there. Ivy Gladstone wrote how local traders arranged transport for the VADs to get through the floods:[1]

> All the nurses and cooks going on duty that day had various rides in coal carts- which did not add to the cleanness of their uniform – and were greeted with cheers from the boys in blue as they arrived at the hospital steps and to their remarks and jests of derision an answer was; Yes we were all but torpedoed!

Staff Shortages

THE SHORTAGE OF VADs, both locally and nationally, remained a constant problem as women left for other war work and the numbers of wounded grew. In May 1918 the VAD Department made a further appeal for women between the ages of 21 and 48 to come forward, but added that women should come forward regardless of experience. In Chippenham it appears the problem was not as serious as in many other areas as the Commandant kept the wards fully operational often with additional help from those in the town.

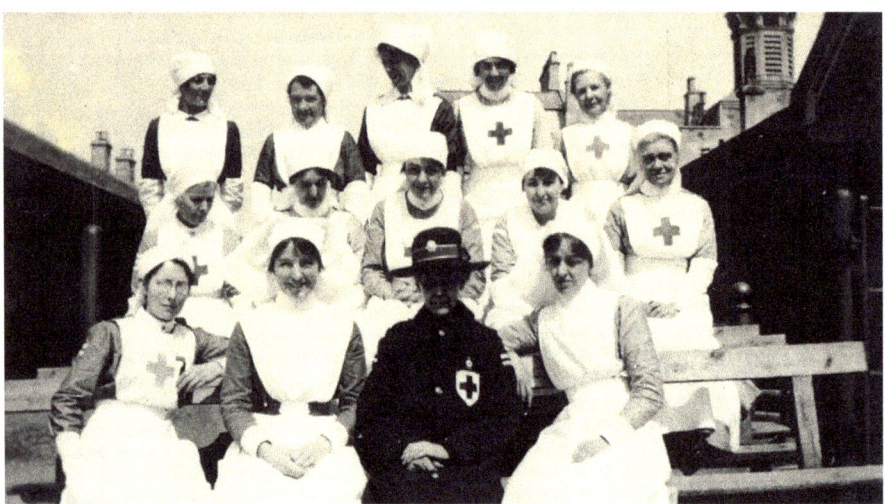

A group of VADs at Chippenham in 1918. Despite a national shortage of volunteers Mrs Wilson was able to keep the hospital fully operational

The Men's Detachment in Chippenham, which during 1917 had reported a full complement of 40, had reduced numbers. By March 1918 they had a complement of 30 having lost ten men to Conscription over the previous year. To cover the shortage they were able to call on Boy Scouts for some duties.

1   Chippenham Museum - *Ivy Gladstone Scrapbook*.

The Story of Chippenham's Red Cross Hospital

Elsewhere in Wiltshire the picture was gloomier as detachments were decimated by Conscription. In July 1917 the Military Tribunal in Bradford on Avon recognised the problem and gave partial exemptions to Herbert Bull and George Brown conditional on them remaining active members of the Ambulance Corps.[1] In December they were still short-handed and advertised for Bradford men to join the Ambulance Detachment.

In Trowbridge an advert was placed in the papers to recruit volunteers, intended to prick the conscience of fit older men:[2] *'It will be necessary for those joining to put in 10 drills per month, but this is surely little to ask of those who remain at home in safety and comparative comfort.*

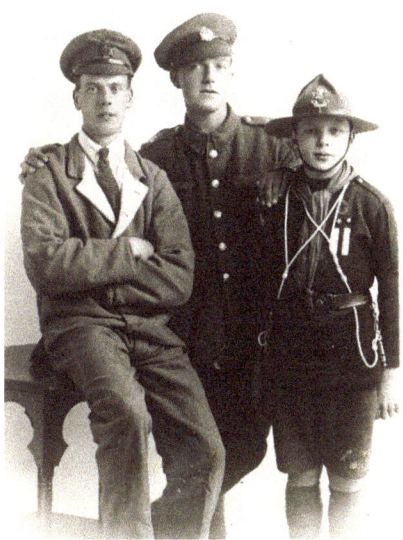

A Scout with patients from the hospital. Scouts were called on to perform duties at the hospital

Ministry of Pensions

THE EVACUATION CHAIN[3] FOR a wounded soldier was a well-trod path: evacuate, treat the wound and return the man to his unit as quickly as possible. What had never been contemplated was the numbers of permanently disabled men resulting from this industrial scale of warfare: men who had lost limbs and suffered serious injuries caused by shellfire and high explosives.

Traditionally the care of the military disabled fell to the Admiralty and the War Office. The award of disability pensions, death benefits and grants for dependants was assessed by the Royal Patriotic Fund Corporation.[4] This was a voluntary fund instigated by Queen Victoria during the Crimean War and awards were decided by a discretionary committee, with much of their income relying on public subscription.

By 1915 this discretionary pension awards system, based on donations, became unsustainable with the high numbers of permanently maimed and the Government passed legislation to standardise the awards to war disabled.

The Naval and Military War Pensions Etc. Act 1915 specified that the award committee was to be a non-discretionary statutory body and the payment of disability

1 *Wiltshire Times* -7 July 1917
2 *Wiltshire Times* - 8 December 1917.
3 *Medical Services in the First World War* – Susan Cohen. Describes the Evacuation Chain, based on the memorandum on the treatment of injuries in war.
4 The National Archive - The Royal Patriotic Fund was created in 1854. Queen Victoria, concerned for the well-being of the widows and orphans of British servicemen dying in the Crimean War, made an appeal for public donations.

pensions and death benefits to widows was to become a state responsibility overseen by a Pensions Board established in September 1916.

In addition to being accountable for the award of allowances the Pensions Board took responsibility for the welfare and rehabilitation of the disabled man after his discharge from the military. The 1915 Act: *'To make provision for the care of disabled officers and men after they have left the service, including provision for their health, training and employment.'*

Further legislation in December 1916 saw the Board become a Government Ministry with the passing of the Ministry of Pensions Act 1916 and by March 1917 the organisation was engaging with existing agencies caring for the disabled war wounded.

The voluntary agencies the Ministry of Pensions worked with included; the Blinded Soldiers' and Sailors' Care Committee, commonly known as St Dunstan's;[1] the Star and Garter Home, which had been established in 1916 for the care of the paralysed; and Roehampton for the care of limbless men.

In 1917 George Barnes, the first Minister of the newly formed Ministry of Pensions, appointed a committee called the Joint Committee of the Ministry of Pensions on Institutional Treatment (JCITMP). The Committee's purpose was to work with existing organisations to provide: *'appropriate institutional care for discharged men to ensure suitable treatment, aftercare and employment appropriate to their disability'*.[2]

The Red Cross, via the Joint War Committee, placed a large sum of money at the disposal of the JCITMP to acquire and equip establishments, while the Ministry of Pensions was responsible for general maintenance and management of the institutions via local boards.

The Red Cross continued to support many of the organisations after the War and the local Red Cross work parties were asked to help by knitting and sewing for many months after the Armistice. In the Chippenham area some of the work parties were still doing needlework for St Dunstans in July 1919 and, as these sewing and knitting groups were wound up, they often donated their surplus funds to the institutions.

With the passing of the Acts of Parliament in 1915 and 1916 there were now clearer lines of responsibility between the War Office and the Ministry of Pensions on the treatment of wounded and disabled.

The War Office were responsible for treating wounded men, with the intention of returning them to their regiments and the War as quickly as possible. A man considered unfit for further war service[3] was discharged from the service and became the responsibility of the Ministry of Pensions. The separation of responsibilities became blurred however when a man discharged from the military as unfit for war service remained at a hospital administered by the War Office because there was no available bed for him at an appropriate civilian institution.[4] An appropriate institution was considered

1 The committee formally adopted the name St Dunstan in 1923
2 The British red Cross Society – Information sheet, *Rehabilitation after the First World War* describes the various schemes for disabled men.
3 Kings Regulations Paragraph 392(xvi)
4 *Hansard* - House of Commons debate 6 March 1917. The Minister of Pensions spoke about

The Story of Chippenham's Red Cross Hospital

to be a civilian hospital or a specialised rehabilitation unit.

The Pensions Minister, George Barnes, negotiated with the Secretary of State for War that a less rigid scheme should be adopted and men could remain at military hospitals for a reasonable time subject to accommodation availability and, where appropriate, provide some outpatient treatment.[1] The fact that the Financial Secretary to the War Office was at the negotiations suggests the debate was as much about which Department would pay for a man while in a military hospital.

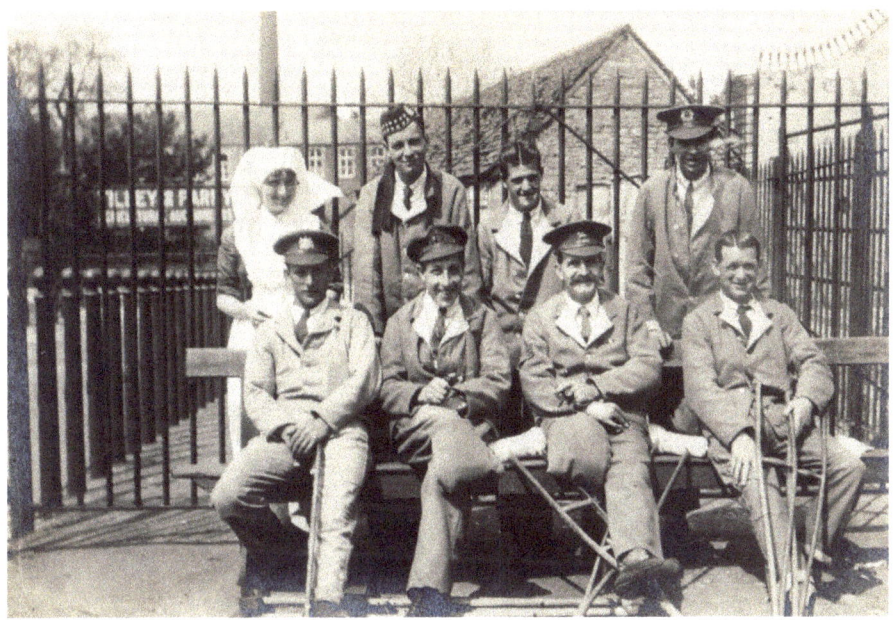

Wounded men at Chippenham. The two men in the front row having suffered amputations were awaiting discharge from the military and further treatment would be provided at a civilian institution

Depending on his disability, once a man was discharged from the services and placed in the care of the Ministry of Pensions he could spend several months in rehabilitation learning a trade such as woodwork, basket-making or boot-making.[2] Other men were so badly injured or paralysed that they remained in institutions for the rest of their lives, while others, perhaps the lucky ones, underwent treatment in a civilian hospital and discharge to their homes. The Ministry of Pensions remained responsible for outpatient treatment and helping adapt to disability.

To administer the care of the disabled and those rehabilitating at home every county was obliged to set up a local committee, usually under the County or Borough Councils, to assist the central committee of the Ministry of Pensions in the award of pensions,

the disputes regarding lines of demarcation.
1   The National Archive – *The Cabinet papers War Series paper G-125*
2   The British red Cross Society – Information sheet: *Rehabilitation after the First World War*.

Unity and Loyalty

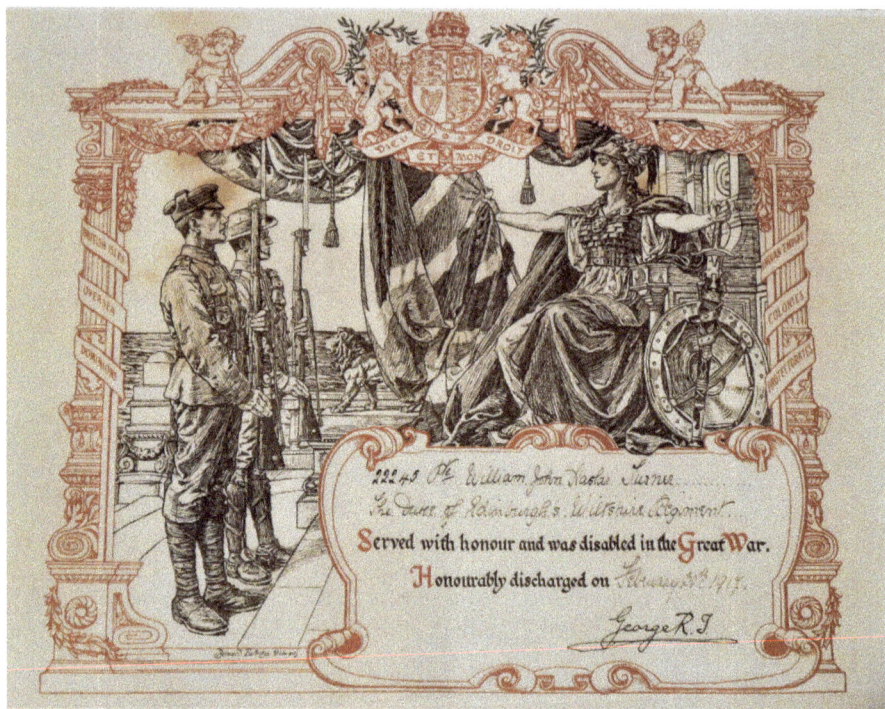

Certificate awarded to a disabled man on his discharge from military service

expenditure of public funds and coordination of continuing treatment.

In Wiltshire the committee was called the Wilts War Pensions Committee with administrative offices at Wicker Hill in Trowbridge.

In March 1918 the Secretary of the Disablement Sub-Committee of the Wilts War Pensions Committee summed up the increased burden on the civilian hospitals following a change in attitude to disabled patients by the War Office. The agreement made by the Pensions Minister and the War Office in 1917 applying a flexible approach regarding the treatment of discharged men was to end: [1]

> Owing to the War Office Order that no further cases of discharged men were to be received by VAD Hospitals for either indoor or outdoor treatment, it had become necessary to circularise Cottage Hospitals in the County to ascertain whether they were willing to take such cases.

The War Office Order gave instruction to adhere more strictly to the legislation on the discharge of men who were unfit for military service. The process had become fairly relaxed, allowing a man to remain in a VAD or military hospital with his comrades as long as possible. Even after discharge from the service it was often a number of weeks before he transferred to another establishment under the Ministry of Pensions. This relaxed

1 *Wiltshire Times* – 28 March 1918

The Story of Chippenham's Red Cross Hospital

attitude clearly had financial implications for the War Office and caused frustration within the military hospital authorities when they were told it was impossible to accept the large numbers of serious cases from the front, as beds were still occupied by men waiting to transfer to a civilian institution.

The stricter instruction reduced the pressure on the military organisation, including the VAD hospitals, but correspondingly increased the demand on the Ministry of Pensions. Inevitably civilian hospitals, such as the Cottage Hospital in Chippenham, would have to deal with more patients.

A sick nursing at home scheme was introduced to provide nurses to visit disabled men in their own homes.[1] The Wilts War Pension Committee engaged with the civilian hospitals in the County to ask if they were able to deal with men as out-patients including those previously dealt with at the VAD hospitals.

Mr Hankey, the Director of the Wiltshire Red Cross, met the Wilts War Pension Committee to discuss how the War Office Order would affect discharged disabled men returning to their homes in Wiltshire.

He told them the Red Cross were keen to help and said the Wiltshire branch of the Red Cross had decided not to adhere too strictly to the instruction from the War Office as he understood that there was still a little flexibility to allow for out-patient treatment to be offered at a VAD hospital if facilities allowed.

He told the committee he thought some of the VAD hospitals in the county had capacity to assist the Ministry of Pensions and relieve the civilian hospitals of some of the additional work they were asked to do.

He went on to say that the Commandant of the Chippenham VAD Hospital had already agreed facilities were available to see some out-patients from the local area, although he did add that it should not interfere with the Hospital's other work.[2] With the numbers of discharged men in need of medical care returning to their homes it was clear whatever the VAD hospitals could offer the bulk of the burden would still fall to the civilian hospitals.

The VADs at Chippenham were totally in support of the decision to provide out-patient facilities, but thought that additional premises were needed due to the expected numbers. In May 1918 Lady Margaret Spicer approached the Chippenham Board of Guardians to ask if part of the Workhouse Infirmary[3] could be used to treat disabled men. The Board of Guardians responded that at the present time they were unable to help.[4]

The Cottage Hospital in Chippenham was able to provide additional accommodation to treat some ex-soldiers and sailors in their out-patient department and also worked with the VADs to set up out-patient clinics in the Red Cross Hospital. It is thought rooms were also rented in the town for clinics and as a result all returning patients in the area received the treatment they needed.

1   This was only provided on recommendation and through the County Nursing Association.
2   *Wiltshire Times* - 28 March 1918
3   Now St Andrews Hospital at Rowden Hill
4   *Western Daily Press* - 14 May 1918

Unity and Loyalty

The Red Cross financial accounts for Wiltshire give some detail of the out-patients treated at Chippenham.[1]

During 1917 there were no Ministry of Pensions out-patients treated at the Hospital indicating that it treated all the men as serving soldiers, but the following year there were 18 Ministry of Pensions out-patients attending. Each man averaged over 24 visits during the year, over 400 appointments in total. The Ministry of Pensions paid the Red Cross an allowance of £62 13s 6d for this work.

The Road to Peace

IN MARCH 1918 the Germans launched their Spring Offensive: an all-out push with the intention of breaking through the Allied lines and reaching the Channel ports. The push was held back and five months later on 8 August the Allies opened the Battle of Amiens with what became known as the 100-day Offensive, ultimately leading to the end of the War.

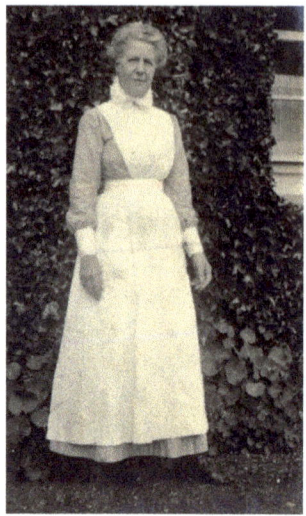

Sister Stevens of Chippenham Cottage Hospital worked with the VADs to arrange outpatient clinics for disabled men

The newspapers were increasingly positive. The Western Daily Press, read by many in Chippenham, reported that the Prime Minister, David Lloyd George, had said he thought that victory was in sight and repeated as much when he wrote to the Mayor of London about his campaign for more War Bonds in September 1918:[2]

> It is not enough to reach the heights where we can see the plains of victory at our feet. We must occupy them. This will cost much patient effort, but it is worth it. We must put *victory through and we cannot do so unless all do their best and give their utmost.*

The Lord Mayor of London responded: '...*the dawn of a brighter day was rapidly approaching and the prize of victory was in our grasp.*'

The Prime Minister's letter coincided with Bulgaria's unconditional surrender and further setbacks for the enemy followed. On 9 November the Western Daily Press summed up the dramatic events of the past months:[3]

> Although it has often been predicted that peace would come as suddenly as the war, no one could have foretold four months ago, or even a month ago, that the collapse of the Central Powers and their subordinates would have been so rapid and complete.

---

1 Red Cross Archive RCB/2/14/2
2 *Western Daily Press* - 1 October 1918
3 *Western Daily Press* - 9 November 1918

Part 3
How Chippenham made the Wounded Welcome.

Chapter 10
A Happy Home Hospital

Caring for the patients

WHEN NORMAN BROOK of the Royal Garrison Artillery left Chippenham in February 1918 he wrote thanking the VADs for their care saying 'A remembrance of a happy time spent in the Chippenham Red Cross Hospital.* Ralph Lethbridge of the Royal Flying Corps wrote in November 1917: *'May I here take the liberty of expressing my sincere wishes and thanks for the kindnesses and innumerable favours shown to me during my stay in Loyalty Ward of the Chippenham Red Cross Hospital.'*

Company Sergeant Major Scott spoke on behalf of the patients in 1917 when he thanked the citizens of Chippenham for their kindness shown to them during their stay. Commandant, Helena Wilson summed it up when she spoke of the sympathy and generosity to the wounded shown by the people of the district, saying: *'It was greatly this spirit of unity and loyalty which made the buildings a happy home hospital.'*

The recurring theme throughout the War was how the whole town came forward to ensure the men at the Hospital were cared for and made to feel welcome.

The Commandant of course also had responsibility to ensure smooth running and maintain discipline. Mrs Wilson successfully balanced the care and needs of the patients against the strict rules she set for the organisation of the wards.

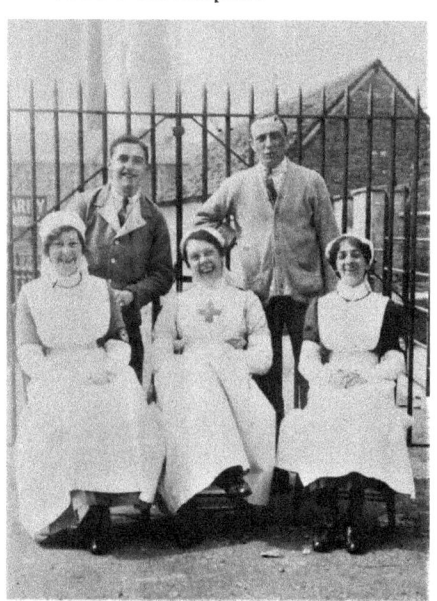

Laughing VADs and patients. The recurring theme was of a happy home hospital

Hospital Routine

IT WAS NEVER forgotten the Hospital remained under military command. A typical day started at 6 a.m. when men would be woken, dress and prepare for the day. Those unable to leave their beds were attended by VADs.

The Story of Chippenham's Red Cross Hospital

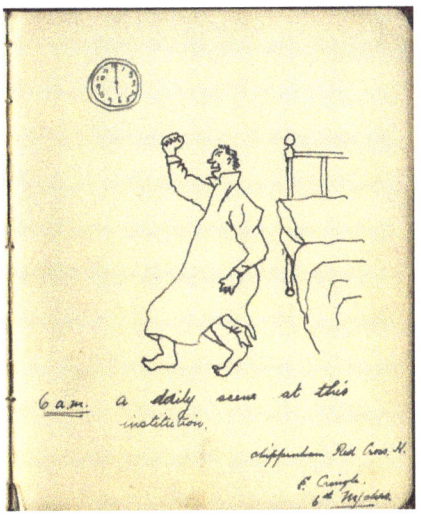

Private Edward Cringle's impression of Chippenham at 6 a.m.

The cleaning staff arrived during the morning: Thekla Bowser, in her book the Story of the British VAD[1] wrote '*These women lead hard lives at all times but they ungrudgingly give hours from their nights in order to get up at five in the morning and go to the Hospital to scrub and clean until they are due at the factory.*' In Chippenham munitionettes from Saxby and Farmer were known to come and help. In the kitchen there was also constant activity as meals were prepared resulting in endless washing up.[2]

After breakfast dressings were changed, treatments given and the doctors usually visited. Later in the afternoon the men were allowed recreation time, singing, a lantern slide display or simply reading and writing

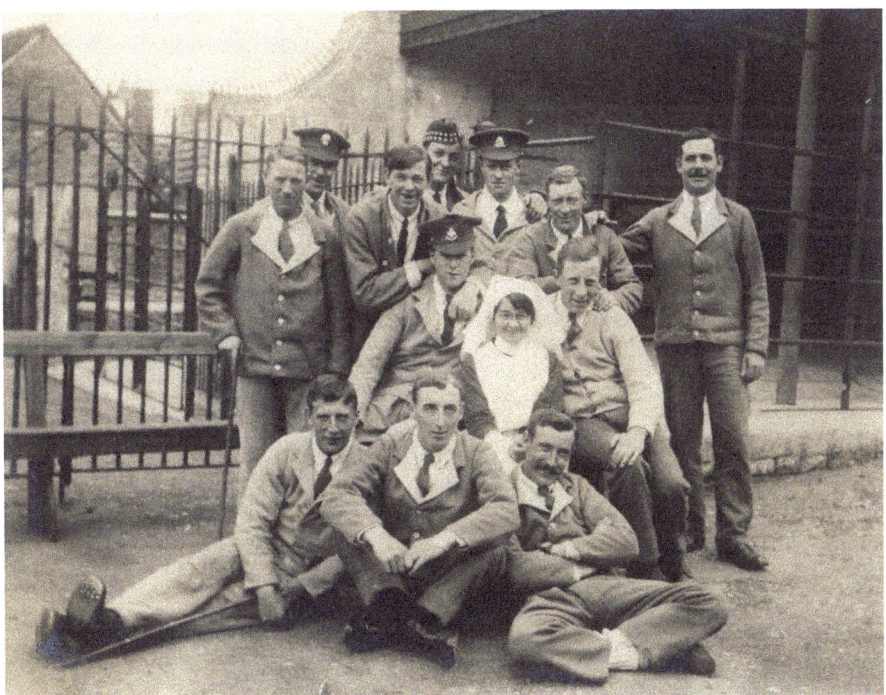

A group of patients with Sister Ethel Vicborn at one of the benches provided by the town for the use of the men

1   *The Story of British VAD work in the Great War* - Thekla Bowser
2   In the book *Observations of an Orderly* by Lance Corporal Ward Muir he dedicated a whole chapter to washing up.

Unity and Loyalty

letters. The men were also encouraged to spend time outdoors in the Market Yard and the High Street where benches were provided for them to sit on.

Convalescent Blues

THE MEN WERE easily recognised in their uniform, known as hospital (or convalescent) blues. The uniform jacket and trousers were made of blue flannel and worn with a white shirt and red tie. To identify his unit each man retained his cap with its regimental badge. The uniform was designed without pockets and in just a few sizes. This standardisation, although saving money, meant the suits were generally a poor fit and men complained that trousers were either too long or too short and sleeves had to be turned up. Apart from this, the outfit was practical and hard wearing and easier to keep clean than the military uniform. Issuing a clean hospital uniform when a man arrived maintained the standard of cleanliness.[1]

The uniform also had a propaganda effect. The public immediately recognised the men as heroes who had given service to King and Country. Strangers would warmly greet them in the street and offer gifts of cigarettes and sweets.

A verse called The Hospital Suit, written by Kate Rawlins, was published on postcards sold in aid of the Red Cross featuring a wounded man dressed in the Blues:

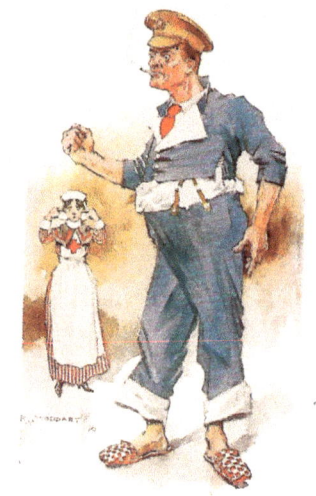

Strafe the Tailor—A Bad Fit of the "Blues."

Comic post card showing the badly fitting blue uniform

> Here's to the suit of light grey and blue,
> Which the richest on earth may not buy!
> And here's to the cap of a nondescript hue!
> And here's to the loose red tie!
>
> The jacket's not cut on the smartest of lines,
> And the trousers may bag at the knees!
> While the shoes, perhaps, show unmistakable signs
> That they're fashioned entirely for ease.
>
> But the knuttiest knut, as he strolls down the Mall,
> With the latest in spats and in ties,
> Cannot vie with T. Atkins, when out with a pal,

1 The Wellcome Collection Archive

The Story of Chippenham's Red Cross Hospital

In the suit which his country supplies.

In these fashions for men there is little that's new,
But the one which is worn with most pride,
Is surely the jacket with one sleeve in view,
And the other pinned down to the side.

Fellow Britons, whom age or misfortune debars
From a share in your country's release,
Who never can earn, by the right of your scars,
The thanks of a nation at peace.

Does the sight of these lads (there are thousands about)
Call to mind that they've suffered for you?
Then your hats will come off, and your hearts will go out
To the boys in the light grey and blue.

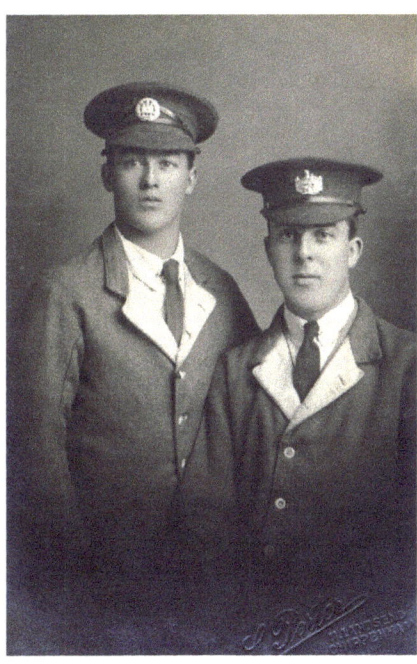

Studio portrait of Chippenham patients Privates Crick and James wearing their blues

Private W Parkin of the 6th Yorkshire Regiment penned his own verse when he wrote in Ethel Brinkworth's album in November 1917:

> They say that we are winning
> But how can that be true
> The time I have been in Chippenham
> With a miss fit suit of blue
> With best wishes to nurse Brinkworth

The blue uniforms became a common sight in Chippenham. Cecil Martin, who was a child during the war years recalled seeing a lot of wounded men in their 'blues' on the streets of Chippenham:[1]

Countless stretchers being ferried to the Neeld Hall, numerous soldiers gathering around the Town Bridge wearing hospital blue uniforms. The limbless and the disabled were to remain an indelible memory.

---

1 Chippenham Civic Society - *Buttercross Bulletin*

Unity and Loyalty

Discipline

BEING EASILY RECOGNISED in the blue uniform also meant that discipline could be maintained. While a man was in hospital he was not allowed to wear any other clothing and if he wore his army greatcoat, he was instructed to wear a blue armband.

In Melksham the magistrates heard the case of a patient who changed out of his 'blues' in order to obtain an illicit drink. The Commandant of Melksham Hospital was quite adamant that the man must have done this in a 'clandestine manner.'

She explained in a letter the strict procedures regarding the issuing of 'hospital blues' and storing uniforms:[1]

> All patients are deprived of their (military) uniform on entry to the hospital and given their 'blues', the uniform being kept under lock and key until the day they leave again.

The government had introduced measures to limit the sale of alcohol, as they feared intoxication would hamper the war effort. The restrictions included reducing public house opening times,[2] John Best, the landlord of the Little George in Chippenham was fined £5 in 1917 for breaching the legislation.[3] The rules for wounded men were even stricter as they were strictly forbidden to consume alcohol, or even enter a public house. This ban was often flouted as drinks were offered to patients as an act of kindness. It became such a problem that a letter was sent to every Chief Constable:

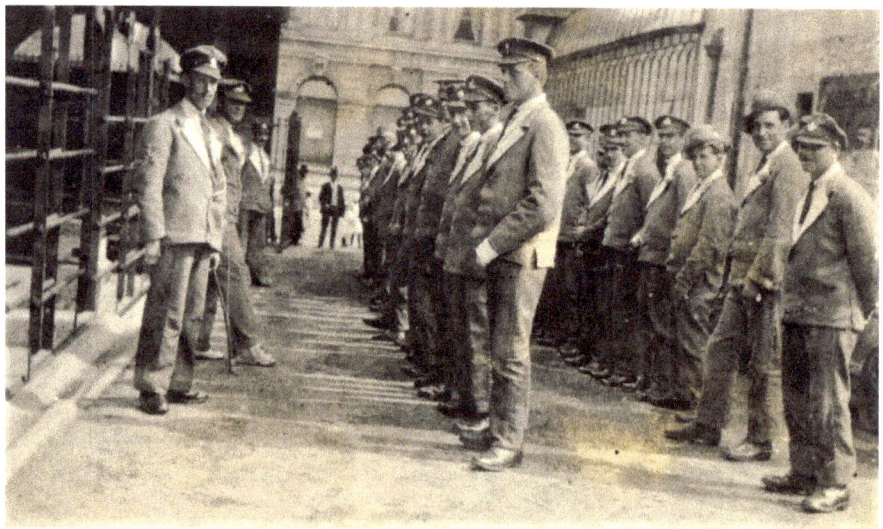

Patients on parade in the Market Yard

1 *Wiltshire Times* - 14 December 1918
2 *Western Gazette* - 9 April 1915, The Royal family lead on the restrictions on alcohol.
3 *Swindon Advertiser* - 8 June 1917

The Story of Chippenham's Red Cross Hospital

Sir.—I am directed by the Secretary of State to say that he has been asked by the Army Council to obtain the assistance of yourself and other Chief Constables in the steps the Council are taking to protect soldiers undergoing treatment in hospitals and convalescent homes from the dangers involved in the consumption of intoxicating liquors. In the case of convalescent soldiers, the consumption of intoxicating liquor may, even if it does not lead to drunkenness, be prejudicial to their recovery.

The Chippenham magistrates received several complaints that men from Chippenham Division were seen in licensed premises and they asked the police to investigate. Any man found to have been drinking risked being confined to quarters by the Commandant,[1] while persistent offenders were referred to the military court.

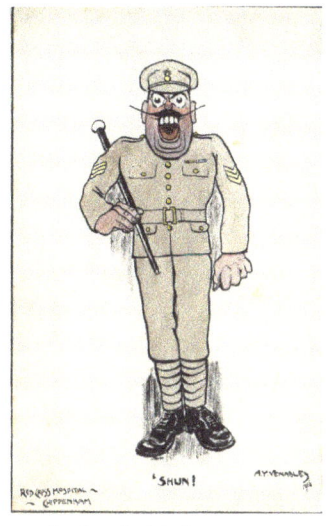

The dreaded drill sergeant as drawn by Private Venables in 1916

Although efforts were made to keep the patients entertained boredom could easily lead to misbehaviour. Those men fit enough were required to attend parades and undertake some training. Despite these activities VAD hospitals were considered more relaxed than the strict regime of the military hospitals. One patient wrote of a VAD hospital: '*It is like the very best boarding house at the sea-side, with everyone charming and anxious to please.*'[2] The Commandant had authority from the War Office to deal with minor offences and enforced a strict curfew. In Chippenham a pass was needed for any man with reason to leave the Hospital during the evening. No doubt, when he returned, it was checked that he was sober.

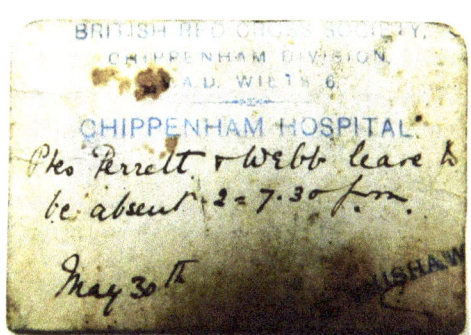

Chippenham Hospital pass signed by the Assistant Commandant

---

1   *A Life Revealed. The Diaries of Herbert Spackman* – Ernest Hird. The Commandant at Corsham found a man to be drunk and confined him to barracks.
2   *The British Red Cross in Action* - Dame Beryl Oliver

Chapter 11
Entertaining the Patients

Visitors

From the outset members of the public were generous with donations and gifts to keep the men amused. There were board games and a library was set up. Well-wishers called regularly with gifts of new books and magazines. Popular authors were Arthur Conan Doyle, Bram Stoker, H.G. Wells and John Buchan's the Thirty-Nine Steps, first published in Blackwood's Magazine in 1915. The popular cartoons of Heath Robinson's *Hunlikely!* ridiculed the Germans.

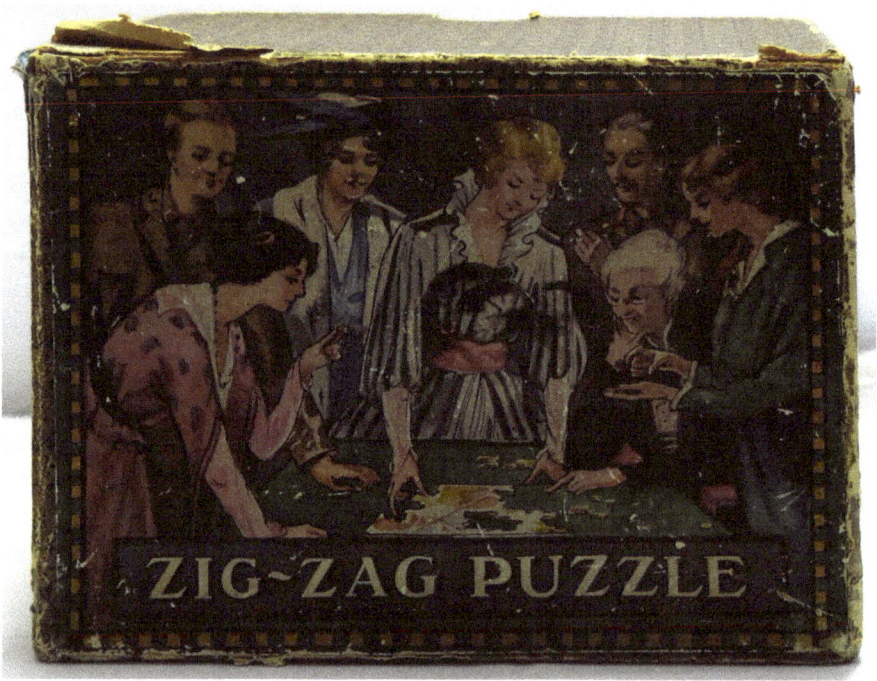

A puzzle enjoyed by the patients in Chippenham

There were so many callers keen to help entertain the men that the Commandant had to restrict visiting hours. Members of the Church of England Men's Society called on Fridays to provide spiritual support and general help, while other visitors usually

The Story of Chippenham's Red Cross Hospital

visited in the afternoon to spend time in conversation or playing games with the patients. A welcome sight was visiting young munitionettes from Saxby and Farmer who helped serve afternoon teas and entertained the men.[1]

The most welcome visitors, however, were family and friends from home. The patients at Chippenham came from all corners of the country, which meant a visit from a family could mean a lengthy journey and an expense that could be ill afforded. To help the families of seriously wounded men financial assistance was available from the Government and by 1918 there was a call for the Government to be more generous and issue more Rail Warrants for families of wounded men.[2]

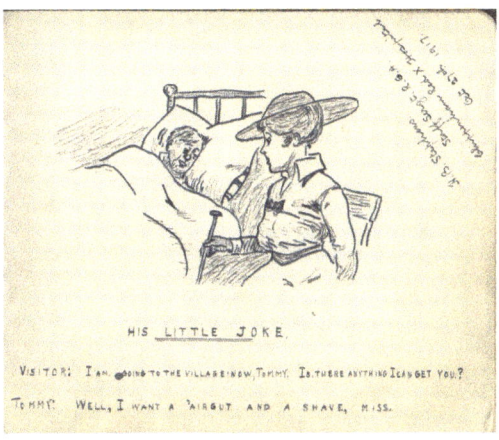

Young ladies were always popular visitors at the hospital. Staff Sergeant Stephens drew 'His Little Joke' in October 1917

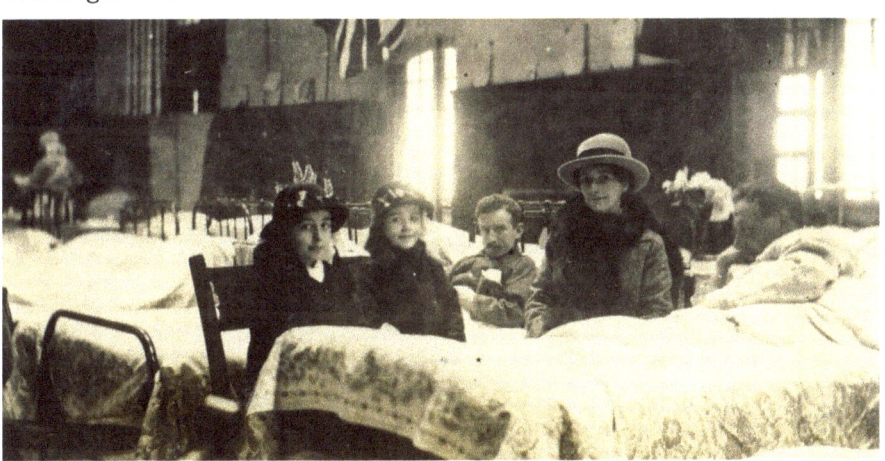

A soldier in Loyalty Ward receives a visit from his family

Music

MUSIC WAS ALWAYS a popular distraction. Arthur Spencer, the owner of the music shop in the Market Place, donated a piano to the Hospital.[3] There was always

1 Recollection of the family of Gladys Treweke
2 *British Widows of the First World War* - Andrea Hetherington.
3 *North Wilts Herald* - 7 January 1916.

Unity and Loyalty

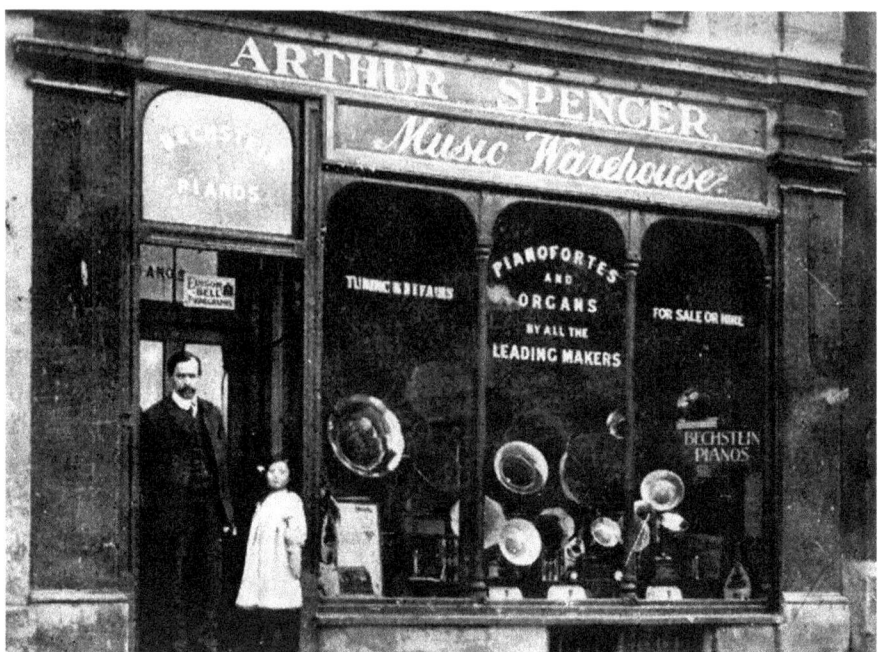

Arthur Spencer's music warehouse in the Market Place

somebody amongst the patients or VADs who could produce a good tune and the men would sing along.

Mr Spencer also gave a gramophone and a regular supply of records. The popularity of the gramophone in hospitals was described in the magazine 'The Great War' when a reporter wrote about a ward full of men enjoying the music: [1]

> Even as I sat there, they began singing comic songs. A chorus they were in a mood for music, the ward Sister disappeared, and in a few minutes an orderly appeared carrying a gramophone and some records. Some light music and songs were played, and the men listened from their beds with keen attention. The orderly put on a record of a little violin and piano piece. The Sister had said it was getting too late for more music; it was bed-time. But in answer to several pleadings she had said they could play one more record if they chose a 'quiet one' that would not disturb men who by now were ready for sleep.

Chippenham Military Entertainments Committee

AT THE OUTBREAK of war Chippenham saw many young men in uniform arrive in the town awaiting instructions to mobilise. With so many men with time on their hands, the people of Chippenham feared that bored troops would result in rowdy

---

1   The Great War, Edited by H W Wilson- *Part 132 How the wounded were brought home.* 24th February 1917

The Story of Chippenham's Red Cross Hospital

behaviour.

The Chippenham Military Entertainments Committee was established to offer recreation for the soldiers. The Committee included members of the music and theatre societies, the churches and local businesses. To entertain the troops they arranged dances, evenings of popular music and whist drives where the soldiers could socialise with people from the town. A typical evening organised by the Committee was described in the newspaper:[1]

> The Chippenham Military Entertainments Committee on Thursday invited all the soldiers billeted in the town to a dance, and every soldier was asked to bring a friend, if possible a lady. The committee had secured the co-operation of the officers and permits were issued to stay out to midnight.
>
> Dancing took place in the old Armoury Bath Road. The Drill Hall was used for the Dance. It was tastefully decorated with flags and bunting lent by Col Neeld and the Anglo Swiss Milk Company.
>
> The party which numbered over 100 included Major McKay of the Wilts Yeomanry. The MC for the evening was trooper Atkinson.
>
> Supper was provided by lady members of the Committee, Mesdames G H Williams, W Ashby, H Daniels. Garnet, and Crofts.

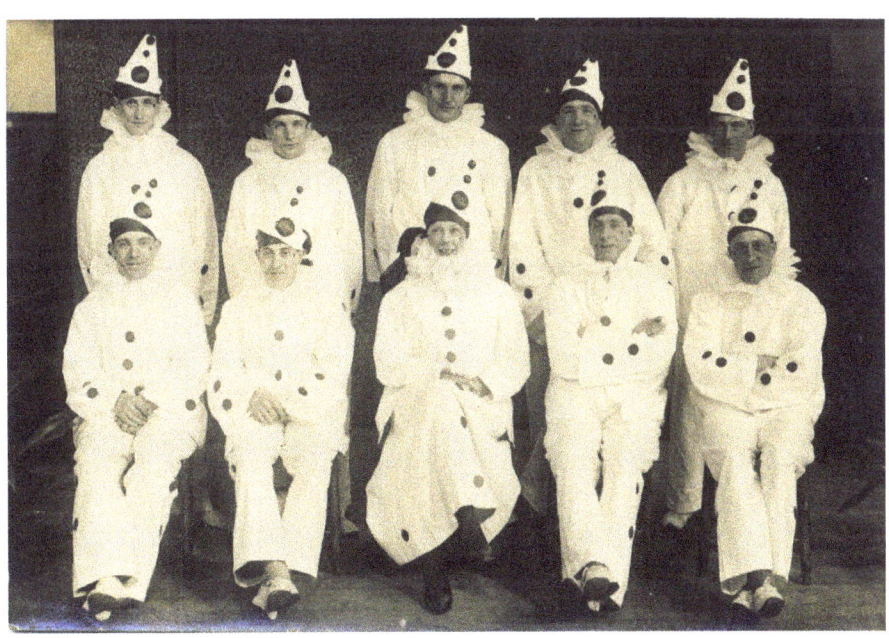

Patients in Pierrot costumes, an act at a Chippenham variety show

1   *North Wilts Herald* - 22 January 1915

Unity and Loyalty

Entertainment was a morale booster for the troops at the front and it proved to be equally effective in the recovery of the wounded.[1] Shows were arranged especially for the wounded heroes. In London's West End, theatre seats were reserved for the 'boys in blue' and shows were adapted to be more suited to the tastes of the ordinary tommy. In the intervals the entertainers greeted the men and served tea and buns.[2]

In November 1915 the Chippenham Military Entertainments Committee followed the lead of the London theatres, organising special musical and social evenings with the patients treated as guests of honour. At Christmas the men were invited to join the town in an evening of music and comedy followed by a whist drive and dancing in the Neeld Hall.[3]

Many of those involved with the Chippenham Military Entertainments Committee also volunteered as VADs and it wasn't long before they encouraged the patients to join them in impromptu performances.

These joint performances became popular with the public, especially when the musical societies in the town had suspended productions as the male members had joined up and ladies were busy on war work.

Hospital helper, Dorothy Hiscock's rendition of 'The Soldiers Toast' was a favourite with the audience, whilst sisters Dora and Evelyn Belcher, both VADs, performed musical excerpts from popular shows accompanied by the wounded soldiers.

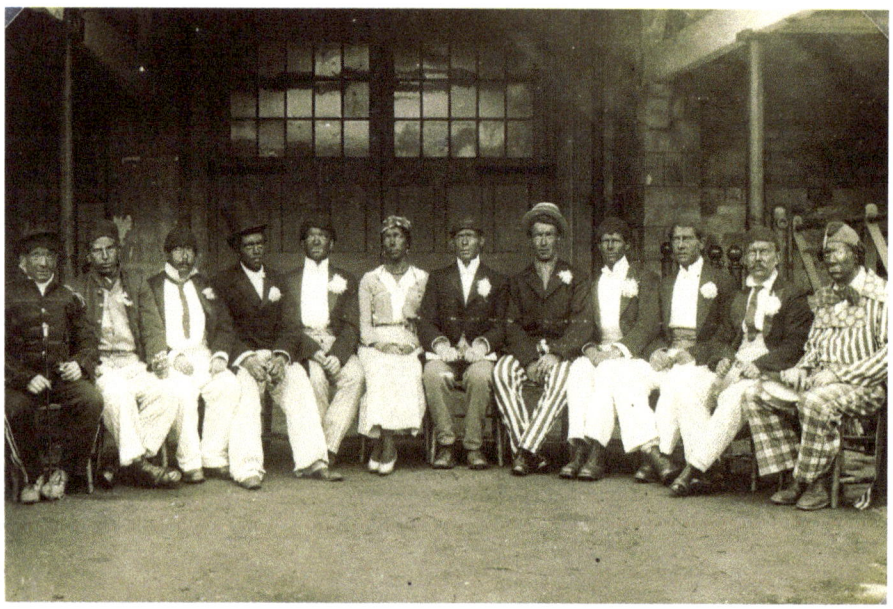

Some of the cast from the Christmas show 1916. Ethel Williams is centre flanked by Sergeants Coombs, Cole, Holland, Norman and other patients

1 Imperial War Museum. Article - *Voices of the First World War: Wartime Leisure and Entertainment*
2 *The Weeping and the Laughter* - Viva King
3 *Western Daily Press* – 28 December 1915

The Story of Chippenham's Red Cross Hospital

By 1918 these joint productions by VADs and patients had become so popular that newspapers reported on the Hospital's Concert Season:[1]

> On Tuesday evening the musical friends of the patients in the Red Cross Hospital, assisted by the patients, gave the last concert of the season in Loyalty Ward as a farewell to 24 of the men who were leaving the following day. There was a large attendance of friends and an excellent programme was well rendered and greatly appreciated. The promotors were greatly assisted by Miss Stinchcomb (Bristol), a young lady possessing a well cultured voice, who delighted the audience with her songs. Ivy Shipp (Foxham) also gave songs and Miss Houlston gave a recitation.

Both Miss Shipp and Miss Houlston were VADs at Chippenham. The collection at the end of the evening raised £3 4s 2d which went towards the summer outing fund.

One of the patients, Private Walter Munday, was a well-known professional singer in his civilian life. His talent and popularity ensured even greater attendances at the shows, the papers reporting: '*his vocal and histrionic talents were always readily given.*' The Hospital even commissioned its own productions. Private W B May, who before the War was a member of a professional opera company, wrote a musical playlet called 'A Stolen Melody' which was performed by the VADs and the men.

The company also ventured into theatrical and comedy pieces and gave special shows at Christmas.

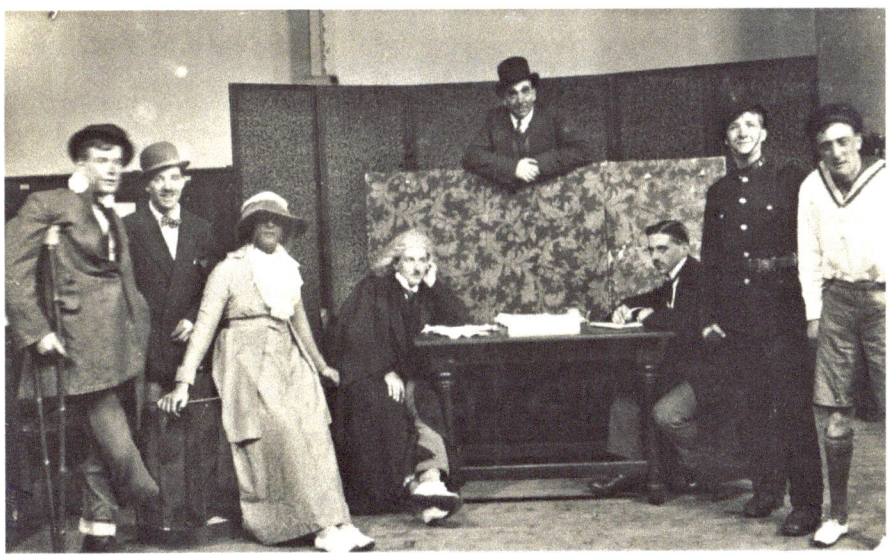

A theatrical production by the men at Chippenham Hospital. Amongst the cast was L/Cpl Frank Seeney. He was discharged from the Army in June 1918 due to his wounds.

---

1   Chippenham Museum - *Garlick Scrapbooks*.

Unity and Loyalty

Touring Concert Shows

As the War dragged on the opportunity to see a show of light hearted revues, songs and sketches was always popular.[1] Professional concert parties were established and toured the country providing shows to the public and the troops.

William Burridge Snr, the proprietor of the Angel Hotel in the Market Place, invited the touring parties to stay at his hotel and provided a driver and vehicle to allow the entertainers to visit hospitals in the surrounding area. Mr and Mrs Llewellen Palmer of Lackham House paid for a party to travel from the Angel Hotel to a concert in Trowbridge Town Hall.[2] William Paddock, who was employed as a taxi driver at the Angel Hotel, recalled how he would often drive for the entertainers. He described one journey:[3]

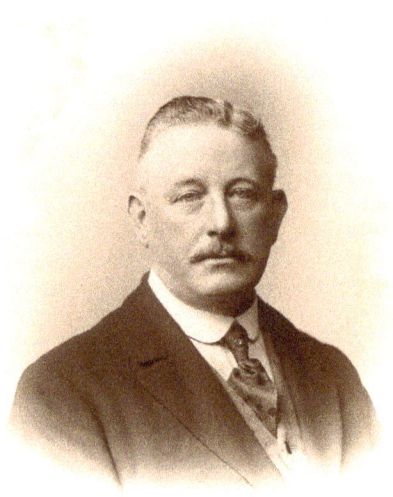

William Burridge senior, the proprietor of the Angel Hotel

> At the Angel Hotel were two gentlemen and three ladies who were entertaining the wounded soldiers at various hospitals. I took them to Malmesbury which had been turned into a hospital. They were practising during the journey — the song I remember well was Keep the home fires burning.

In Chippenham concerts were performed at the Palace Theatre in Station Hill and inevitably the proceeds went to the Red Cross Hospital. The VADs provided refreshments for the interval and patients sold programmes. Joe Buckle and the Military Entertainment Committee made arrangements with Mr Hooper, the manager of the theatre, to ensure seats were reserved for the wounded and help was provided for those men unable to walk.

One group of entertainers to come to the area was Victor Lloyd's famous London Concert Party with entertainers from the London Stage. They appeared in Chippenham on 15 September 1916 as part of their North Wiltshire tour of towns. The newspaper described the show:[4]

1   Imperial War Museum. Article - *West End or Western Front?*
2   *Wiltshire Times* - 30 September 1916
3   *A Country Boy* - W.J. Paddock
4   Chippenham Museum- *Buckle scrapbook collection*

ENTERTAINMENT BY A LONDON CONCERT PARTY

One of a series of entertainments, which were given throughout various parts of North Wilts by Mr Victor Lloyd's London Concert Party, in aid of funds to provide comforts for the wounded soldiers in the places visited, was given at the Palace, Chippenham on Friday evening and like all other concerts held for the same object, was an overwhelming success, and it is expected that the profits of the evening will amount to something over £50. Much of the success of the week's tour was due to Mr H V Lloyd, of Corsham, who acted as business manager. Since he has resided in the locality he has been energetic in any scheme to help a worthy object. As far as Chippenham was concerned, Mr J Buckle acted as local secretary and he was assisted by a small committee, and the arrangements were successfully carried out. The hall was crowded to its utmost capacity and the programme went with a swing throughout. A large number of wounded soldiers from the local Red Cross Hospital were present and thoroughly enjoyed themselves. Decorative ferns for the stage and the hall were lent by Mr Richardson, and scenic effects by Messrs E N Tuck and Affleck. Programmes were sold by Assistant Quarter-Master D. Belcher, Nurse Awdry, Nurse Pearce and Nurse King, and sweets by Nurses Spinke and Hetherington. All the sweets were given by the staff of the Red Cross Hospital.

The programme was delightfully varied. Miss Dorothy Fry was at the piano, Miss Winifred Mansfield, the comedienne of the company, was very popular, and she established herself a favourite from the start, especially with the soldiers. Her songs, 'Willie, will you leave off winking', 'Whistle and I'll wait for you' and 'Blighty' were especially good. The contributions to the programme by Miss Gladys Haysack (soprano) was another treat, and she was greatly appreciated. Mr Jerome Murphy was clever and at the same time funny with his Irish songs and stories. Messrs Wilkin and McGowan provided a marionette performance which proved the most laughable part of the performance. Mr Arthur Mortimer, the tenor, showed considerable ability. His duets with Miss Haysack were very commendable. The duets 'They didn't believe me' and 'If you were the only boy in the world' proved very popular. Flowers were given by Mr W Ball and Mrs Garnett and arranged into bouquets by Private Stevens one of the patients at the Red Cross Hospital, who handed them to the three lady artistes.

In November 1916 the Concert Party returned to Chippenham and performed at the Constitutional Hall for two nights. Once again the wounded men from Chippenham, Bowood, Corsham and Melksham Red Cross hospitals were invited to attend free of charge.

Local Entertainers

EQUALLY POPULAR WERE local amateur entertainers. The Spackman family of Corsham were accomplished musicians arranging evenings of Music Hall

Unity and Loyalty

entertainment and were regular visitors at the Red Cross Hospitals in the district.[1]

At Bowood Lady Lansdowne organised open-air fetes and concerts in the gardens of the house. In 1917 the August Bank holiday was celebrated with music in the Italian Garden to which over 150 patients from the neighbouring hospitals were invited.[2]

Schoolchildren visited Chippenham Hospital to entertain the men. Miss Morgan, a music teacher at the Secondary School often arranged for a group of boys and girls to sing popular songs and give recitals.

A group of ladies in Chippenham formed their own Concert Party to entertain the troops in the area. Their popularity spread and they were asked to visit hospitals in neighbouring towns, where they provided evenings of 'enjoyment and merriment'. Amongst the members of the Concert Party were Miss Alfreda Parry, Mrs Elinor Davis, Mrs Beatrice Hetherington, Mrs Sarah Mackness and Miss Elsie Watts, all VADs at Chippenham.

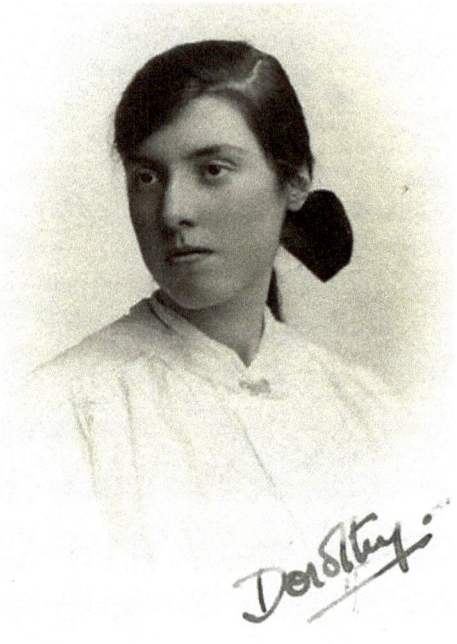

Dorothy Spencer was only 15 in 1918 but sang regularly for the patients. Her parents were Arthur and Kate Spencer owners of the Music Warehouse

Saxby and Farmer

As one of the largest employers in Chippenham, Saxby and Farmer boasted an active social and musical society including many women recently recruited as munitionettes. They produced a number of variety shows to entertain the wounded men. In March 1917 they visited Corsham:[3]

> On Saturday evening a party of munition workers from Chippenham visited the hospital and entertained the soldiers with a programme of vocal and instrumental music, action songs in costume etc. which was much enjoyed.

1 *A Life revealed. The Diaries of Herbert Spackman* – Ernest Hird
2 *Daily Mirror* – 9 August 1917
3 *Wiltshire Times* - 24 February 1917 gives an account of concerts at Melksham and Corsham hospitals.

The Story of Chippenham's Red Cross Hospital

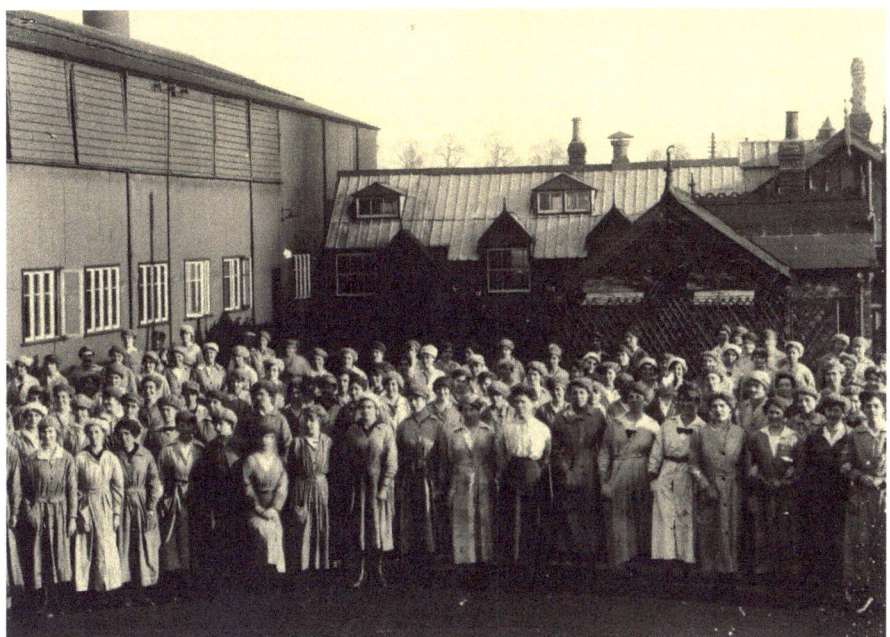

The munitionettes of Saxby and Farmer

A week earlier they had entertained the patients and staff at Chippenham with an evening of songs and sketches.[1] The newspaper gave a full account of how much the soldiers enjoyed the show:[2]

> In the enjoyable entertainment given by the employees of Messrs Saxby and Farmer Ltd on Saturday to about 100 wounded soldiers in the Chippenham Red Cross Hospital there was something more than appeared to the eye – happy and inspiring a scene as that was.
>
> There was a symbol of the spirit that is going to win, the typification of the united effort of both sexes in one common aim. The soldiers in their blue hospital uniforms, the women munitioners in their regulation overalls, the nurses in their familiar costume – it was a pretty picture, one that none of the participants will forget.
>
> If these young ladies in the overalls have left the house for the factory they shewed they had lost none of the feminine accomplishments. Thoughts of machines and whirring wheels were put aside and these simple acts of attention that come so naturally from a woman were substituted. The net result was a truly happy evening and one that all desire to be repeated.
>
> The arrangements were admirably carried out by a committee of the lady munition workers of the firm, the misses Carr and Goulding having proved themselves capable Hon. Secretaries. The proceedings commenced at 5.30 when the soldiers found

1   Chippenham Museum - *Garlick Scrapbooks*.
2   Wiltshire Times - 10 March 1917

Unity and Loyalty

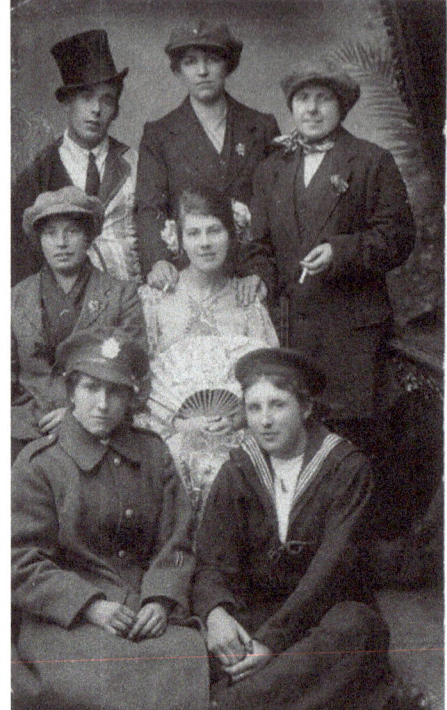 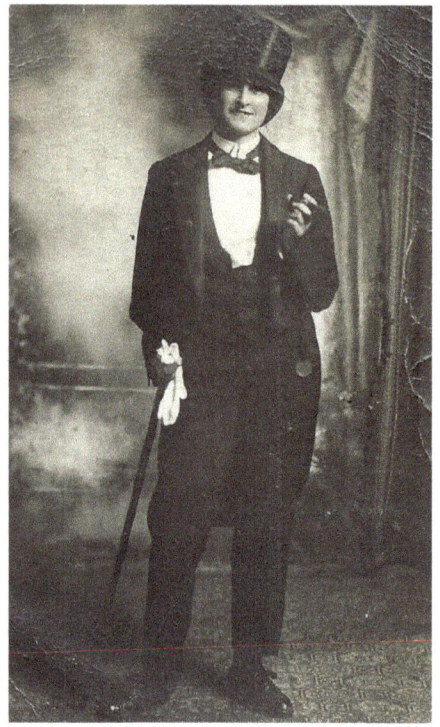

left: After the show one of the patients joined the performers. He wears a top hat and one of the munitionettes is wearing his cap and greatcoat. right: Gladys Treweke in costume for a show.

the tables artistically laid out for a tempting tea. The large number of young ladies acting as waitresses attired as stated in their working overalls were most assiduous in their attention to the 'Tommies' several of whom intend to work at Saxby and Farmer after the war.

An excellent programme comprising vocal and instrumental items had been provided for the guests and they were well satisfied with their tea, which they greatly enjoyed. It was a stroke of genius to open the programme with 'Popular Choruses' for these were heartily taken up by the soldiers and the right spirit was obtained to ensure the success of the remainder of the programme. It would not be fair to select any individual part of the programme as each contribution was asked for again but time would not permit.

During the interval the hostesses again flitted amongst the soldiers this time laden with cigarettes fruit and crackers. Amongst the closing items Saxby and Farmer Ladies Band (Conductor Mr C Scammell) and the 'Street Vendors' met with a tremendous reception and altogether the programme was fully enjoyed not only by the entertained but by the entertainers.

The following was the programme:
Popular Choruses - Ladies Choir
Clarinet solo - Mr M Pecher

The Story of Chippenham's Red Cross Hospital

Wonderful Rose of Love - Mr C Hulbert
Over the waves - Misses Baker and Kirkham
I can't come out today - Mr C Scammell
Back home in Tennessee -Misses Carr and Jenning
Dialogue - Miss K Brewer and Mr Merriman
Always - Miss M Tanner
The Bing Boys - Misses G Baker and Perry
Sketch 'wedlock' - Misses Bodman, Baker, Lessiter and Brewer
Street Criers - Ladies Choir
'Zammy and Zusan' - Misses Gardner and Davis
Mignon - Miss B Pennez
The trail that leads to home - Mr A Tyler
Selection by the Ladies munitions Band (Conductor Mr C Scammell)
Violin solo 'Romance' - Master Archard
A little bit of heaven - Miss E Carr
The Twins - Miss E Brewer

The evening was arranged by Ernest Scammell, who worked in the machine shop of Saxby and Farmer. He lived in Tugela Road and arranged a number of further concerts financed by subscriptions from the workers at the factory. The men in the machine shop even made their own drums and formed a novelty drum band.

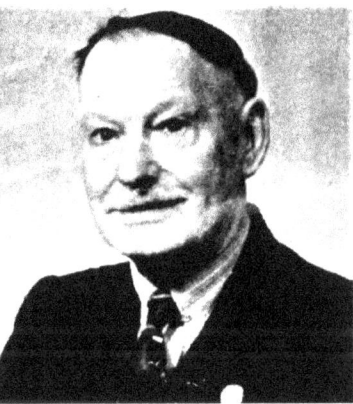

Ernest Scammell at his retirement in 1951

Chapter 12
Sport and Amusement

Pastimes

A MAN'S TREATMENT COULD be lengthy and gave the opportunity to think about the pastimes he had enjoyed before the War. Men were invited to join local societies such as the angling clubs and allotment societies. Others joined the Church of England Men's Society while the Literary and Scientific Institute was a regular destination for men who wanted to make use of the reading room and billiard table. The President of

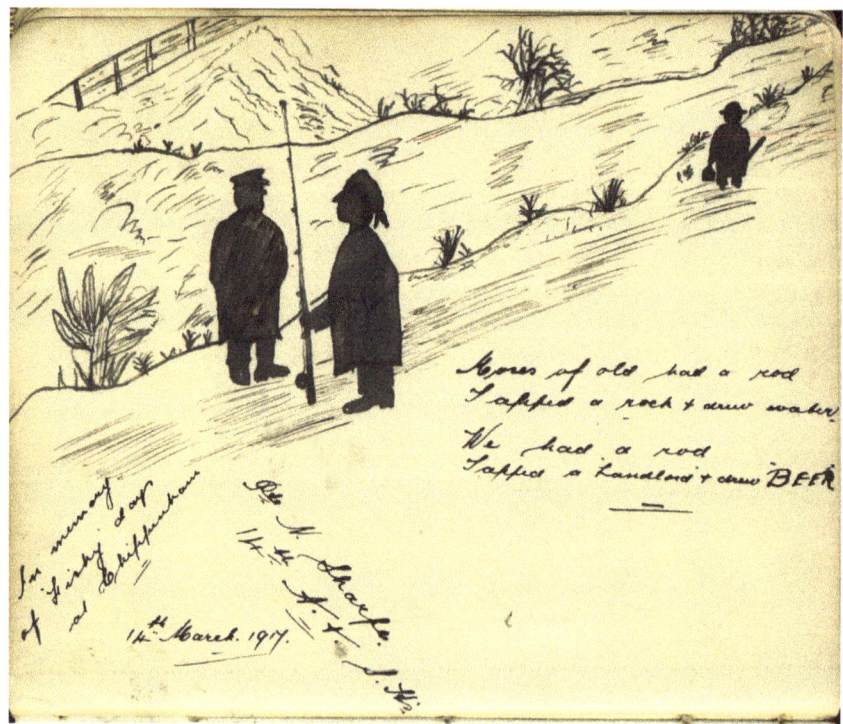

Private Sharpe of the Argyll and Sutherland Highlanders remembers 'fishy days' in Chippenham. The local angling club organised fishing competitions for the men

the Institute, Charles Garnett, ensured that a wounded man could always get a game of billiards as he had pre-paid the table costs for the patients.[1]

1 *Wiltshire Times* – 12 April 1919. Annual meeting of the Institute.

The Story of Chippenham's Red Cross Hospital

Football

FOOTBALL WAS A passion for many of the men. With players away at war the town's clubs had been suspended but as patients became stronger they joined the clubs and managed to raise an occasional team. The games were adapted to take account of men with crutches and amputations and matches were often played against neighbouring hospitals.[1]

Increasingly popular was football played by women. Teams were raised in the munitions factories and matches attracted thousands of spectators.[2] On Easter Monday 1917 munitionettes of Saxby and Farmer challenged a team of ladies representing Chippenham Town to a match at the Saxby and Farmer sports ground.[3] The match, which was in aid of the Red Cross Hospital, was well attended and enjoyed by the spectators. Chippenham Town won 4-2 and the sum of £7 was raised.

The teams were:

Chippenham Town; Misses Warrilow, Burgess, Alsop, Knight, Tompkins, Jones, Tompkins, Davis, Anstis, Dorwell and Guy.

Saxby and Farmer Ladies; Misses Granger, White, Neate, Davis, Mustoe, Davis, King, Perry, Beamish, Milford and Shorland.

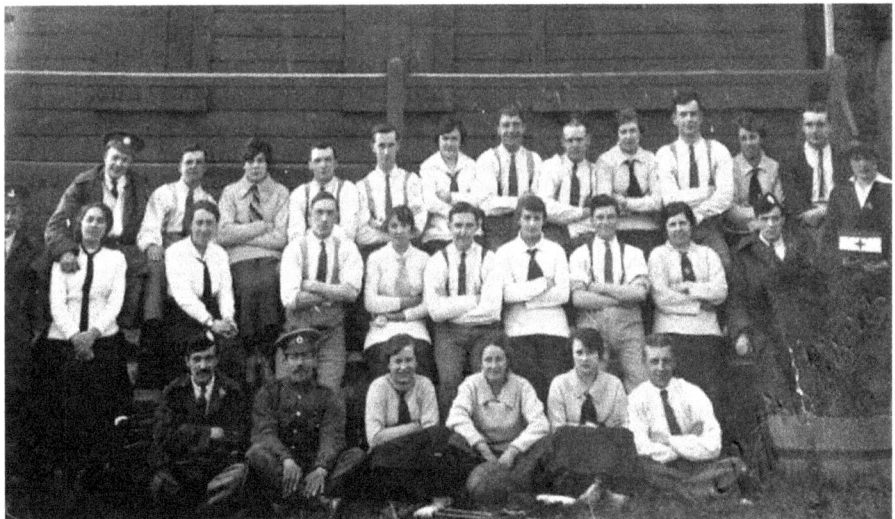

After the football match between patients and Saxby and Farmer Ladies. Alice Granger front row third from left

1   Royal Pavilion Museum Brighton and Hove holds the archive of the *Pavilion Blues*, a newspaper produced by patients at the Pavilion Hospital in Brighton. There are numerous articles about sport including photos of football matches. These games between hospitals became the early inspiration for the Paralympic Games.
2   Imperial War Museum. Article - *9 Facts about football in the First World War*
3   *Wiltshire Times* – 14 April 1917

Unity and Loyalty

The ladies from Saxby and Farmer team were regular visitors to the Hospital and knew the men well. A few days after their defeat at the hands of Chippenham Town they challenged the patients to a match. The photographs taken after the match show how enjoyable the game was for both teams.

Alice Granger, known as Kathleen, was a member of the Saxby and Farmer team and sent her brother William, who was in France with the 6th Battalion Wiltshire Regiment, the pictures. She wrote:[1]

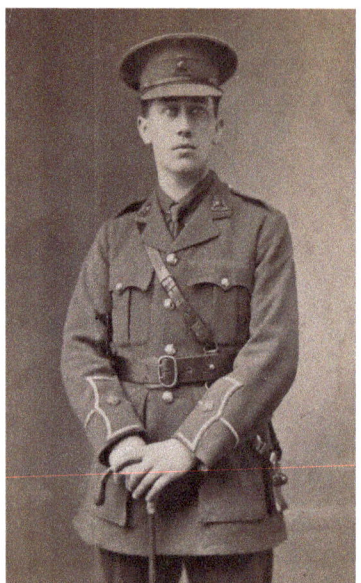

William Granger

Dear Billy

I expect you think it funny that I have not written before but I have not had time. I hope you will like both these photos that I am sending. We played football with these wounded and then had our photos taken. The other one is really the best of the two. Well dear I must close now so I remain your loving sister.

Kath

P.S. I am getting on fine with my singing with best love Kath xxx

Billy received his sister's letter and no doubt enjoyed the photos and the thought of his sister playing football. On 21 September 1917 Lieutenant William Granger died of wounds near Ypres.

Sports Clubs

AS THE WAR continued sports clubs struggled financially. The Chippenham Sports Club showed a deficit of £20 for 1916 at their AGM due to the loss of subscriptions from men away on active service.[2] When the patients were invited to join the public became enthusiastic to help, especially when blue uniforms were conspicuous at fund raising events.[3]

In Corsham the Cricket Club arranged a match where the players, including wounded men, wore fancy dress. The ground was packed with spectators and a healthy collection was shared between the Club and the hospitals.[4]

The cricket pitches at the Chippenham Sports Club were used by patients to practise their batting and during 1917 a team was raised by the Hospital to play teams in

---

1 Caroline Saye- Family archive.
2 *Western Daily Press* - 28 February 1917
3 *Wiltshire Times* – 5 February 1916. Mrs Pinfield organised a Jumble sale that raised £26 for Chippenham Sports Club.
4 *Gazette and Herald – From the files* - 15 September 2016

The Story of Chippenham's Red Cross Hospital

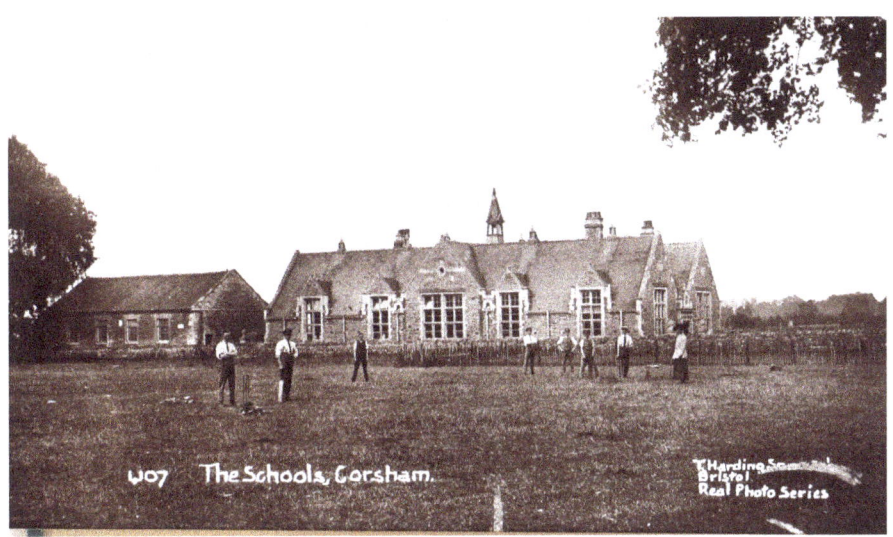

Cricket match in Corsham

the town. On Whit Monday they played the local Fire Brigade.[1]

The members of Chippenham Sports Club were particularly interested in helping the patients. Many on the committee were closely involved with the VAD Hospital. The President of the Sports Club was Charles Garnett, also chairman of the Hospital Finance Committee.[2] The Chairman of the Sports Club was Mr Hathaway the husband of Margaret, who served as a VAD. Other members of the Committee included Frank

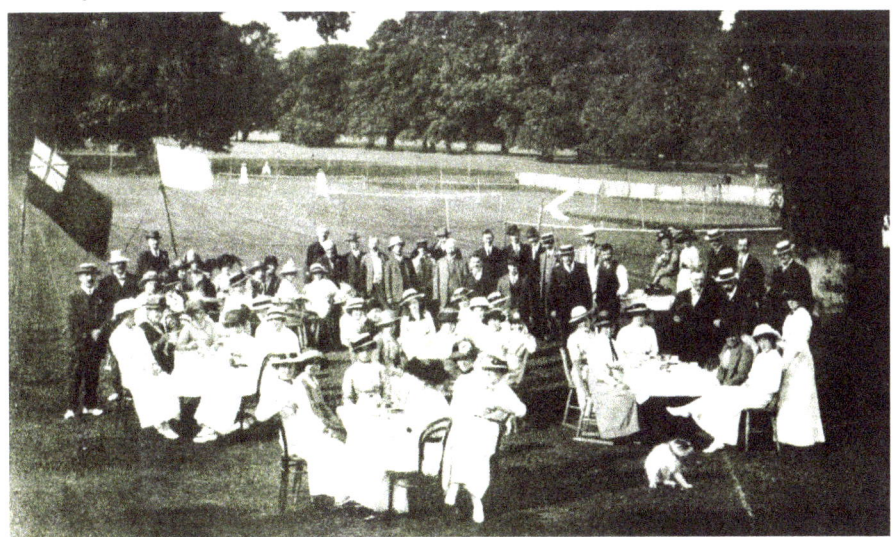

Members of Chippenham Sports Club, summer 1914

1. *Wiltshire Times* -2 June 1917
2. Charles Garnett was also the President of the Literary and Scientific Institute and the honorary Commandant of the Chippenham Ambulance Detachment.

Unity and Loyalty

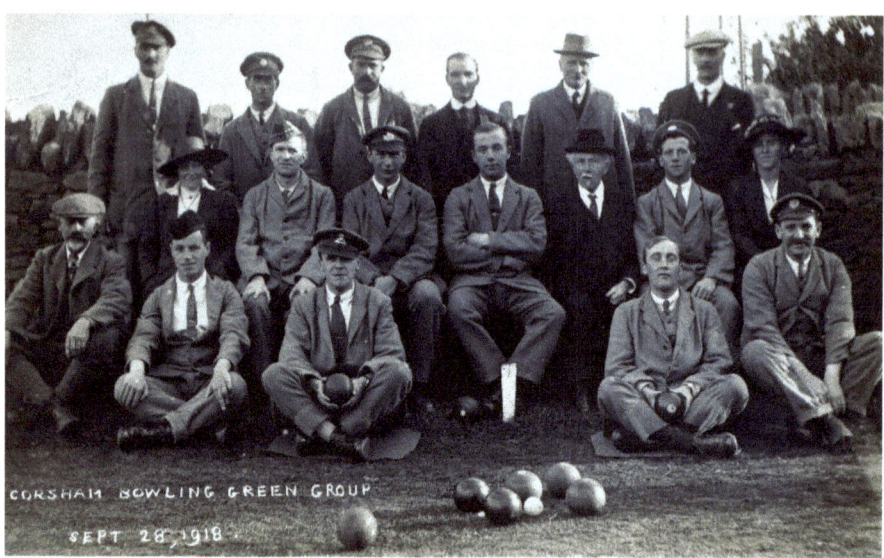

Patients join the local bowls clubs.

Buckland, George and Emily Pinfield, Mr Burridge, Mr Slade and George Hunt all active supporters and workers at the Hospital. As a goodwill gesture the committee decided patients should have free membership and use of the facilities of the Sports Club including the pitches, clubhouse and bowls green.[1]

Bowls was particularly popular and matches were arranged between club and hospital teams.

Special fun days were arranged for the wounded men. The Saxby and Farmer Recreation Club invited the patients to the company's sports ground where the clubhouse was decorated with flags and bunting. To ensure all the men could take part arrangements were made that stretcher and wheelchair cases were brought to the ground by Mr Burridge and men from the Ambulance Detachment.

A typical afternoon began with a short musical programme organised by VADs Emily Pinfield and Elinor Davis. The men were then encouraged to join the members and their families in an afternoon spent playing games taking part in competitions with the emphasis on fun and enjoyment. The games were arranged to take account of the men's injuries and included skittles, egg and spoon races, bowls, musical chairs and 'thread the needle' races. To ensure that men in wheelchairs and on stretchers could join in the games they included hat making competitions, memory races and a bath chair championship. All the prizes were donated by members of the club. In the interval tea was served by Mrs Pinfield with a group of assistants from the hospital kitchen often serving over 100 people.[2]

The afternoon ended with the men listening to songs performed by local singers. Maud Parry, a school teacher and part time VAD, sang for the men, accompanied by her

1   *Wiltshire Times* - 2 March 1918. Annual meeting of the Chippenham Sports Club
2   *Devizes and Wiltshire Gazette* – 13 July 1916

The Story of Chippenham's Red Cross Hospital

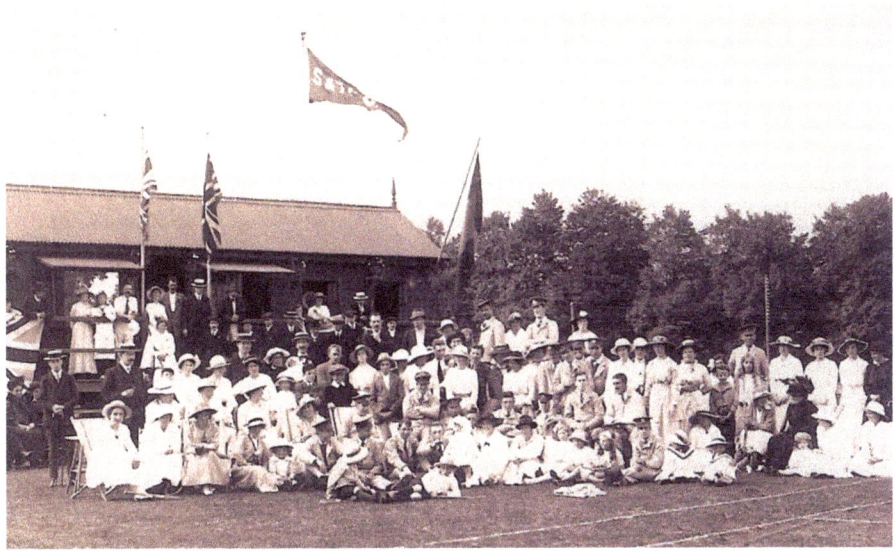

Fun Day at the Saxby and Farmer sports ground

pupils. When nine year old Greta Slade[1] sang the finale the men joined in with a rousing chorus of 'Keep the Home Fires Burning.'[2]

Hilda Taylor of Steinbrook House, at Kington Langley, was a regular supporter of the Red Cross in Chippenham, both contributing to funds and supplying produce from her garden. In August 1917 she hosted a 'Grand Sports Day' at the Sports Club grounds for the patients and staff. To add to the fun, she invited 200 guests from the town to join the proceedings.[3]

Mrs Taylor was assisted by Mr Hathaway, Mr Slade and Miss Whishaw the Assistant Commandant. Refreshments were arranged, as usual, by Mrs Pinfield and a group of volunteers.

A cricket match was organised between a team captained by Julian Spicer, the husband of Katherine the Quartermaster of Wilts 38 VAD, and a team of patients.

A series of races took place for those well enough to take part and for less mobile men the bowls green was available. There was a fancy-dress competition which caused 'much merriment' as the patients paraded around the club as Red Indians and female impersonators.

At the end of the afternoon the prize giving was followed by speeches. Sir George Helme spoke on behalf of the Red Cross Hospital thanking Mrs Taylor for an enjoyable afternoon. Company Sergeant Major Scott then stood up and spoke on behalf of the patients. The newspaper reported his speech:[4]

1   Thought to be Edith Greta Slade daughter of Harry and Annie Slade.
2   *Wiltshire Times* – 29 July 1916
3   *Wiltshire Times* – 2 March 1918. Annual meeting of the Chippenham Sports Club
4   *Wiltshire Times* – 1 September 1917

It gave him pleasure on behalf of his comrades to acknowledge Mrs Taylors thoughtful kindness. He could assure Mrs Taylor that they had all thoroughly enjoyed themselves and that they were full of gratitude to her for her kindness. They were also deeply grateful to the sports club for allowing them the free use of the ground for cricket matches croquet and bowls. Personally, he should like to thank the citizens of Chippenham for their kindness to him during his stay in the charming old town, and he knew that his feelings in that respect were shared by every man in the Hospital.

Mrs Taylor responded to the speeches:

She did not think she had ever done anything that gave her greater pleasure than in welcoming them all that day and to see everyone heartily enjoying themselves. She felt that they could not do enough for men who had done so much for us.

Despite all the enjoyment at the Sports Club the realities of war were lurking in the background. In early October 1917 the news was received that a town sportsman had been killed in action. Bert Pinfield was a well-known footballer and referee for the County Football Association and member of the club.[1] He was the son of Committee member George and his wife Emily, who faithfully arranged the teas and music for the sports afternoons.

A few weeks later another Committee member, George Hunt, received the news his son Percival had been killed in action. George and his wife Matilda lived in Langley Road and were very active in arranging the fun days. Matilda was also a volunteer and was described as a keen worker in the VAD and helped organise outings for the patients.[2]

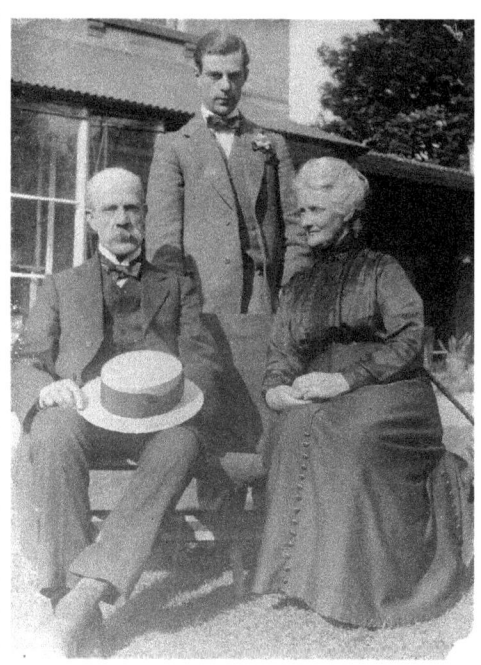

Percival Hunt with his parents George and Matilda

1   *Wiltshire Times* - 13 October 1917
2   *Wiltshire Times* – 4 June 1932 – Matilda Hunt obituary.

Chapter 13
Fund Raising

Our Day

MUCH OF THE funding needed came from public donations. The War Office paid the Red Cross a Capitation Grant for each bed occupied, but this was barely enough to cover a man's food and domestic needs.

To cover the additional expenses and provide the men with 'comforts' a special day to collect donations and highlight the work of the Red Cross and Order of St John was arranged. Known as 'Our Day' the first national fundraising day was organised on 21 October 1915.

As well as receiving gifts and donations the Red Cross sold small flags: paper ones were sold for a penny and silk ones for sixpence.[1] In Chippenham Division the fund-raising committee arranged for flags to be sold door to door. In the High Street collectors included patients. By the end of the day the Division had raised a total of £510 16s 7d in sales and donations.[2]

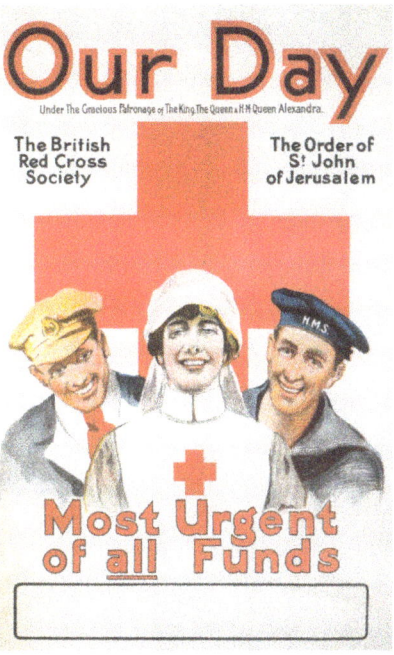

Red Cross Our Day poster

The day was so successful that it was repeated annually throughout the War.

Wiltshire Farmers

NATIONALLY THE BRITISH Farmers Red Cross Fund raised over one million pounds in support of the Red Cross both at home and abroad. Locally farmers raised money and gave practical help.

In a rural community like Chippenham it was inevitable that wives and daughters of farmers were involved with the Red Cross and naturally the farmers had a particular

---

1   The British red Cross Society – Information sheet: *Fundraising during the First World War*
2   *Wiltshire Times* - 25 March 1916

Unity and Loyalty

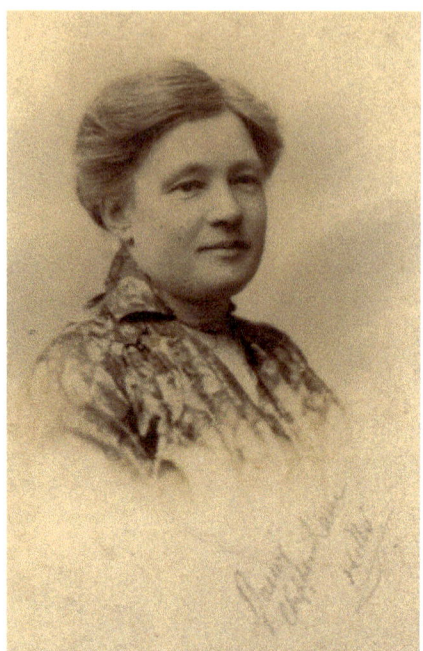

Farmers wife Myra Ferris helped organise fundraising by Wiltshire Farmers. She was also a member of a Red Cross work party

interest in supporting them. Walter Ferris farmed in Tytherton and organised the collection of equipment when the wards opened; he also helped organise a number of Farmers Red Cross fund raising days. His daughter, Fanny, served as a VAD at Bowood and Chippenham and his wife, Myra, was joint organiser of the Red Cross work party in the village of Tytherton.[1] She ran the work party with Alice Collett the wife of another farmer, William Collett.

In the years before the War the farmers of Chippenham and North Wiltshire had formed a farming co-operative called Wiltshire Farmers Ltd. This association, through its members, raised thousands of pounds locally for the war effort, much of which was donated to the hospitals in Chippenham Division.

The farmers organised a number of events to raise money, a particularly successful one was the Farmers Red Cross day in Chippenham in April 1916.

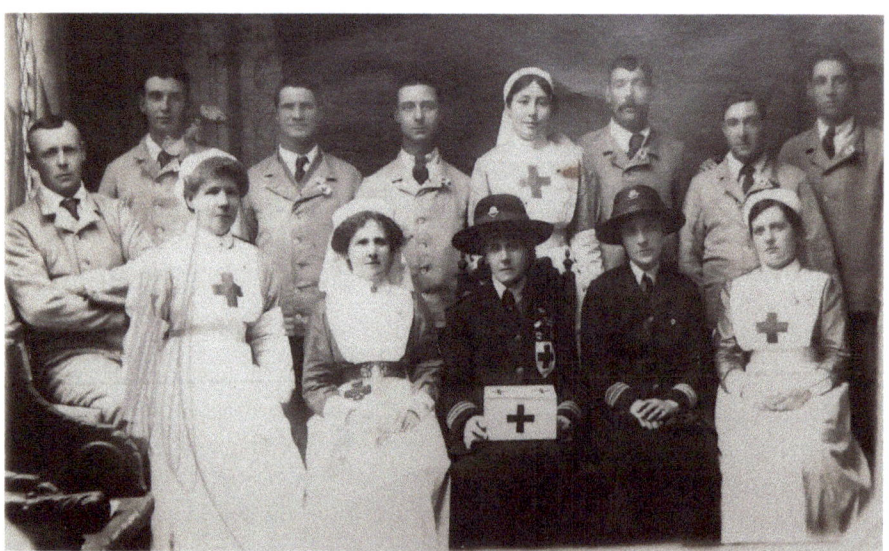

The Chippenham Hospital Red Cross collectors. The men are wearing paper flags

1   *The Bremhill Foxham and Tytherton Newsletter*- February 2016. Article about the Tytherton Work Party.

The Story of Chippenham's Red Cross Hospital

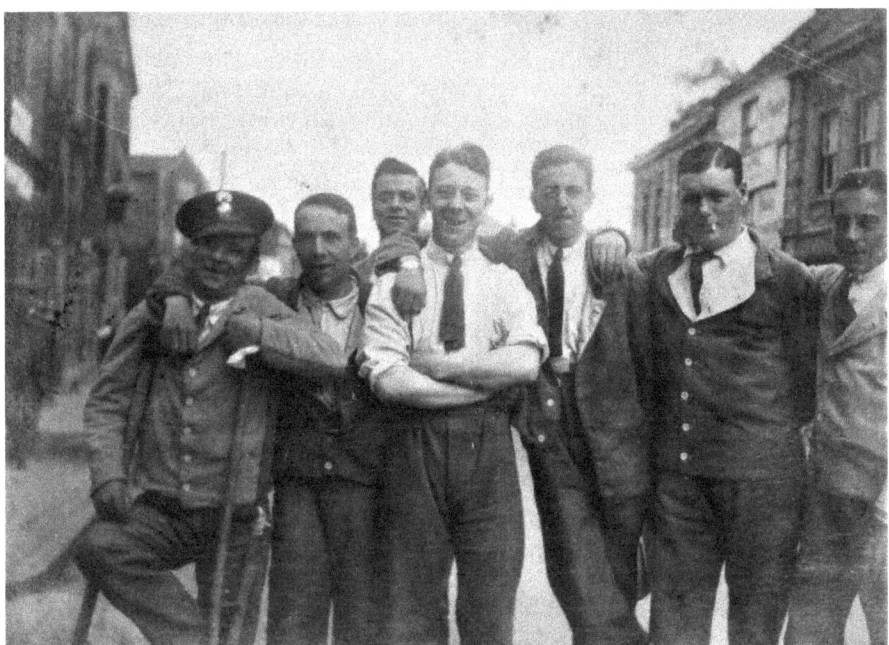

Patients were recruited to play the barrel organ

The day started with VADs and patients selling Red Cross Flags in the High Street. The sight of the blue uniform often meant an extra penny was donated. Another group of wounded joined Edwin Duck and Walter Archard, members of the Ambulance section, collecting money around the town by playing tunes on a barrel organ.

One of the patients, Corporal James Cox, who in peace time had been the Town Cryer in Burnham, went round the streets encouraging the public to give generously and announcing the programme of entertainment due to take place later that day at the Palace Theatre on Station Hill.

The acts for the matinee and evening performances were local celebrities. Popular singer Ursula Luce,[1] a VAD at Malmesbury Red Cross Hospital, was joined on stage by

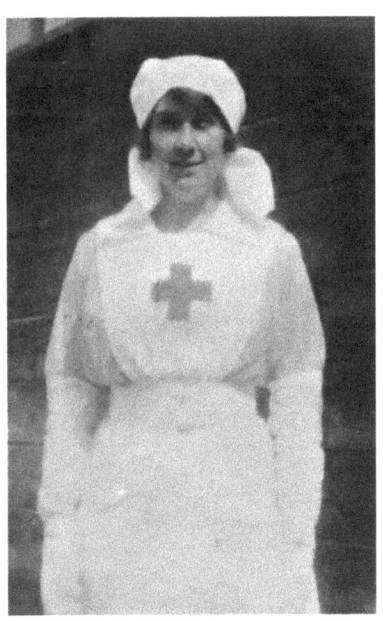

VAD Joan Spicer was one of the popular singers

1   Evelyn Luce, known as Ursula, was a popular singer and appeared at concerts from Lacock to Cirencester. She lived at the Knoll at Malmesbury

Chippenham VADs Joan Spicer and Gertie Pinfield. The singers were accompanied on the piano by cook Ethel Williams.

Harvey Brinton, a professional entertainer, who was appearing at the Bath Palace Theatre, joined the VADS during the day and helped raise a total of £84 17s 6d for Red Cross funds.

The day ended with an auction where it was reported a lady's hat was sold 52 times, such was the enthusiasm to give money. Over £1,100 was raised from the various events held during the day.[1]

Chippenham Fete

IN 1917 THE Wiltshire Farmers decided that reinstating a Fete would be good for the town, both boosting morale in the town and raising additional funds for the Red Cross.

Before the War Chippenham had traditionally held a number of fetes and shows during the summer. One of the biggest and most popular was the flower show that took place at the end of August. The show in 1911 was described as the most pleasurable event of the season. Since 1914, however, these shows had been abandoned because the organisers were either on active service or involved in other war work.

The farmer's committee made arrangements with Chippenham Sports Club to use their Hardenhuish Park grounds to host a fete and on 5 September 1917 the gates opened at one p.m. As anticipated, the crowds flocked in: it was estimated there were over 3000 visitors during the afternoon.

The band of the Wiltshire Regiment, based at the barracks in Devizes, played throughout the afternoon and the galloping horses and fairground rides provided by Mr Jennings[2] proved very popular. There were competitions for all the family including a fancy-dress parade and baby show with the centre of the show ground reserved for sporting events. The patients were encouraged to enter the fancy-dress parade.

At the end of the judging for the fruit and vegetable competition all the produce was auctioned in aid of Red Cross funds with many of the successful bidders in turn donating their purchases to the hospitals.

Advertisement for the Wiltshire Farmers Fete

> **WILTSHIRE FARMERS, Ltd.**
> Red Cross Day—Wednesday, Sept. 5th 1917.
> **GREAT FETE & SALE**
> ON THE SPORTS GROUND.
> **Hardenhuish Park, Chippenham.**
> Grand Programme of Attractions!
> **BAND OF THE WILTSHIRE REGIMENT**
> Sale of Produce, &c.   Novel Weight-Judging Competitions.
> J. JENNINGS' GALLOPING HORSES, SWINGS, ETC.
> **SPORTS FOR WOUNDED SOLDIERS.**
> SPECIAL COMPETITION FOR MALE MEMBERS OF V.A.D.'s, FOR A VALUABLE SILVER CUP
> Presented by the "News of the World."
> Judged by DR. LESLIE BEATH, M.R.C.S., L.R.C.P., (Chief Examiner of St. John Ambulance Association).
> **Show of Roots, Fruit, and Vegetables,**
> Open to Farmers, Allotment Holders, and Cottagers.
> For Schedule and Conditions of Competition apply to Mr. W. Swatz, Market Place, Chippenham.

1   *Wiltshire Times* – 22 April 1916
2   James Jennings World Fair of Devizes were regularly seen at shows around the district before the War.

The Story of Chippenham's Red Cross Hospital

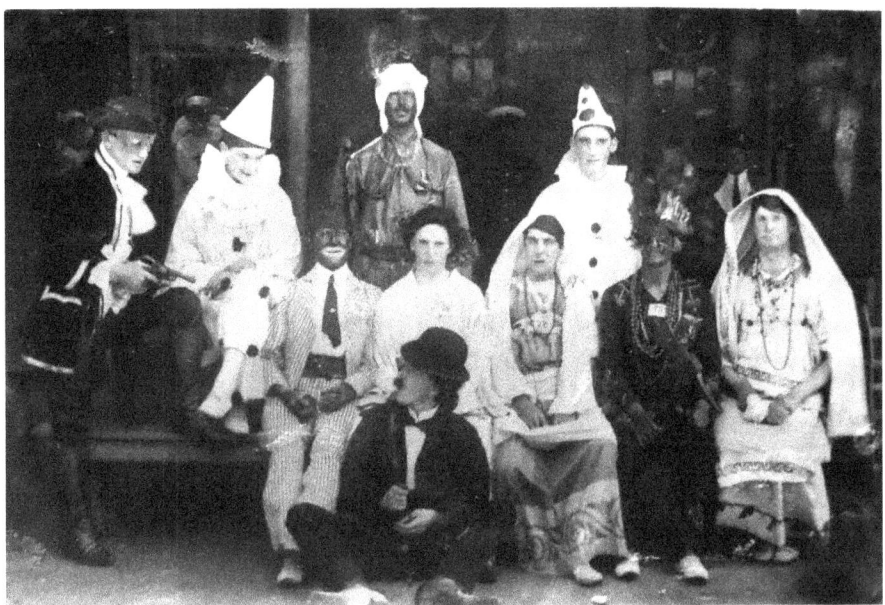

Patients in fancy dress at the Red Cross Fete

Men and women from all Red Cross detachments in the area were enlisted as helpers for the afternoon. VADs Dora Hart, Rachel Anstee and the Spinke sisters were in charge of a stall where the prize was a load of coal. The winner was Miss H Burridge who donated the coal to Chippenham Red Cross Hospital.

The VADs from Chippenham, Corsham and Box took part in a First Aid Competition for a silver cup presented by the News of the World newspaper. Box Detachment were the eventual winners.[1]

By the end of the day nearly £2000 had been raised and, after expenses were deducted, the Wiltshire Farmers distributed the proceeds to various branches of the Red Cross:

> £45 – to Basil Hankey for an X-Ray Ambulance for Wiltshire Red Cross[2]
> £20 - Men's VAD for uniforms.
> £100 - Chippenham Cottage Hospital
> £524 - Chippenham Red Cross Hospital
> £188 – Corsham Red Cross Hospital
> £173 - Calne Red Cross Hospital

---

1 *Wiltshire Times* - 8 September 1917
2 The British Red Cross Society - VAD index card record – In November 1917 John and Louisa Dutton of Sutton Veny Military Hospital operated the VAD portable X Ray equipment in a converted ambulance. They visited 11 VAD hospitals across the County, usually on a Sunday.

Unity and Loyalty

The balance of £441 14s 5d was added to the British Farmers Red Cross Fund.[1]

In November the National Farmers Fund gave the Central Office of the Red Cross £10,000 for the provision and upkeep of recreation huts at hospitals at home and abroad, the Wiltshire Farmers were listed amongst the contributors.[2]

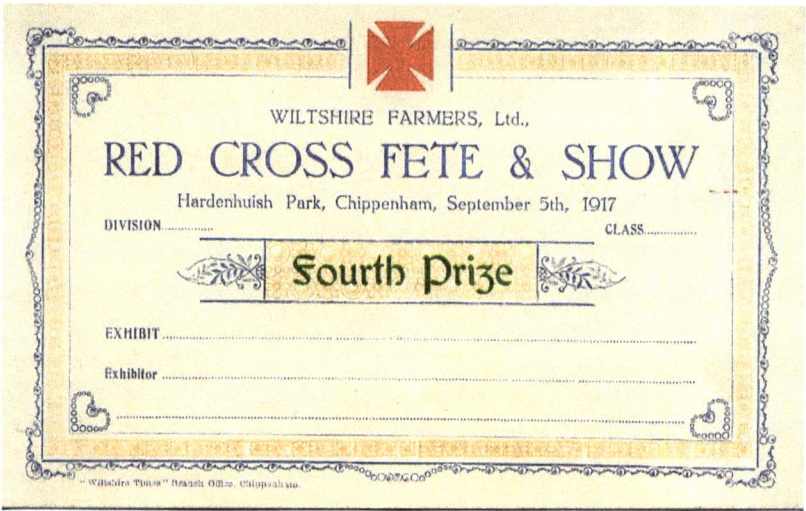

A prize certificate from the Red Cross Fete

1 *Wiltshire Times* - 17 November 1917.
2 *The Times* – 26 November 1917

Chapter 14
Ambulances

Shortage of Vehicles

From the first days of the War there were too few vehicles to transport patients and the men of the detachments used their skills to improvise. In North Wiltshire the men of the Malmesbury Detachment requisitioned farm wagons and converted them to rudimentary ambulances ready to receive patients at the railway stations of Hullavington and Somerford.[1] When Chippenham VAD Hospital first opened there was no ambulance available and the local laundry loaned a vehicle to transport stretchers. The battles of the Somme in 1916 emphasised the shortage of ambulances. There was conflict between the immediate needs at the front and the supporting role conveying patients at home. Red Cross transport sections in Britain were told their ambulances were to be requisitioned by the military in France. Early in 1916, at Southmead in Bristol, a vehicle had been donated by a Reverend Portman to be used by the local Red Cross. By mid-July it had been requisitioned by the military for use in France and an appeal was put out for a replacement vehicle.[2]

In Chippenham, since 1910, the police relied on an Ashford Ambulance or Litter, a wheeled stretcher, to convey accident victims to the Cottage Hospital. This vehicle was also used by the VADs at their training events.

Several of these ambulances were used at Chippenham VAD Hospital. Arthur Phillips, who joined the Chippenham male section in 1916, worked for Hinders Cycle shop in the town and used his skills to make and repair them by fitting bicycle wheels to stretchers.[3]

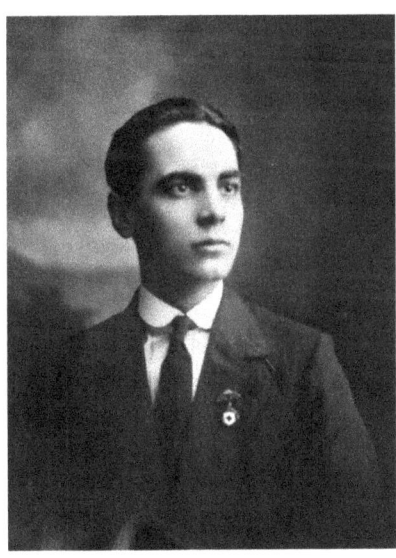

Arthur Phillips wearing his Red Cross lapel badge

These vehicles were satisfactory for use close to a hospital but for longer journeys and carrying wounded from the station a motor ambulance was essential. A motor

1   Western Daily Press - 20 August 1914. Hullavington station probably served Draycot House
2   Western Daily Press - 24 July 1916
3   As told to family members Betty Bird and Rae Whitney by Arthur Phillips.

Unity and Loyalty

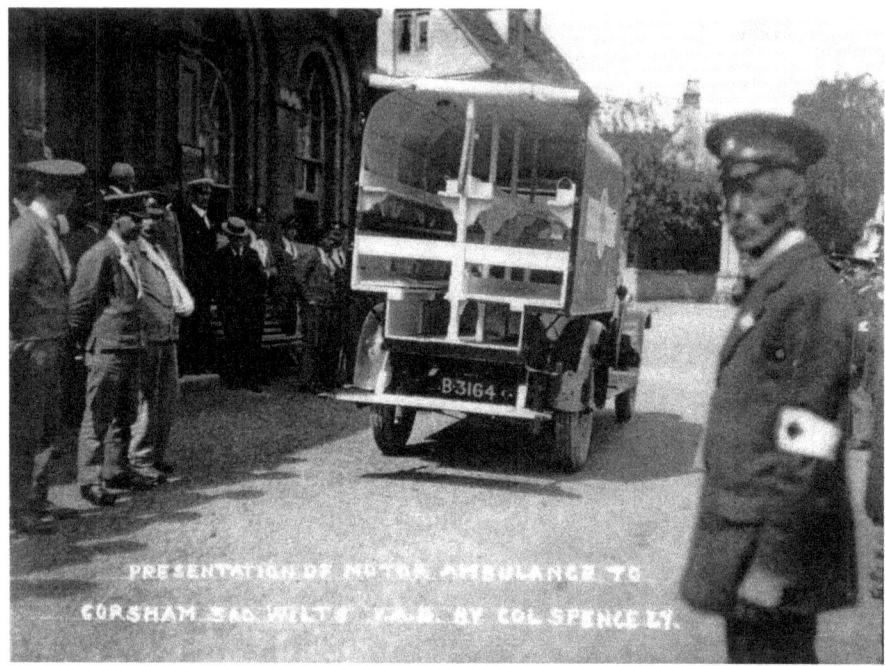

The ambulance presented to Corsham, Wilts 3, by Colonel Spencely

ambulance could carry four stretchers at greater speed and in greater comfort. In Chippenham Mr Garnett loaned his ambulance during the early months of the Hospital.

As the War progressed donations were given to buy more ambulances. By 1919 Chippenham had the use of at least three motor ambulances. In Corsham a second ambulance was donated in 1917:[1]

> GIFT OF A MOTOR AMBULANCE
>
> On Saturday afternoon, Lieutenant-Colonel Spencely, of Ashley House, Box, presented to Lady Goldney, Commandant of the Corsham Red Cross Hospital, an 18.25 horsepower Wolseley motor ambulance for service by the 3rd Wilts Men's Voluntary Aid Detachment attached to the Corsham Hospital. The handsome vehicle was driven up to the Hospital entrance where Lady Goldney, Sir John Goldney, Lieutenant-Colonel Spencely, Commandant P. J. Gane, Mr. A. C. Kinneir, J.P., the Matron and Staff and members of the 3rd Wilts Voluntary Aid Detachment (including Box) and wounded soldiers had assembled.
>
> Colonel Spencely, in presenting the Ambulance, said: On behalf of my wife and myself I formally present this motor ambulance to Lady Goldney, the Commandant of the Corsham Red Cross Hospital, and dedicate it to the 3rd Wilts Voluntary Aid Detachment for the transport and comfort of wounded soldiers, and other Red Cross and First Aid work.

1   *Wiltshire Times* - 21 July 1917

The Story of Chippenham's Red Cross Hospital

The men from Corsham and Chippenham Detachments often worked together and ambulances were 'pooled' to attend Bowood, Corsham and Chippenham hospitals as needed.

Cecil Martin, described how he saw ambulances parked in Chippenham awaiting the next train bearing patients.

> Hospital trains were often seen. Army lorries with their solid tyres, were parked along the frontage of the Town Mill, waiting to transport war casualties from the station to the temporary hospital set up in the Neeld Hall.

The Army Service Corps may have loaned military vehicles to assist when a large allocation of stretcher cases arrived.

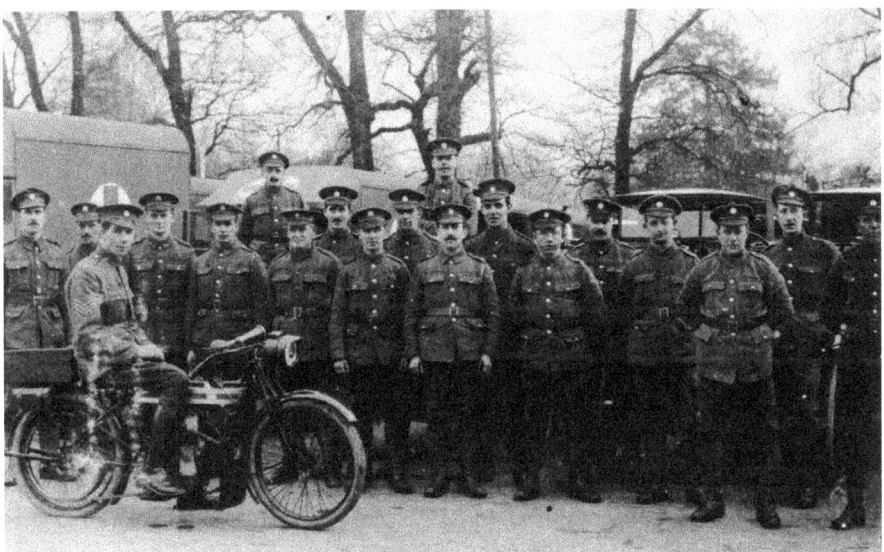

The ASC in Chippenham with military ambulances destined for the front. It is thought they were loaned to the Red Cross when large numbers of patients arrived

Ambulance Funds

AS SOON AS war broke out various schemes were introduced for the public to subscribe toward the purchase of vehicles. Early in 1915 Lady Bushman started an ambulance fund on behalf of the Red Cross and St John Ambulance. Her idea was that every ambulance donated should bear a female name and every woman in the country with that name should contribute to its cost. The idea was engaging and women came forward to volunteer as collectors for their name. Ivy Gladstone of Bowden Park, one

Unity and Loyalty

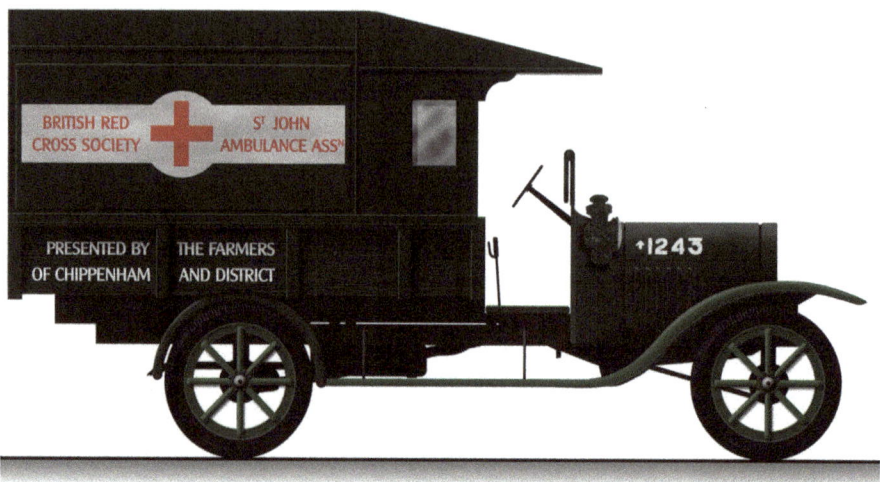

Artists impression of the ambulance presented to the Red Cross in Chippenham by the Wiltshire Farmers

of the VADs at Chippenham, put her name forward and soon ladies around the country called Ivy sent in donations towards the ambulance. 'Ivy' was soon seen in France alongside Dorothy, Agnes and a host of other names.

In November 1915, the Mayor of Calne handed over an ambulance to the Red Cross purchased with money raised in the town. Businesses were keen to help: The Brewing Industry initiated a subscription to purchase two convoys of motor ambulances for use in France while the British Sportsman's Fund raised sufficient money to buy 16 ambulances for the Red Cross.

Following the successful Chippenham 'Red Cross Day' organised by the Wiltshire Farmers in April 1916 proceeds amounted to over £1000. It was decided to use this money to buy an ambulance for the Red Cross.

On 7 July 1916 there was a large gathering in Chippenham Market Place where the ambulance was presented to Mr. E. M. Clark, the official head of the Ambulance Department of the Society. The cost of the ambulance was £400 and £320 was given towards running costs. It was described in the Devizes and Wiltshire Gazette:

> ...being substantially built, capable of accommodating four stretchers or eight sitting cases, completely equipped, including first-aid appliances, heating apparatus, and electric light. On the outside there is the Red Cross in the centre of the inscription in red letters on white ground, British Red Cross Society, St. John Ambulance Association, and underneath the words painted in white letters, 'Presented by the farmers of Chippenham and District.

The Story of Chippenham's Red Cross Hospital

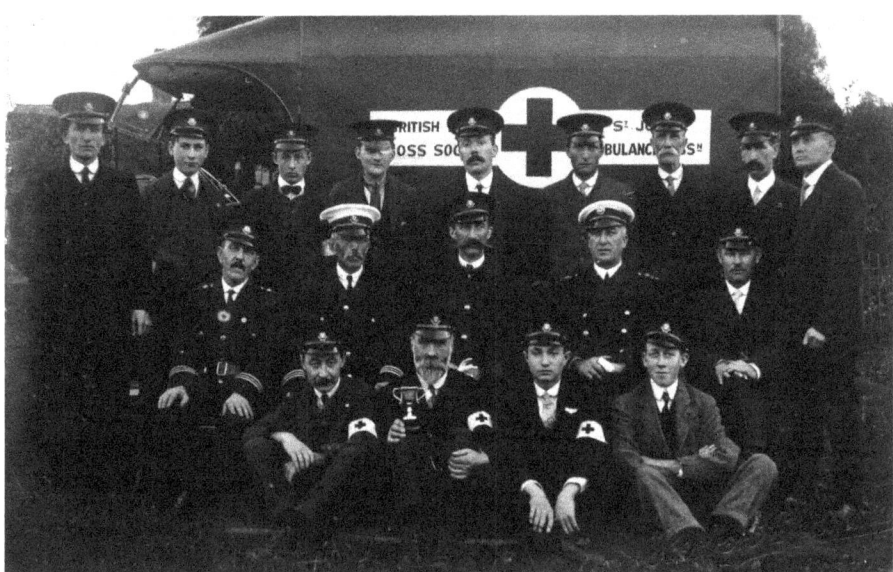

Corsham Wilts 3 Detachment with an ambulance, probably taken some time after the war

Percy Gane, the Commandant of Corsham Men's Detachment, and a member of the Committee of Wiltshire Farmers, arranged for the vehicle to be displayed in Chippenham, Calne, and Corsham, where it was: *'inspected with interest and pride by the inhabitants, who regarded it as 'Our Car.'* It is understood this ambulance was later sent to France as part of an ambulance convoy.

The Ambulances were engaged in transporting patients but, when free, also helped the civilian population. A particularly nasty road accident took place at Chequers Hill, between Chippenham and Corsham, when a vehicle lost control and the five occupants were injured. An ambulance crew attended together with two nurses from Corsham. The injuries were treated at the scene, but one man was transported to Bath for an urgent operation.[1] In March 1916 Mr and Mrs Garnett were travelling back from Bristol when their car skidded and overturned. Badly shaken they were taken by ambulance to Chippenham VAD Hospital where their injuries were treated.[2]

---

1 *Bath Chronicle* - 15 July 1916.
2 *Devizes and Wiltshire Gazette* - 9 March 1916.

Chapter 15
Outings and Friendships

Firm Friends

THE RED CROSS Hospital became an established part of life in the town. Sunday became a popular day with the public to pop in and socialise with the patients over a cup of tea.

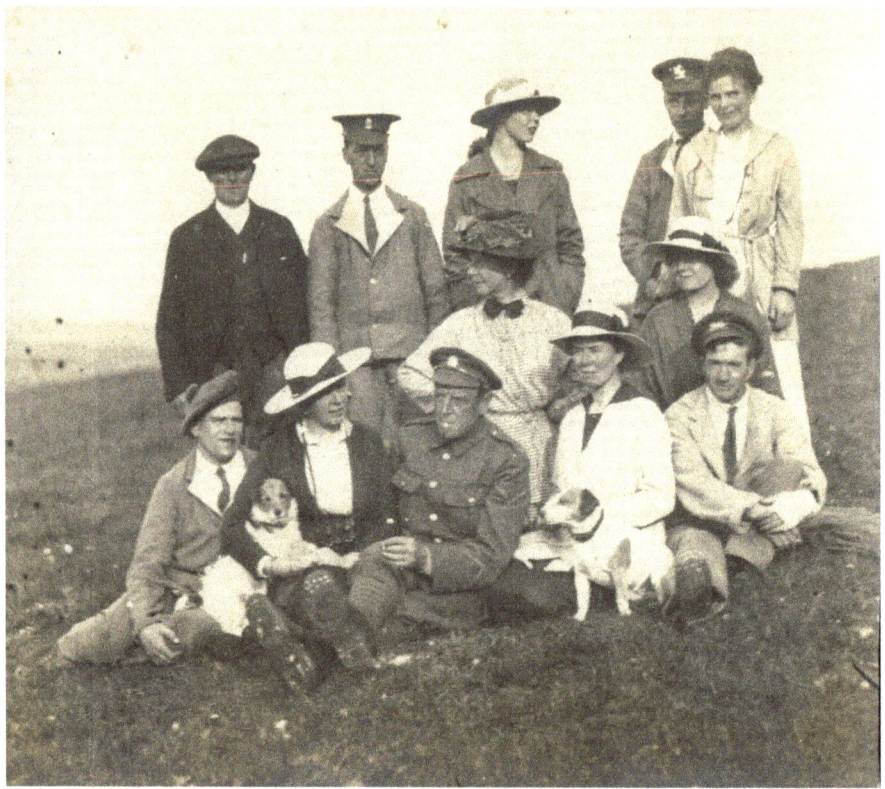

Patients enjoying a sunny afternoon with friends

At the beginning of 1918 there were complaints, that due to the recently reduced train timetable, visitors who lived outside Chippenham found it difficult to travel. Corsham Parish Council met with the railway company to ask for more trains to stop

The Story of Chippenham's Red Cross Hospital

at Chippenham, Corsham and Box in the evening. The Chairman of the Council said there was a need for more trains: *'so that hospital people could come back after visiting their friends.'* The Railway Company did little to improve the timetable, so the local MP, Mr Terrell, took up the case and wrote to the Board of Trade asking for improved services on a Sunday.[1]

When a man left hospital photos and addresses were exchanged. The VADs, of course, got to know the men well and would hear about their families, even meeting them when visits were made. They often kept in touch and corresponded as friends. Mrs Souter, the wife of a patient, kept in touch with Ethel Vicborn and when her husband was discharged, she wrote: *'With kindest regards to dear Sister Vicborn for her great tenderness and sympathy shown to my darling husband.'*

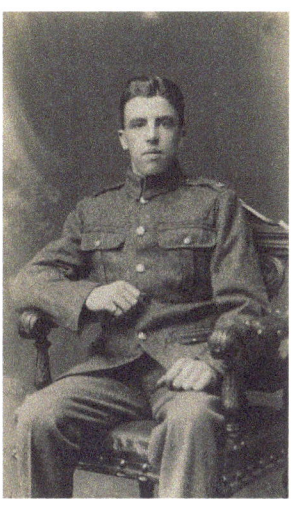

Private Souter

Ethel Williams' address book included several patients and their families and she corresponded with them for many years after the War.[2] She regularly arranged parties in her garden where the men could enjoy the company of her friends and family. At the end of 1917 Ethel Williams left the Hospital for personal reasons: she was expecting a baby. Despite this she continued to invite patients for afternoon tea.

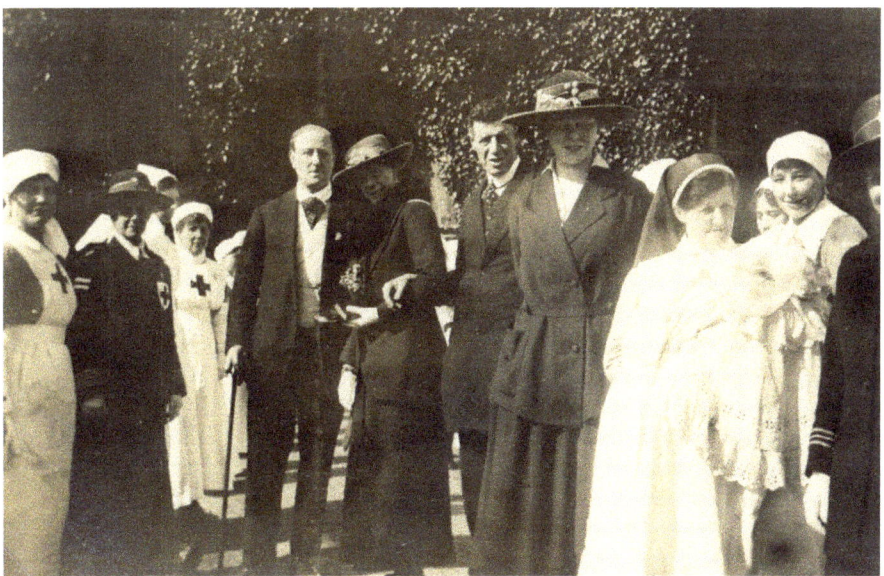

VADs at the christening of Ethel Williams' son John

1 *Wiltshire Times* – 5 January 1918.
2 Avice Wilson told how her grandmother, Ethel Williams, kept in touch with her friends, VADS and patients, for many years after the War.

Unity and Loyalty

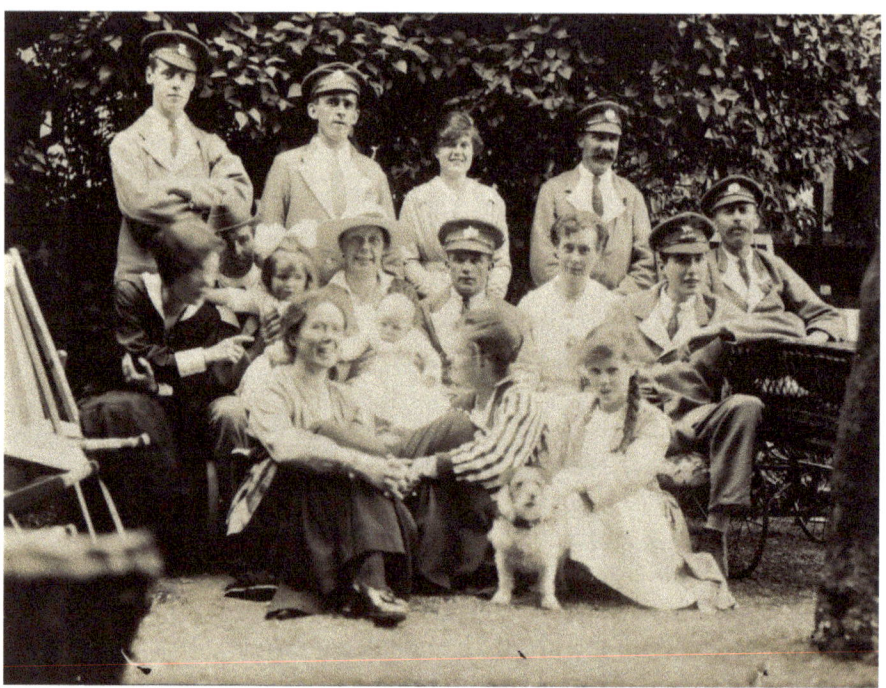

Patients and friends in Ethel Williams' garden in 1918.

When her son John was born in February 1918 her fellow VADs gathered at his Christening at St Paul's Church in Chippenham and no doubt the men raised a non-alcoholic toast in honour of the baby.

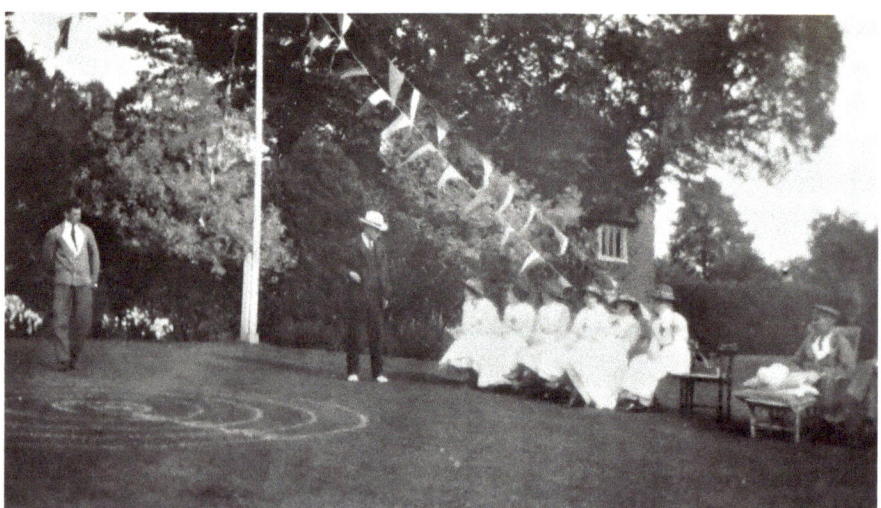

VADs and patients enjoying an afternoon at Grittleton House

The Story of Chippenham's Red Cross Hospital

Despite the convention of the time for mothers to remain at home with baby, Ethel was keen to get back to work as soon as possible and returned to the kitchen for a few hours each week. She continued her tradition of inviting patients to her home until 1919.

Well-wishers from the town and surrounding area also opened their homes. George White, a solicitor in Chippenham, invited the men to spend time in his house in the High Street to simply sit quietly and read or play a game of croquet in his garden.

Colonel and Lady Neeld, who supported the Red Cross in numerous ways, invited large groups of patients and VADs for refreshments and a game of bowls to their home Grittleton House.

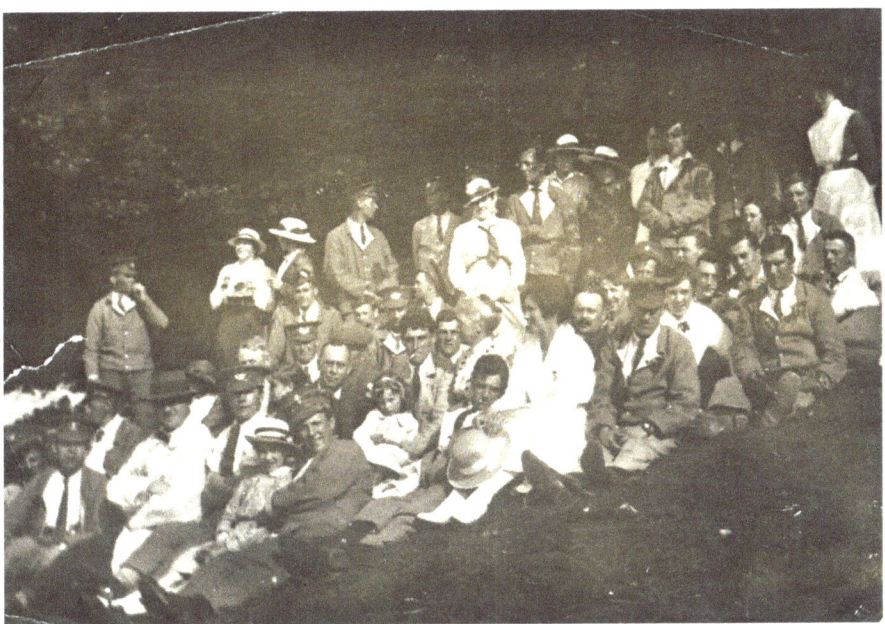

Hospital outing to Cherhill

The Entertainment Committee organised outings for the men when a picnic was made up by the ladies in the kitchen. The trips became real family affairs with the VADs bringing along their children and friends to share the day with the patients. Transport was arranged by Mr Burridge, Mr Buckle and others on the committee. Colonel Neeld used his car to take groups of VADs and patients for visits to Bath and other towns and trips were arranged to visit nearby VAD hospitals to meet comrades and take part in inter hospital sporting fixtures.

Part 4
Peace and the Hospital Closes

Chapter 16
After the War – November 1918

THE WAR IS over and the country rejoices. The VAD hospitals remain busy as the wounded in Europe are returned to Britain. Spanish Flu strikes Chippenham. Christmas festivities are enjoyed at the Hospital for the last time.

The Armistice

ACROSS THE COUNTRY everybody anxiously awaited the news that the War was over. Shortly before 11am on Monday 11 November 1918 news came through that the Armistice had been signed.

An immediate relaxation of some wartime measures was announced; all military recruiting was suspended; limits on the opening of hotels and places of entertainment were lifted; the lighting of bonfires was allowed; and restrictions on the ringing of church bells withdrawn.[1] Across the country there was celebration.

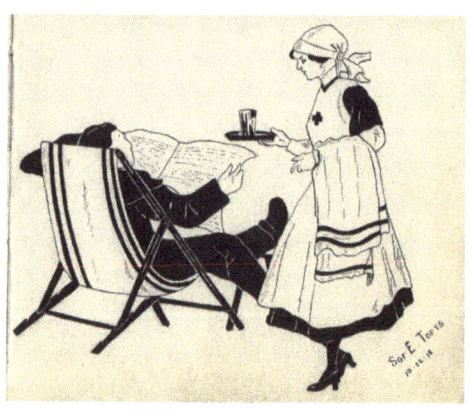

Now the war was over Sergeant Tofts jokingly suggested Chippenham VADs become waitresses

In Chippenham, with the news confirmed, workers took to the streets and the rest of the day was spent rejoicing. The streets were soon decorated with bunting and flags, cheering crowds thronged the Market Place and the church bells sounded throughout the afternoon. The Salvation Army band led the street parades and, in the evening, there were services of thanksgiving.

Two days later a hastily organised torchlit procession left the Market Place and paraded through the streets of the town. The torches were made from empty tins nailed to wooden handles and stuffed with paraffin-soaked material; the condensed milk factory was short of a few hundred tins the next day.[2] The Wiltshire Times described the event:

> Chippenham had a second joy day, or rather joy evening, on Wednesday expressive of all their feelings at the fact that the war is at length over. A torchlight procession hurriedly

1   *The Times*- 12 November 1918
2   Chippenham Civic Society - *Buttercross Bulletin issue 80 and 81, 1996* – Cecil Martin remembers

The Story of Chippenham's Red Cross Hospital

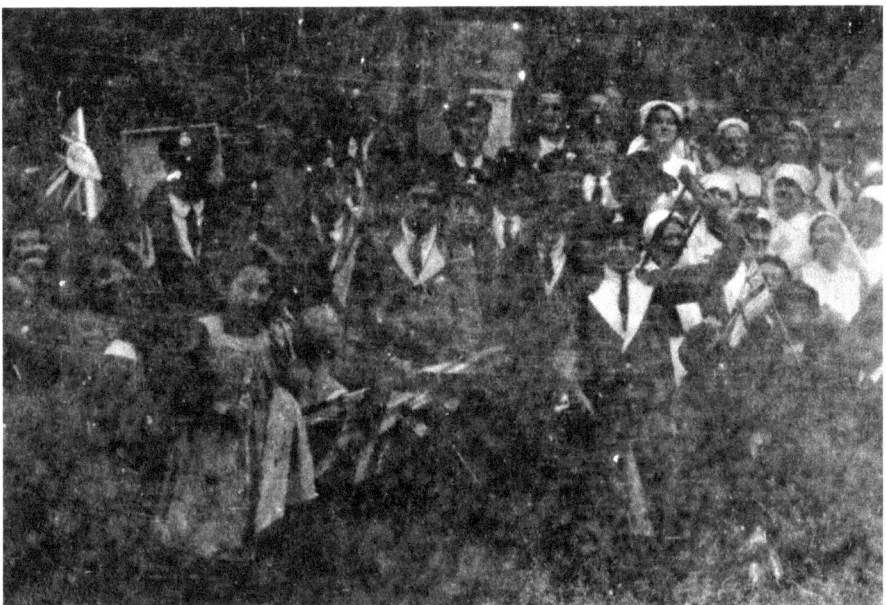

Despite the poor quality of the image smiles and flag waving at the Armistice are clear

arranged, but excellently carried out was held. The proceedings were organised by Capt. Mills, Mr J H Buckle and Mr F J Burden.

The procession formed up in the Market Place, where a large concourse assembled, those taking part including the Volunteers, under Capt. Mills, the Boy Scouts with Scoutmaster Dear, the nurses from the Red Cross Hospital, the members of the VAD, the convalescent soldiers from the hospital, the munitionettes, munition workers and employees in other industries of the town.

The march around the town was started about 7 o'clock, at which hour the Salvation Army Band, which has rendered such valuable service in many ways during the war, played the Volunteers into the Market Place to the strains of 'La Marseillaise'. The procession moved off in splendid order, and as it passed down the High Street it extended from the Market Place away over the Town Bridge, and presented a pretty sight in the clear moonlight. It made its way amid densely crowded streets to Landsend as far as the West End Club, then through Park Lane, New Road, back through the Market Place and St. Mary Street through the Butts into London Road and through the Causeway to the front of the Angel Hotel. Excellent order was preserved throughout and the crowds continuously gave vent to their joyous feelings. The band played selections for a time in the Market Place and the National Anthem concluded the display.

When the crowds returned to the Market Place the wounded soldiers and VADs were invited into the Angel Hotel and were taken onto the balcony where the crowds cheered the men in blue and their nurses.

The whole town took part from the youngest to the oldest. The schools organising

Unity and Loyalty

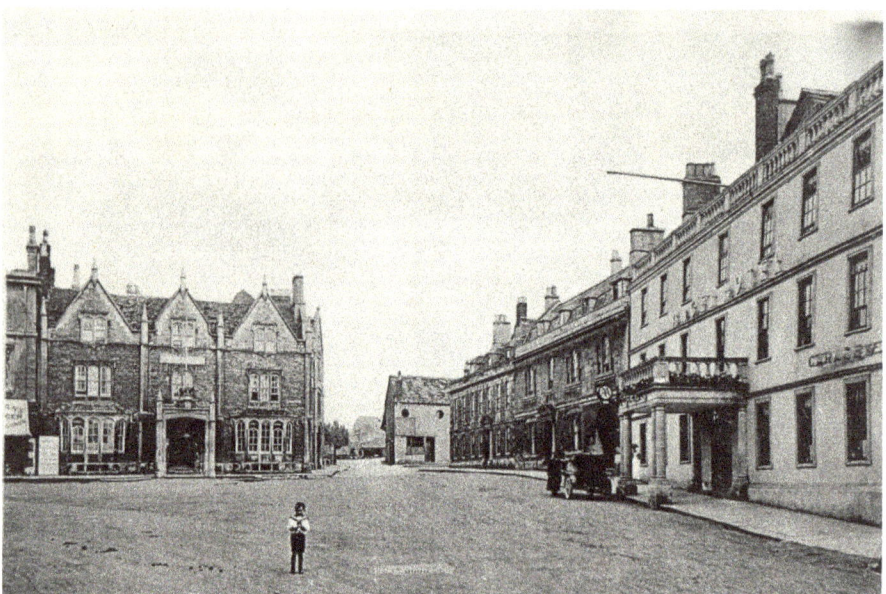

The Market Place Chippenham where the crowds gathered to celebrate the Armistice. On the right is the balcony of the Angel Hotel where the VADs and wounded were cheered

their pupils. Arthur Garlick was seven years old when he joined his teacher and schoolmates in the parade. His mother couldn't afford to buy a Union Jack, so he simply tore up an old red petticoat to represent the flag.[1]

From War to Peace

WITH THE SIGNING of the Armistice a cloud was lifted across the country. Everybody hoped for a return to normality as soon as possible. On 13 November the Ministry of Munitions published instructions to munitions factories, including Saxby and Farmer in Chippenham, on how to transfer from a war to a peace footing as efficiently as possible.

To deal with the large war workforce, mostly now redundant, the Ministry gave the following guidance:

> The great task before the country Is the transformation of industry from war to peace. This necessarily involves the disturbance and dislocation of industries and workshops, and very large numbers of workpeople will have to change their employment, and in many cases their present abodes. This must be faced.
>
> In order that the change may be made with the least possible hardship and the minimum of waste, exceptional arrangements are necessary. The Government intend to recognise in these arrangements the good work which has been done by munitions

---

1 *Chippenham Times and News* – 2 September 1966, Personality Arthur Garlick

workers in helping to bring the war to a victorious conclusion.

The following instructions are hereby issued to all factories and firms engaged on work for the Ministry of Munitions:-

There should, so far as possible, be no immediate general discharge of munitions workers. All workers however who desire to withdraw from industry or to leave for any reason, and all workers who can be absorbed elsewhere should at once be released. All overtime should be abolished.

Two weeks after the Armistice the Daily Mirror highlighted the opportunities for women, now that munitions workers were no longer needed, saying that single women with or without experience should consider returning to domestic service as there were many opportunities for servants.

For married women the expectation was they should resume their duties in the home and the pre-war social order.

For many this was unacceptable and five thousand women munition workers paraded in Trafalgar Square to demonstrate against their sudden dismissal from munitions work at Woolwich. In response they were told by the Ministry of Munitions that where possible suitable alternative work would be offered, but this did not materialise and by the end of the year there were many thousands of unemployed war workers.

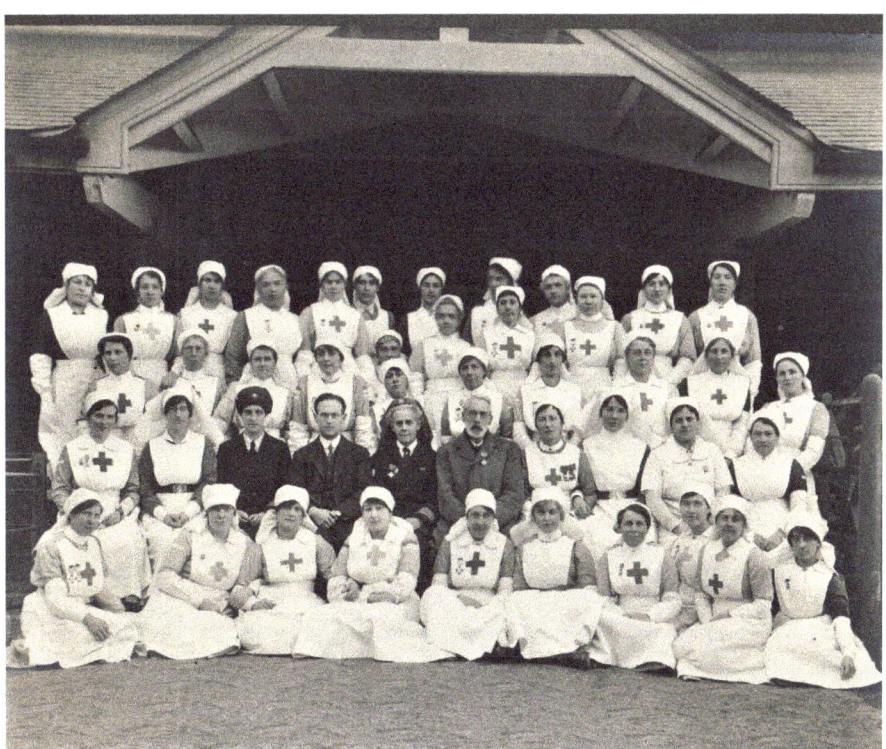

The VADs and doctors at Chippenham in 1918 around the time of the Armistice

Unity and Loyalty

For the VADs, both men and women, there was no question of their work ending with the War. Although they were volunteers the VADs were told the prospect of their demobilisation should not be expected for some time. Men in the detachments, especially those who had joined the Red Cross as a condition for exemption to military service, had hoped to be released as soon as possible. The task of returning the wounded from overseas had just started and was expected to last for many months. After the excitement of the Armistice, the VADs returned to their duties and carried on as usual.

In the first few weeks following the ceasefire there was little change to the VAD's routine as convalescent patients continued to arrive. In Bristol trainloads of wounded still arrived but gradually, by the end of the year, the flow reduced.

Unexpected Casualties

On the 14 of November 1918, three days after the signing of the Armistice two young RAF[1] officers climbed into their aircraft at Filton airfield near Bristol. The pilot, Second Lieutenant Leo Edwin Aldrich, and his passenger, Second Lieutenant Edward John McDougall, were about to fly to the RAF training camp at Yatesbury, near Calne.

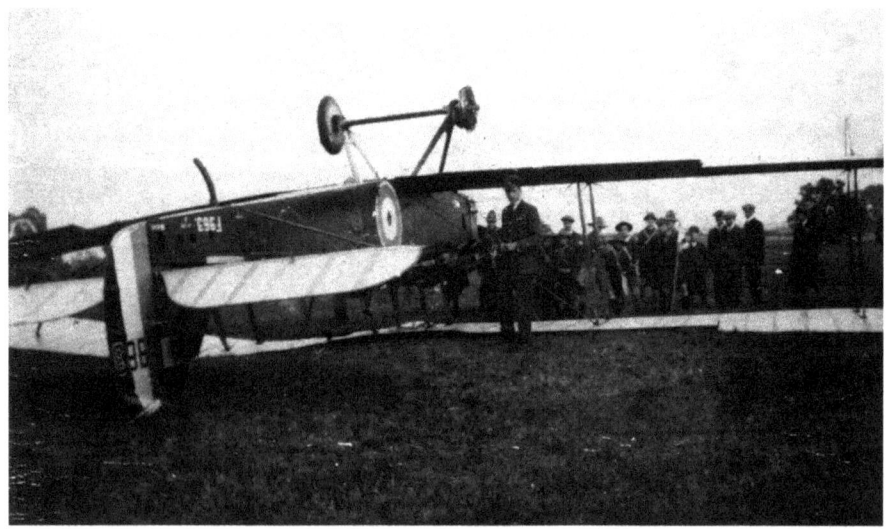

The crashed Aircraft on the outskirts of Chippenham

Leo Aldrich was an American and Edward McDougall a Canadian. They had both enlisted at the RFC depot in Toronto, Ontario in January 1918.

The weather was fair with a little rain expected later in the day. The flight was uneventful until, flying over Chippenham, a fault developed and the aircraft spiralled out of control crashing near New Leaze Farm on the outskirts of the town. Farmer Pryor

1 In April 1918 the Royal Flying Corps became the Royal Air Force

The Story of Chippenham's Red Cross Hospital

Glass and some of his men rushed to the wreckage and pulled the pilots clear, but they had both suffered serious injuries.

Mr Glass telephoned the Red Cross for help and Doctor Laurence and VAD Fanny Ferris were despatched to administer first aid.

Men of Corsham Detachment arrived with their ambulance and prepared to transport the pilots to the Chippenham VAD Hospital After assessing the injuries however it was decided to take the two men directly to the Bath Military Hospital. Leo Aldrich died later in the evening, while McDougall was found to be less seriously injured and although in a critical condition, was later described as doing as well as expected.

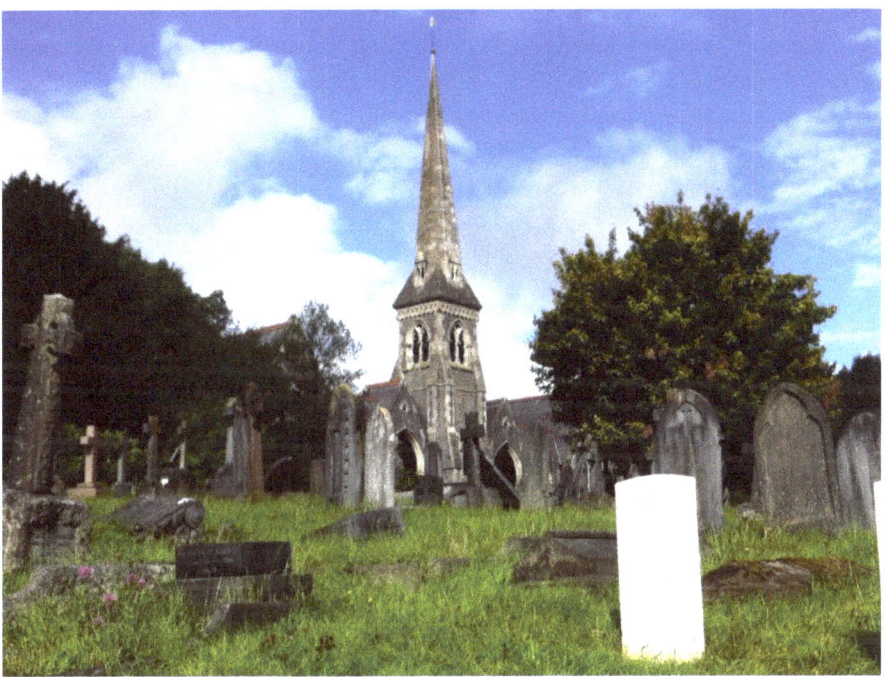

The Aldrich war grave, Locksbrook cemetery Bath.

Second Lieutenant Leo Edwin Aldrich was laid to rest in Locksbrook Cemetery in Bath on 19 November, his coffin carried by his fellow officers from Yatesbury. His family in America erected their own memorial to him in Ridgelawn Cemetery, Elyria, Ohio. Edward McDougall survived his injuries and was discharged from the service in 1920, returning to his home in Toronto.

The Influenza Crisis

WHILST THE COUNTRY looked forward to peace a new enemy was threatening. The Spanish Lady was gripping the nation.[1] Early in 1918 the first cases of flu

---

1 *Pandemic 1918* – Catherine Arnold. The Spanish Lady was a common name for influenza.

Unity and Loyalty

had been reported. Winifred Spencer, the daughter of a Wiltshire farm worker, recalled the atmosphere around her: [1]

> Everyone was getting worn down, low spirited. Food was rationed now and there were queues everywhere. Then in spring 1918 came the first of the flu epidemics and thousands died all over the country.

In the first few months of 1918 soldiers in the trenches complained of sore throats, headaches and a loss of appetite. As the men returned home wounded or on leave they unwittingly spread what would became known as Spanish Flu. Increasingly there were reports of sickness in the civilian population. By June it started to spread rapidly across the country and by October the whole country was affected. The newspaper headlines announced *Influenza Plague – Spreading at an alarming rate.*[2] Hospitals were overwhelmed and in some districts theatres, dance halls, churches and other public places were shut to avoid the spread of the illness. The flu pandemic claimed 228,000 lives in Britain and 50 million worldwide.

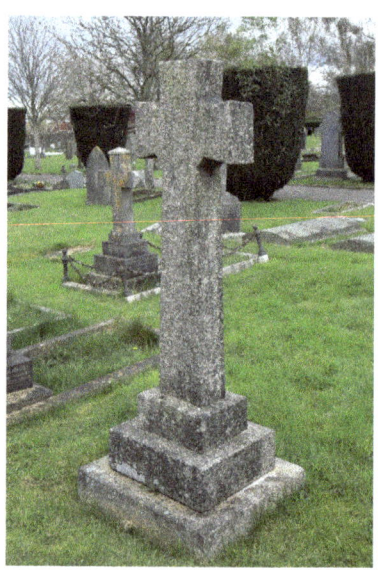

The memorial to the Rooke sisters in Chippenham cemetery

In early October 1918 Captain Wallace Rooke, of the Wiltshire Yeomanry returned to Chippenham from France on sick leave having contracted flu at the Front. The son of Mortimer Rooke, a Solicitor, the family lived at The Ivy in Bath Road. Within a few days Wallace Rooke's condition deteriorated and he died at home on 8 October.

His sisters Doris and Ellen, volunteers at the Red Cross Hospital, helped nurse their brother. With flu being so infectious they both inevitably fell ill within days of his death. Doris, who was 17 years old died on 14 October and 20 year old Ellen succumbed two days later.

There were many cases of flu in the town with whole households affected. In early December 1918 the Stevens family of New Road were struck down. William was the owner of Gowen and Stevens, plumbers and decorators. His wife Lilian, known as Annie, was the daughter of Samuel Spinke, who had championed the opening of Loyalty ward in 1916. Annie was also a VAD working alongside her sisters.

Within a few days of contracting the illness the family slowly started to recover but Annie suffered a setback and died. Her funeral took place on 11 December 1918 at St Paul's Church and amongst the mourners were many VADs and patients.

1 *Winifred. A Wiltshire Working Girl* – Sylvia Marlow. Winifred grew up on Salisbury Plain
2 *Western Gazette* - 25 October 1918.

The Story of Chippenham's Red Cross Hospital

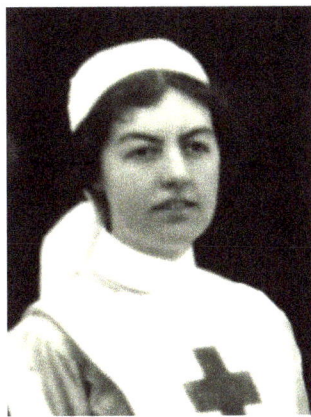

Annie Stevens

Joan Spicer the daughter of Lady Margaret Spicer, the Vice President of Chippenham Division, was a VAD at Bowood and Chippenham and one of the regular performers at hospital concerts. She contracted flu in February 1919 and died a few days later at the family's London home, aged 23.

Christmas 1918

BY MID-DECEMBER, AS fewer patients arrived from Bristol, Chippenham was at half its capacity with fifty patients. Over the festive period twenty of those men were allowed to spend the holiday at home with their families.[1]

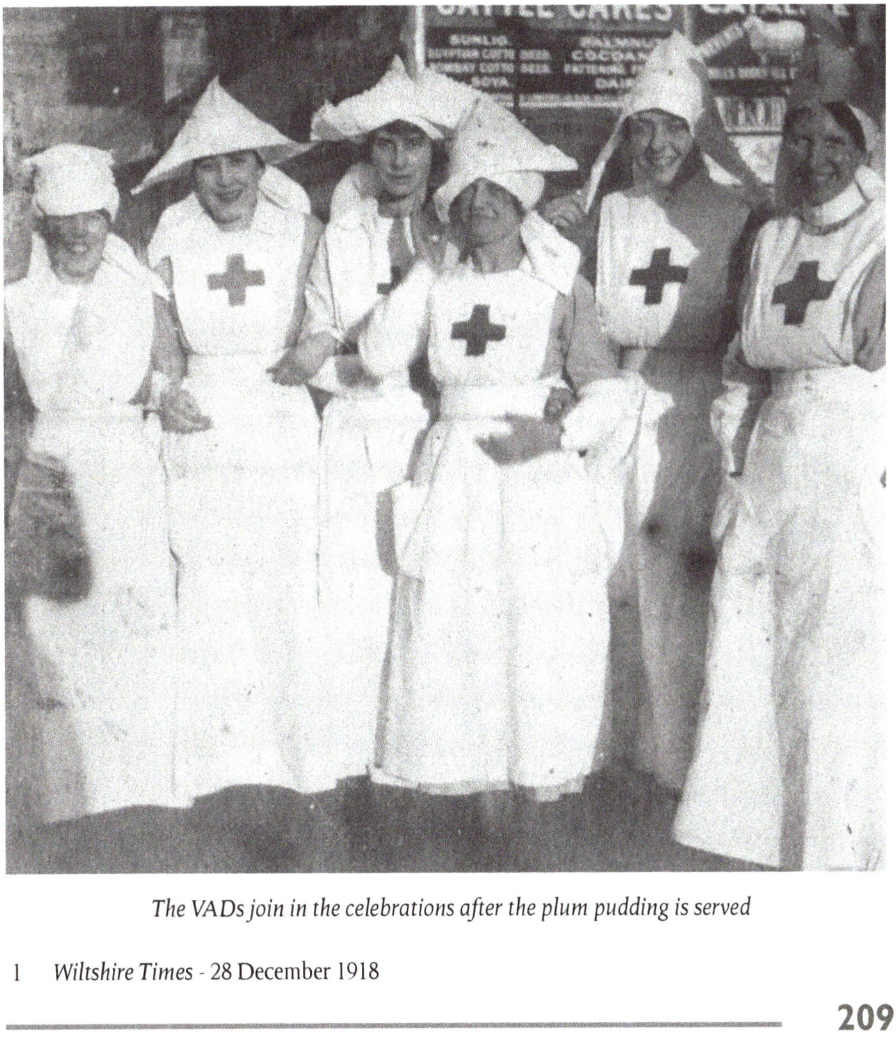

The VADs join in the celebrations after the plum pudding is served

1 *Wiltshire Times* - 28 December 1918

Unity and Loyalty

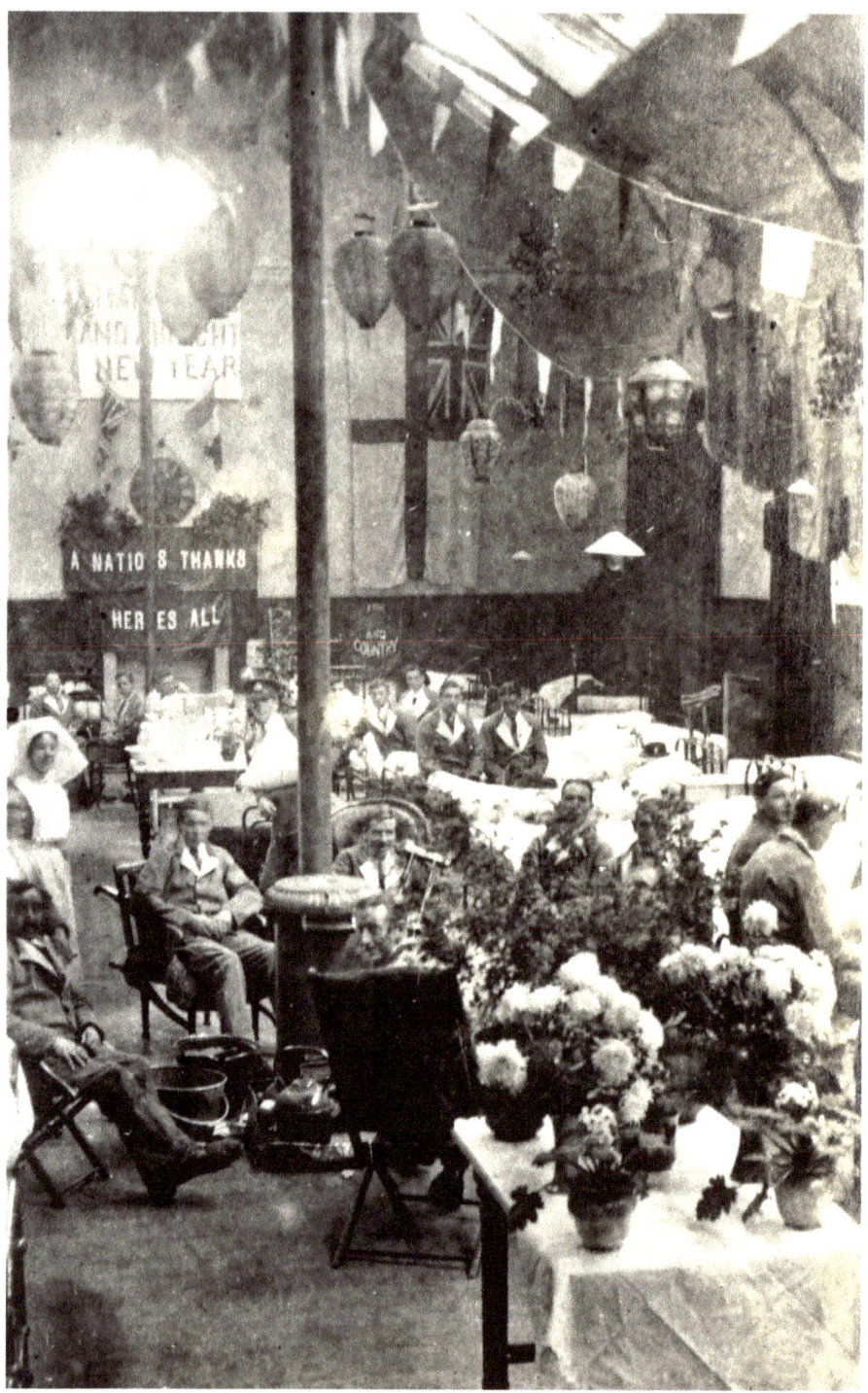

The last Christmas in Loyalty Ward. The banner on the wall says A Nations thanks. Heroes all

The Story of Chippenham's Red Cross Hospital

This would be the last Christmas celebrated in the auxiliary hospitals and the VADs decided to make it a memorable time for the men who remained. Mrs Warren the Commandant of Melksham Hospital summed up the feeling within the Chippenham Division when she placed an advert in the newspaper: [1]

> For the fourth time I am making a special Christmas Appeal for the men of this Hospital. It will probably be the last Christmas that we shall have our Australian Troops with us and we would like to give them such a good time they will always look back with pleasure on the Christmas spent in Melksham.
> Will everyone help us? Gifts of every kind and description welcomed.

At Chippenham the wards were beautifully decorated by the staff with flags, lanterns and bunting. A large Christmas tree was donated by Lady Margaret Spicer and was laden with gifts given by friends in the town.

On Christmas Day the staff and men gathered around the tree and Doctor Laurence, disguised as Father Christmas, called to distribute more gifts. Christmas dinner of roast goose was then served to the men and their friends. Despite shortages the Christmas puddings were described as '*all that could be desired.*' [2]

During the afternoon games were played and friends visited. On Boxing Day the patients were joined by local men who had recently been released from German captivity, for an afternoon of entertainment including singing by members of the VAD. At the close of the festivities Sergeant Byrne, on behalf of the patients, proposed a vote of thanks to the staff and all who arranged the event, his sentiment reflecting the care men had received since the Hospital opened in 1915: [3] '......*the whole population of Chippenham and Neighbourhood had treated the patients of that hospital in the most kindly of manners.*

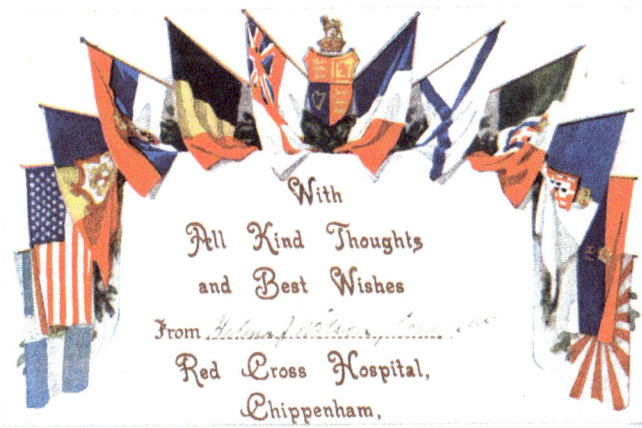

Helena Wilson sent Christmas cards to VADs and friends of the Hospital.

1 *Wiltshire Times* – 14 December 1918
2 Chippenham Museum – *Ivy Gladstone album*
3 *Wiltshire Times* – 4 January 1919

Chapter 17
Return to Peace – 1919

EVERYBODY LOOKS FORWARD to a brighter future now the War is over but economic storm clouds are brewing. Military hospitals are closed as patients are discharged to the care of the civilian authorities.

Chippenham VAD Hospital closes and everybody wants to return to their normal lives. The fallen are remembered and the VADs are honoured.

A Happier Country for All

WITHIN WEEKS OF the signing of the Armistice there was a General Election and for the first-time women were amongst the electorate.[1]

Known as the Khaki Election, the slogans included 'A land fit for heroes to live in' and 'A happier country for all.' The expectation was that after four years of war a brighter future lay ahead for the nation. In fact, there were bleak years to come as the country headed towards an economic slump.

In 1935 the book The Story of Twenty-Five Years, celebrating the silver jubilee of George V, described the period following the conflict:

> But those jubilant crowds of November 11 did not realise that years were coming that would tempt their endurance further, that the country would be wracked again, if not by war at least by civil strife, economic disasters and even more tragedies to face. The Military battle was over. The economic battle had only just begun.

The sheer scale of bringing men back from the battlefields presented its own problems for the Government. At the time of the Armistice over three million British men[2] were in uniform. By the end of January 1919 well over two million were still waiting to be demobilised and return home.

Releasing men from the military too quickly would simply add to the civilian numbers seeking work exacerbating the growing unemployment figures.

In March 1919 there were nearly 10,000 unemployed in Bristol.[3] Amongst them were women who a few months earlier had been working in factories, on buses, on the

---

1   The first election in which women over the age of 30, and all men over the age of 21, could vote.
2   The National Archive - Spotlight on History- *Demobilisation in Britain, 1918-20*
3   *Western Daily Press* – 26 March 1919

railways and keeping the peace in the city. The unpopular advice they were given by the Ministry of Labour was:

> If you are a woman worker who can afford to stay at home instead of working it would be patriotic to do so, and so leave the field open to those who have to work to earn a living.

Returning soldiers came back expecting to step back into their old jobs, but employers had adapted. One man who worked in a gentlemen's outfitters before the War found two women were now doing his job, at a lower wage.

To ease the unemployment situation the Ministry of Labour had published a Guide to Employers and Employees to get people into work and keep the wheels of peacetime industry turning, but in reality there were too few jobs and the only option for most was to simply register at the nearest Employment Exchange.

In Chippenham, as Saxby and Farmer turned their production lines to peacetime work and men were demobilised the town saw increasing unemployment. The Wilts Vagrancy Committee in April 1919 said there were over 300 homeless men in the county who had served in the Army and Navy. They called on the Government to find employment to prevent '*these men who have served the country from lapsing into vagrancy.*'[1]

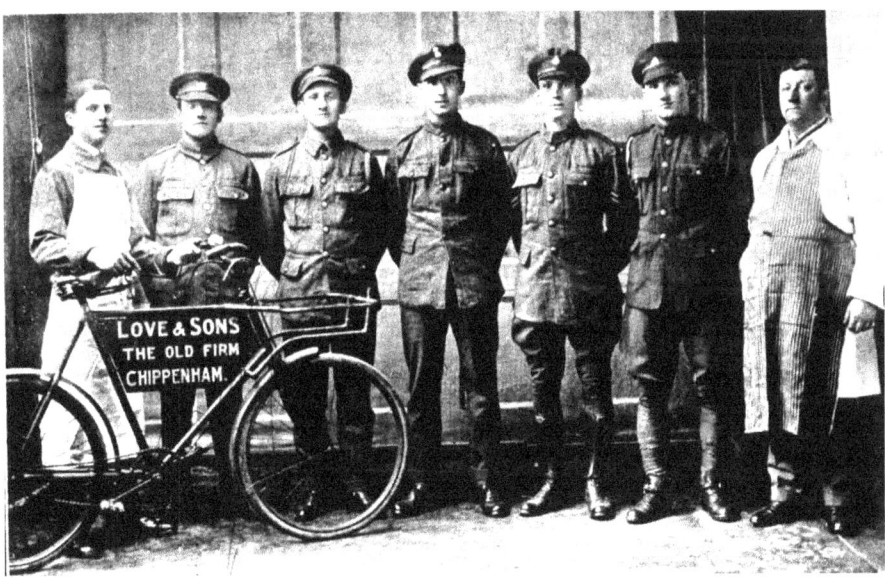

The Love brothers returned to the family business in Chippenham but many men found they were unemployed when they were demobilised

During March 1920 six unemployed ex-servicemen in Chippenham wrote a letter in response to a comment made by Mr Marshall at a Town Council meeting, suggesting that

1   *Wiltshire Times* - 26 April 1919

the unemployed didn't want to work. The letter demanded an apology from Mr Marshall and went on to blame many of the employers in the town, who refused to reinstate men in their old jobs when they returned from the War.[1] The letter was an indication of the underlying frustration felt by the ex-serviceman in the town.

Military Demobilisation

MEN AWAITING DEMOBILISATION from the services were equally frustrated and became increasingly discontent as they waited months, in some cases over a year, to be released. They had been told there was a need for an ordered return to civilian life but there were allegations of unfairness in the system with those conscripted last being amongst the first to be released.[2]

The delays in demobilisation caused unrest and riots broke out at several military camps. Troops from the Empire, anxious to return home, were told there was a shortage of transport. Canadian troops, frustrated at the delay in repatriation and poor conditions, rioted at Kinmel Park transit camp in North Wales where five men were killed.[3] While on Salisbury Plain, at Sling Camp, Bulford, 4600 Australian and New Zealand troops were waiting to return home. Following rioting and looting they were put to work cutting a Kiwi in the chalk hillside.[4]

Wounded Servicemen

TO DEFUSE THE situation the government introduced a more equitable demobilisation scheme early in 1919. As part of this it was agreed returning prisoners of war were to be treated as special cases and released from the military within weeks of their return to Britain. The wounded were also selected for early release: they were entitled to immediate demobilisation once they had recovered sufficiently to be discharged from the military hospital. There was no need to send a man to a VAD hospital to convalesce as he was not needed by the military and would be happier recovering at home in familiar surroundings, therefore the VAD hospitals only received convalescent men who couldn't be treated at home.

The War Office decision to release the wounded from military service and return them to their homes was of course popular and perhaps even seen as generous, but releasing patients also relieved the War Office of their obligations to continue treatment, which passed to the Ministry of Pensions.

The official advice given to military patients from the Ministry of Labour reinforced

---

1 *Wiltshire Times* - 13 March 1920
2 The National Archive - Spotlight on History - *Demobilisation in Britain, 1918-20*
3 BBC Wales Blog - *The Kinmel Camp riots of 1919* – Phil Carradice 4 March 2012
4 *Whanganui Chronicle*. 28 April 2018. Article by Sandi Black, Whanganui Regional Museum New Zealand.

The Story of Chippenham's Red Cross Hospital

Henry Hibberd was classified as no longer fit for military service on his discharge certificate. His ongoing treatment would continue at a civilian hospital

the War Office's desire to discharge as many men as soon as possible;[1] *'If you are sick or wounded get fit to leave hospital. That is all you need to do.'*

By the beginning of 1919 Beaufort War Hospital in Bristol dealt with the last wounded man and in February 1919 it was returned to the civilian authorities, re-establishing its role as a psychiatric unit and renamed Glenside Hospital.

Return to Civilian Life

EVERY TOWN AND village throughout the country was welcoming back its heroes as they were released from the military. The men often arrived still wearing their uniforms[2] and the hope was to return to their civilian lives as quickly as possible.

Amongst the returning men were the recovering wounded, recently discharged from hospitals around the country. Maurice Wicks, a young boy in Hullavington near Chippenham, recalled the soldiers returning to his village at the end of the War:[3]

> Alec Miles coming up past the school in khaki and on crutches, and the other kids saying he was a wounded soldier. Soldiers on the bridges and mother making little rock cakes with lemonade or hops.

For some of these men it would prove impossible to settle back to their old lives. For them there would be lengthy periods of treatment and in some cases coming to terms with disability.

One of these men was Henry Hibberd who returned to Chippenham a disabled man. He had been in various hospitals and was finally discharged in April 1919. In June 1919 he was awarded the Silver War Badge recognising the fact he was considered permanently physically unfit. He and his wife, Alice, continued to live in Chippenham where they brought up a family. Henry found work with a local coal merchant.[4]

Some Chippenham Patients

IN CHIPPENHAM PATIENT numbers dwindled. Men had often asked to be treated closer to their homes and, as there were now far fewer patients, requests to transfer were treated sympathetically.

Forty-one year old William Chivers was discharged from Chippenham VAD Hospital on 6 December 1918. He had enlisted with the Royal Engineers in June 1916

---

1 *Western Daily Press* – 20 December 1918. A Ministry of Labour guide. This was later amended to apply to men who had been in hospital for at least 23 days.
2 While on final leave the man was still technically a soldier and could wear his uniform. He was given a form Z50 to take to his nearest railway station to hand in his army greatcoat. For this he was paid £.1.
3 *Hullavington Memories* –Maurice Wicks
4 *1939 Census*- lived at Sandbrook Place Chippenham

The Story of Chippenham's Red Cross Hospital

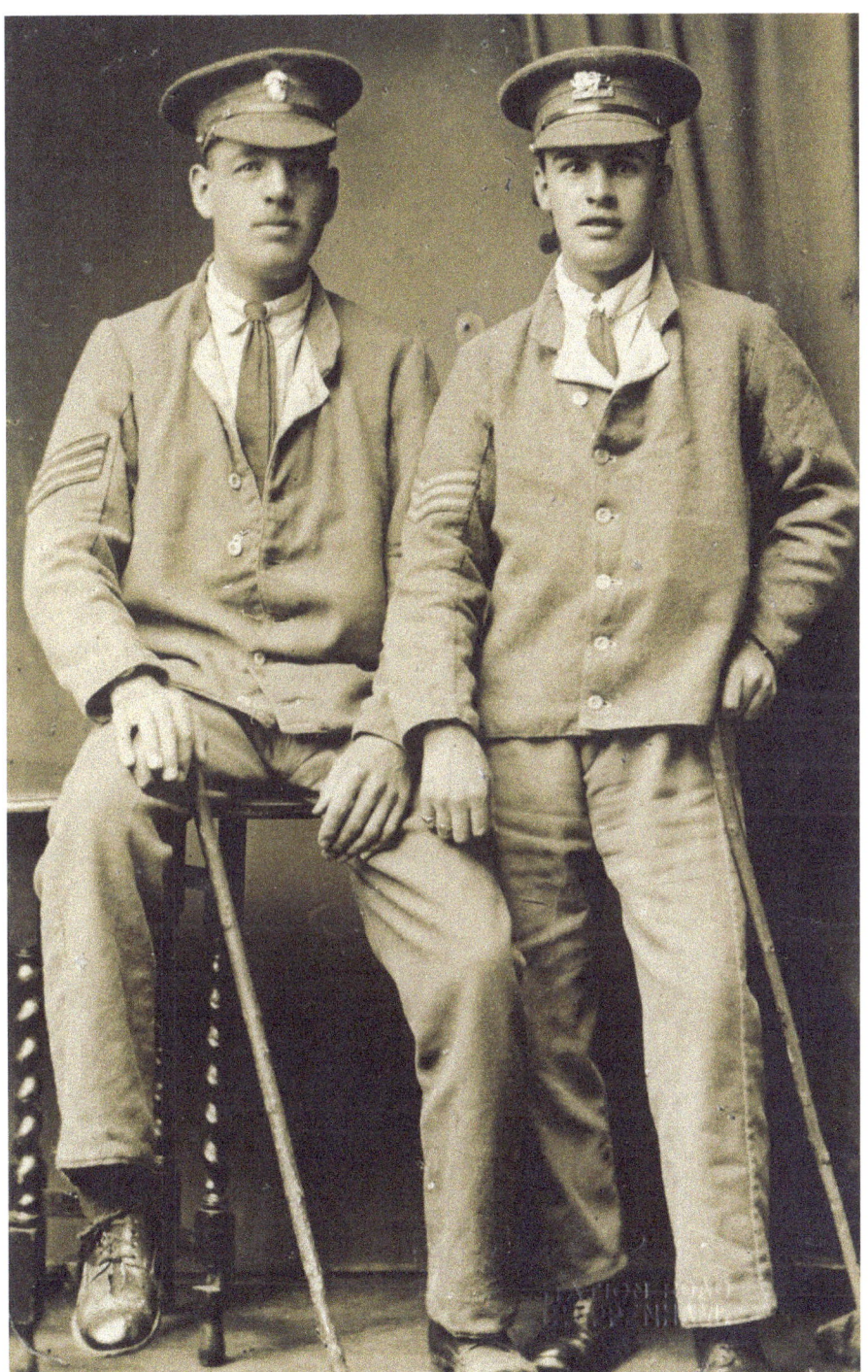

Two sergeants at Chippenham awaiting their discharge from the military.

Unity and Loyalty

and had suffered wounds in action and consequently was awarded a Silver War Badge.

He returned to his family in nearby East Tytherton, where he took up work as a boot maker.[1]

Some of the other local men to be treated as in-patients at Chippenham were Ernest Webb of Lacock,[2] Oliver Pearce of Bremhill,[3] William Thompson who lived in Westmead Lane and Fred Evans of Ashfield Road in Chippenham.

Fred Evans, was employed as a newspaper boy before the War. In 1915 he joined the Wiltshire Yeomanry and saw service with a number of regiments. In 1918 he was injured in Salonika and by November, just as the Armistice was signed, he was invalided home. After his treatment at Chippenham he was discharged in the spring of 1919.

On discharge he returned to his pre-war employer, Wyman's newsagents, who had bookstalls at Chippenham and Bath stations.[4] In 1922 he became the manager of the Chippenham bookstall, where he stayed for fifteen years, until he opened his own paper shop in Chippenham in 1937.

The end of the War also meant changes for William Edwards. William and his family lived in Hornsey in London and he joined the Army in February 1915 seeing service in Egypt. By November of that year he was sick, possibly having contracted Typhus and found himself a patient at Chippenham. His medical condition meant that he was unfit for further war service and, therefore, he was discharged from the military.

Rather than returning home to London, he decided to stay in Chippenham and took a job as the VAD Hospital handyman. In 1919, as it closed, he found himself unemployed but was offered a job as Dr and Mrs Wilsons chauffeur.[5] He accepted the position and arranged for his family to move to Chippenham And they settled in St Mary Street.

During the 1920s Dr Wilson retired and had a villa built in Corsica where he, his wife and daughter spent every winter. Each year they would close their house in St Mary Street and arrange for all their staff, including the chauffeur, to join them in Corsica.[6]

William Edwards remained with the Wilsons until 1933, when Doctor Wilson died. He went on to work for Tilley & Culverwell and Westinghouse, previously Saxby and Farmer, until he retired.

As men left the VAD Hospital there was the opportunity to think about a new future. In January 1919 William Troll, of the Northumberland Fusiliers,

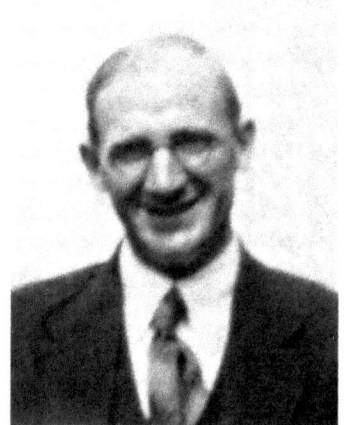

William Troll

1. *1939 census*
2. Lacock History Society
3. David Wood - Bremhill History Society
4. Chippenham Museum – *Miscellaneous scrapbook* - Retirement of Fred Evans
5. *Wiltshire Times* - 17 February 1951 Obituary W T Edwards
6. Chippenham Museum - *Garlick Scrapbooks*. News cutting 11 August 1983.

The Story of Chippenham's Red Cross Hospital

found himself in Chippenham recovering from gunshot wounds to his arm. He had joined the Army in August 1917, aged 18, and described himself as an office clerk on his enlistment papers.

During his stay at Chippenham he became passionate about plans for a war memorial in his home town of Millom, near Barrow-in-Furness. He wrote to his local newspaper, the Millom Gazette,[1] from his hospital bed, concerned that the town couldn't decide what to do to honour his dead comrades. He wrote: '*Now Millom, what are you going to in the matter? Remember it concerns the whole population of Millom.*'

He advocated a public institution, such as a swimming pool or park, be provided to benefit the public and improve the social life of the community. After discharge from Chippenham William decided to give up his career as a clerk and devote his life to the community. He studied theology at Spurgeons College in Croydon and became a Baptist minister in Millom.[2]

A number of Australian patients were at Chippenham at the end of the War. One of them was Vincent Boreham, a Lance Corporal with the Australian 7th Field Company Engineers, who had been admitted to Beaufort War Hospital in Bristol in September 1918. He had enlisted with the Australian Imperial Force in June 1917, when he gave his occupation as an accountant and lived in Sydney.

He was transferred from Beaufort to Chippenham as the Armistice was signed. Whilst recovering at Chippenham he was given leave to break the hospital routine.[3] He left for a few days in London, but during his leave he was diagnosed with Trench Fever; the symptoms being a sudden high fever and severe headache. He was admitted to Endell Street Military Hospital in London for a week and when discharged remained in London continuing his military service in the Army Records Section. He finally returned to Australia in January 1920 on the ship 'Aeneas' and was demobilised on 11 February 1920. In 1922 he married Eleanor Boylson and they continued to live in New South Wales. Vincent died in 1953 in the Sydney suburb of Manly.[4]

Another Australian, Arthur Ashmead, was wounded in April 1918 and arrived at Chippenham in June 1918 having spent time at various military hospitals, including Beaufort, recovering from his wounds. By the time he arrived at Chippenham his injuries were healing, but he was suffering from laryngitis and debility as he had also been the victim of mustard gas poisoning. On 18 November 1918 he returned to Australia still suffering from the debilitating effects of the gas attack. He was discharged from the military some months later. When he died in 1948 his death was attributed to his war service and his grave is now recognised as a war grave.[5]

Throughout Chippenham Division VADs were saying goodbye to patients as they were discharged from the services. A Melksham patient Fred Pullin was a well-known

---

1   *Millom Gazette* - 31 January 1919
2   Margaret Troll
3   Ann Brinkworth research notes
4   Australia index to deceased estates.
5   The University of New South Wales - *The AIF Project*.

Unity and Loyalty

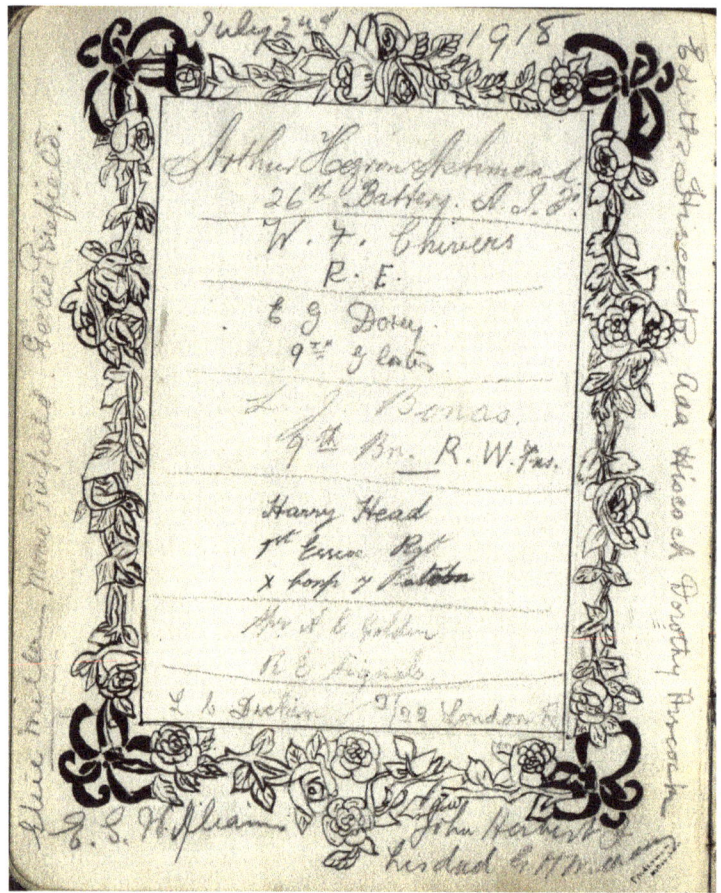

A page from an autograph album dated July 1918. Amongst signatures are Arthur Ashmead and William Chivers, both discharged from Chippenham after the Armistice.

entertainer and on his release he returned to the stage. He joined the Dinkies Concert Party, who were described as a Group of London Artistes providing a 'Merry Mixture of Mirth and Melody.'[1] In March 1919 he returned to Melksham with the Dinkies to entertain his old friends in the town.[2]

Wilts War Pensions Committee

A S DISCHARGED WOUNDED men returned to their homes in Wiltshire it fell to the Ministry of Pensions and the Wilts War Pensions Committee to arrange their continued medical treatment. For men like Alec Miles, William Chivers and Henry Hibberd the Chippenham Cottage Hospital would provide that care.

1 *Thanet Advertiser* – 7 June 1919 Review of the Dinkies
2 *Wiltshire Times* – 1 March 1919

The Story of Chippenham's Red Cross Hospital

The Cottage Hospital had been treating wounded ex-servicemen with the assistance of the VADs since early 1918, but as the War was now over the numbers of discharged men in need of treatment swelled.

The Wilts War Pensions Committee had overall responsibility for the ex-servicemen in the county and they saw the demand for out-patient treatment grow dramatically. By April 1919 nearly 4000 men classified as disabled or in need of treatment had returned to their homes in Wiltshire.[1] In October 1919 the number of men requiring treatment had almost doubled with 7370[2] on the register. The local hospitals in Wiltshire, including Chippenham Cottage Hospital, said their existing facilities simply were not adequate and they could not deal with such an influx.

The Wilts War Pensions Committee, chaired by Lady Radnor, met in January 1919 to discuss how they could provide suitable additional facilities to treat the disabled and injured.

The central item on the agenda was the shortage of money available to help the civilian hospitals deal with so many additional patients. There had been some suggestions nationally that the Red Cross should be able to continue to provide the facilities to treat disabled men and that voluntary donations from the public should be sought. It was also debated in the House of Commons that donations be requested from other charitable trusts such as the Kings Fund to help the war wounded:[3] The Kings Fund had originally been established in 1897 to maintain voluntary hospitals in London.

The suggestion of seeking donations and help from voluntary organisations to treat war heroes was contentious and for many County War Pensions Committees it was considered wholly unacceptable. In Liverpool the Wallasey War Pension Committee felt so strongly they wrote to the Ministry of Pensions saying it should be the responsibility of the state to provide for the war disabled, making the point, that many agreed with: *'anything else had a taint of charity about it and the men deserved better.'*

The Wilts War Pensions Committee agreed with the sentiment and decided not to request help from charitable organisations for the treatment of ex-servicemen although they did make the point that to refuse the offer of help, especially from the VAD hospitals in the county, would be detrimental to the disabled men, saying: *With so many of the VAD hospitals closing the rather serious question arose as to where disabled men were to get efficient treatment. In a great number of cases massage treatment was necessary.*[4]

Many of the discharged wounded men returning to their homes were orthopaedic cases, having suffered gunshot and shrapnel injuries, and part of their care was specialised massage treatment.

1 *Wiltshire Times* - 12 April 1919
2 *Wiltshire Times* - 29 November 1919
3 Founded as the Prince of Wales's Hospital Fund for London in 1897. In 1907, Parliament incorporated the fund as the King's Fund. The fund was originally set up to contribute to London's voluntary hospitals
4 *Wiltshire Times* – 11 January 1919

Unity and Loyalty

Basil Hankey told the Wilts War Pensions Committee that in Chippenham where the VAD Hospital had specialised in orthopaedic cases, the Red Cross were quite prepared to assist by providing a room for out-patients receiving massage treatment whilst it remained open.

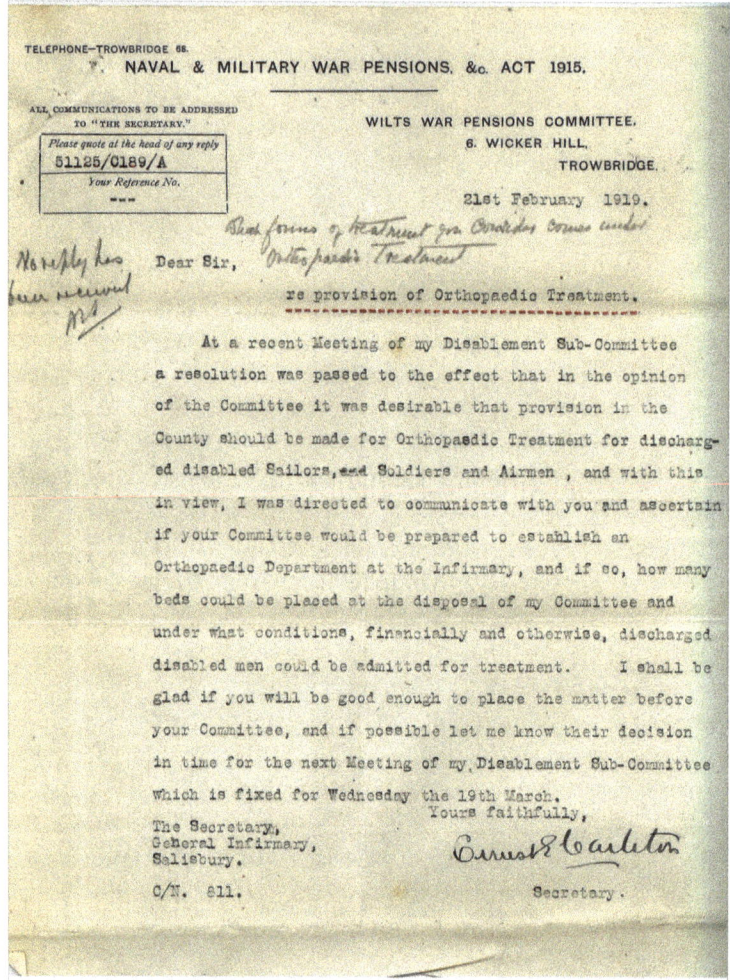

Letter from the Wilts War Pensions Committee to Salisbury Infirmary asking they treat disabled servicemen. A similar letter was sent to Chippenham Cottage Hospital

This offer of help was gratefully accepted, but a more permanent solution was needed. The Secretary of the Wilts War Pensions Committee was asked to write to Swindon Hospital, Salisbury Infirmary, and Chippenham Cottage Hospital to ask that they consider opening their own orthopaedic departments to treat the men returning to Wiltshire.

The Story of Chippenham's Red Cross Hospital

Chippenham Cottage Hospital acknowledged the help they had received from the Red Cross, but responded to the letter saying that to accept further orthopaedic cases they needed more money for specialist staff, treatment rooms and equipment. The Wilts War Pensions Committee said the only solution was to apply to the Ministry of Pensions for a grant, which was a lengthy process as so many Committees were applying for help.

The Chippenham Cottage Hospital Board decided not to wait for the Ministry of Pensions, but saw another opportunity to apply for financial help. Now the War was over and the VAD hospitals were closing the National Joint War Committee found it had surplus reserves of one million pounds. It was decided to use the fund to award grants to institutions who provided help to ex-servicemen in need of medical care.

Chippenham Cottage Hospital, who of course were already treating some war wounded, applied for and received a grant of £1000, under the category of a civilian hospital maintained by subscribed funds whose patients include ex-servicemen.[1]

The Wilts War Pensions Committee were able to secure additional funds to assist with the cost of renting rooms to treat patients and the Ministry of Pensions agreed they would meet the cost of employing specialist masseurs.[2] As a result a number of orthopaedic centres were opened around the county to provide physiotherapy and electrical massage therapy.

During the War a Massage Corps was formed to provide specially trained masseurs in military and VAD hospitals.[3] In Wiltshire there were a number of VADs who were trained and suitably qualified to provide massage therapy. Beatrice Houlston,

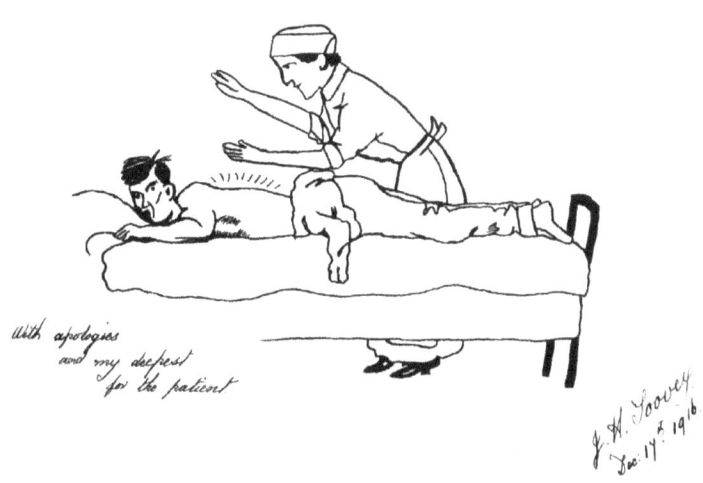

A patient's view of orthopaedic treatment

1 *Wiltshire Times* - 20 September 1919
2 *Wiltshire Times* – 22 February 1919
3 The Almeric Paget Military Massage Corps

the daughter of Robert Houlston, who owned the stationers in Chippenham High Street, had undertaken the appropriate training and was proficient in Swedish and Electrical massage.[1] She treated the men at the VAD hospitals in Chippenham, Calne, Bowood and Corsham. Mr Hankey told the Wilts War Pensions Committee that she was also available to travel to Malmesbury and Swindon to treat men in those towns.

Beatrice Houlston continued with her work after the hospitals closed as part of the Ministry of Pension's commitment to provide staff. A room in the Town Hall was rented for a short time and became a temporary massage treatment room later moving to the Drill Hall in Bath Road.[2]

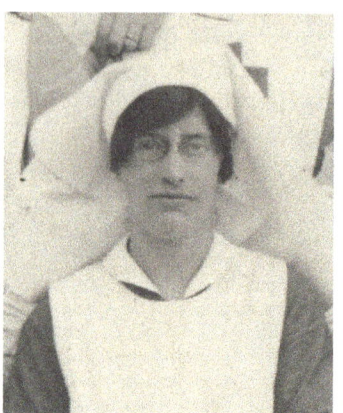

Beatrice Houlston

By November 1920 a permanent treatment room had been established in the Jubilee Institute in the Market Place. Dr Laurence told the Town Council that the disabled ex-servicemen attending for treatment told him that they often found the stairs in the building difficult and would find a handrail of great help. Dr Laurence's request was agreed to and the surveyor was authorised to undertake the work of fitting a handrail.[3]

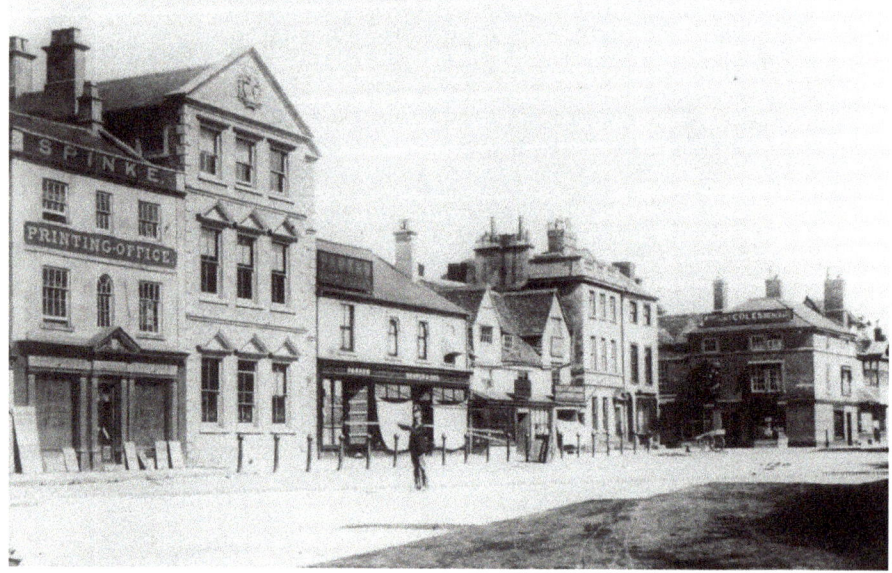

The Jubilee Institute, next to Spinke printing office. The upper floors of the Institute were used as treatment rooms for injured ex-servicemen.

1   The British Red Cross Society - VAD index card record
2   *Wiltshire Times* - 29 November 1919
3   *Chippenham Council minute book 10* - 11 November 1920

Chapter 18
The VAD Hospital Closes

Peace returns to Chippenham

EVERYBODY WANTED TO get back to a pre-war normality. Saxby and Farmer returned to peacetime production and restrictions were lifted.

The Belgians who had settled in the town started to return to their homeland. They remembered the kindness shown by the VADs and the people of the town. Mademoiselle Penniniez placed an advert in the Wiltshire Times expressing her *'sincere gratitude for the great kindness which they (the residents of Chippenham) have shown her from the first moment she obtained refuge among them.*

Chippenham Town Council wanted to reclaim the Town and Neeld Halls as quickly as possible to use for town business. At the beginning of 1919 they raised the matter with the Red Cross and in February Mr Hankey responded, saying a definitive date could not be given to close the VAD Hospital. He went on to say the Ministry of Pensions may make an application to continue to use the Town Hall, on behalf of the War Office, for returning prisoners of war who needed treatment.

The Council's response was that they would be unable to approve such a request as they thought it was important to bring the halls back into public use as soon as possible.[1] It was even suggested the War Office were making every effort to close their own hospitals, at the expense of authorities like Chippenham.

By early March 1919 the Southern Command at Bristol still hadn't agreed a date, but Basil Hankey was able to tell the Council it was likely the Town and Neeld halls would only be needed for a few weeks longer. When the Councillors pressed Mr Hankey he said he could not be precise as he was waiting for a decision. Mr Alderman Neale proposed that a meeting should be arranged as soon as possible between Mr Hankey, a representative of the Military and members of the Council to agree a firm date to hand the halls back.[2]

By the end of the month the matter had still had not been resolved and the Councillors were becoming increasingly frustrated. The eventual response was that Southern Command were unable to send a suitable representative to meet with the Council but wrote:[3]

---

1 *Chippenham Council minute book 9*
2 *Chippenham Council minute book 9 - 4 March 1919*
3 *Wiltshire Times - 5 April 1919 Report of the Council meeting.*

Unity and Loyalty

Whilst they appreciated the desire to obtain the use of the hall for the town, they feared that in view of the scarcity of beds in the district it would not be possible immediately to release the use of the hall, though that would be done as soon as circumstances permitted.

This response was unacceptable to the Council, especially as neighbouring Gloucestershire had reached an agreement to close all their Red Cross hospitals by the end of March. Melksham had also closed its VAD Hospital during March and even Beaufort Military Hospital in Bristol, where many of the patients at Chippenham had originated, closed during February 1919.

The military authority's letter was challenged by the Town Clerk and within days there was a change of heart when it was agreed there was no need to retain the Hospital and it would close.

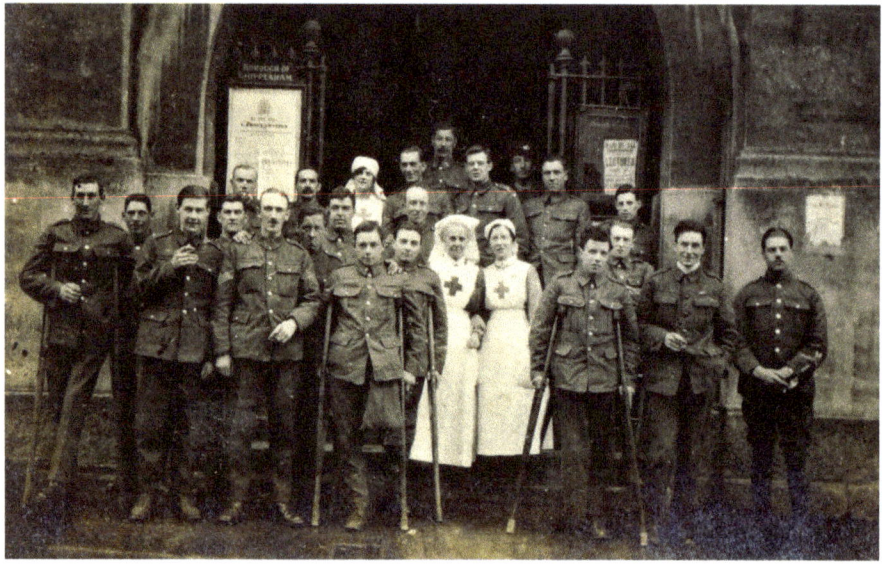

The final convoy to leave the Hospital

Returning the Halls.

ARRANGEMENTS WERE RAPIDLY made for patients to be transferred or discharged and, on 8 April 1919, the final convoy of patients was despatched. The men were transported to the railway station where the VADs and friends from the town were waiting to give the men a good send-off.

With no patients the task of removing the equipment and making good any alterations started.

Items that were on loan were returned to their owners and Mrs Wilson arranged

The Story of Chippenham's Red Cross Hospital

an auction sale on 30 April to dispose of the equipment acquired over the previous three and a half years. Amongst the items listed for sale were:[1]

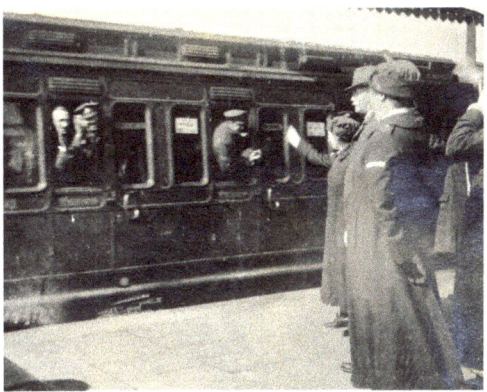

> Bedsteads, mattresses, bolsters, pillows, Blankets and linen.
> 3 large modern gas cookers, described as suitable for a hotel or restaurant, and tea urns, cooking utensils, kitchen, tableware and cutlery
> Lockers, bedside cupboards, screens and invalid bed tables
> 2 Gramophones
> A library of books
> A number of porcelain lined baths and fittings

The VADs say goodbye to the patients at the station

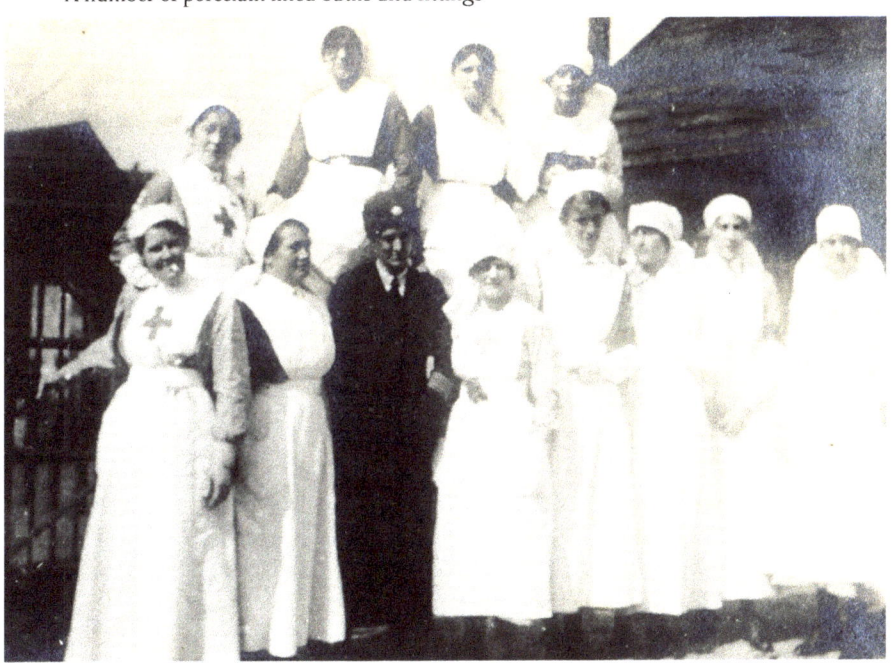

A group of VADs on the last day

It was decided by the Divisional Red Cross Committee that some of the furniture and equipment should not be sold, but would be put aside for use by the Cottage Hospital,

---

1 *Wiltshire Times* – 19 April 1919

Unity and Loyalty

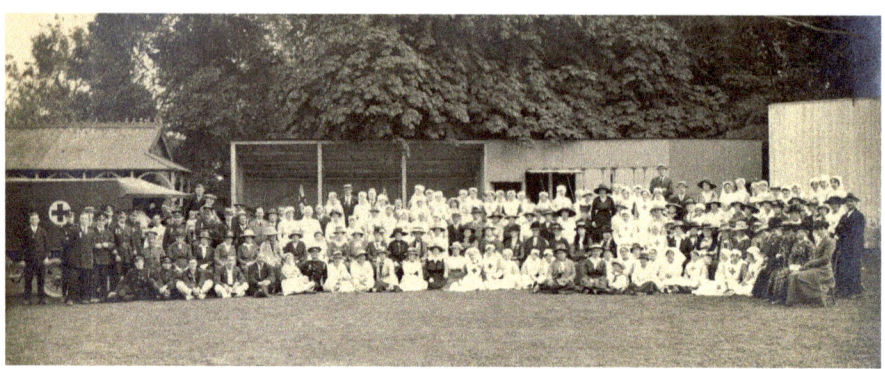

VADs, Ambulance section and helpers probably at the closure of the Hospital

where the Management Committee had for some time been planning a new wing and the surplus items were thought to be suitable to equip it. Mrs Wilson also told the Committee that the Red Cross had agreed any profit realised after the auction would be donated towards the cost of their new wing.[1]

Chippenham and Corsham Detachments also had surplus ambulances and it was proposed these would be best used by the Union Workhouse in Chippenham.[2]

With all the equipment removed from the Town and Neeld halls remedial building work could start. Alterations carried out by the Red Cross had to be made good to bring them back to their original condition. The bathrooms and kitchen in the Corn Exchange were dismantled and temporary treatment rooms demolished. A number of modifications added by the Red Cross, such as the toilets and the corridor between the halls, were considered improvements by the Town Council and were retained.[3] The halls were handed back in May 1919 and the final financial settlement was agreed between the Red Cross and the Council in November 1919.

Before Mrs Wilson handed the halls back she organised a reunion for all those VADs and volunteers who had served throughout the war years. She told the gathering that the Detachment would continue its good work and offer first aid classes and lectures to volunteers, as they had before the War, and she would continue to lead as its Commandant.

Some of the VADs, including the Belcher and Spinke sisters and Mrs Hulbert, continued with their work in the Detachment and helped it return to its peacetime role. Lady Margaret Spicer remained as Vice President of the Division for many years. For many of the volunteers, cooks, kitchen workers, nurses, porters and stretcher bearers however it was time to demobilise and leave the Red Cross.

In the final days before it closed small souvenirs were taken. A blind eye was turned as blankets and tea towels disappeared. A group of young VAD nurses each took a

---

1   *Wiltshire Times* – 3 May 1919. Annual meeting of the Cottage Hospital Management Committee
2   *Wiltshire Times* – 6 September 1919 Board of Guardians monthly meeting
3   *Chippenham Council minute book 10* - 6 May 1919

The Story of Chippenham's Red Cross Hospital

tablecloth and asked friends and patients to write messages on them. Some of the VADs embroidered the messages and the tablecloths became treasured keepsakes.[1]

Once the halls were handed back it seemed appropriate that one of the first public events in the Neeld Hall was the Peace Day celebration in July 1919,[2] when 450 discharged soldiers and sailors were entertained for lunch followed by dancing in the evening.

At the closing of the VAD Hospital there were many words of praise for the Commandant and staff. The local newspapers wrote about the selfless attitude of both the staff and people of Chippenham:[3]

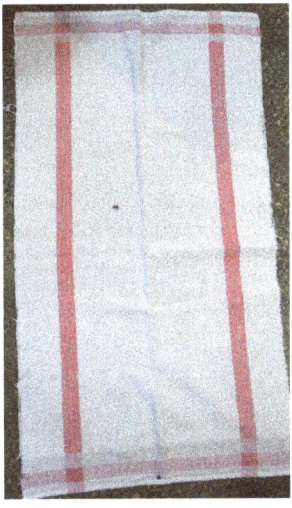

A tea towel taken from the hospital when it closed

> During the time the Hospital was open 1872 patients were admitted, men belonging to all parts of Great Britain and Ireland and from all parts of our scattered dominions, who will make the name of Chippenham known, and will express their gratitude for the skilful and gentle treatment they received from the medical staff, the Commandant, and the nurses at the Chippenham Hospital, and the efforts made by the townspeople to brighten their lives and make them feel thoroughly at home.

Vote of Thanks

IN MAY 1919 the Mayor, Edwin Bowker, said it was only right and proper for the Council to pass a vote of thanks to the Commandant and her staff and he said about those who served the Hospital:[4]

> I cannot speak too highly of the whole staff for their self-sacrifice and devotion, and they had carried out their duties with a spirit of cheerfulness and kindness which had a very beneficial effect on the patients, who would never forget the great attention bestowed upon them by the nurses.

The minutes of the meeting recorded:[5]

> The Council on behalf of the town, should recognise the very valuable work which had

1 The family of VAD Fanny Ferris told how the tablecloth was a treasured memory and regularly used.
2 *Western Daily Press* - 21 July 1919
3 Chippenham Museum - *Garlick Scrapbooks*
4 *Wiltshire Times* – 10 May 1919
5 *Chippenham Council minute book 10*

been carried on at the Hospital and he moved that the best thanks be offered to Mrs Wilson, the Commandant and all who were associated with her in the work, for their services. He also proposed that the town Clerk be asked to have a vote of thanks printed in sufficient numbers to enable the commandant to distribute them among the whole of the staff.

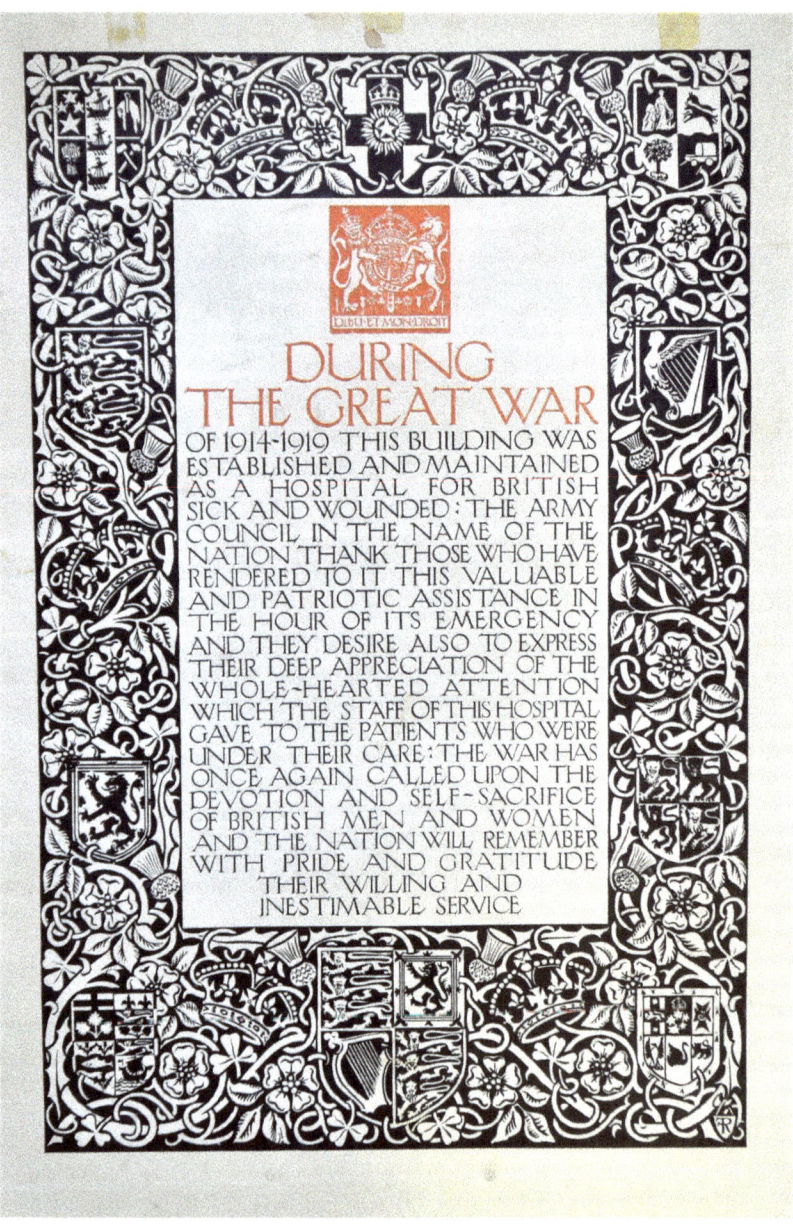

The Testimonial from the War Office

The Story of Chippenham's Red Cross Hospital

The following year it was decided to have a photograph of all the VADS who served at the Hospital hung in the Town Hall as tribute to their work during the War. Councillor Hyatt was given the task of finding a suitable photograph, but in November 1920 he said it was impossible to find a photo of the full complement of VADs. It was suggested that a suitable alternative would be a roll of those who served to be displayed in the Town Hall beside the testimonial received from the War Office. This proposal was rejected by the Town Council. It is not known why.

Awards and Honours

As well as being thanked by the Town Council the VADs were honoured by the Red Cross when on 23 December 1918 Lady Spicer presented Honourable Service and Red Cross Service Certificates. The presentation took place in the Neeld Hall with the patients present. Lady Spicer said to the men and women of the Red Cross at Chippenham:[1]

> ....they (the certificates) will serve to remind you in years to come of what you did in the Great War, and also of the happy days you spent in this hospital. I cannot let this occasion pass without congratulating you all from the Commandant downwards on the way you have worked since this hospital has been opened.
>
> You have all nobly upheld the traditions of the Red Cross. These traditions are symbolised by the badges you wear – the badge of the Great International League of Love and Pity. Perhaps this will be the last time I shall address you before you are demobilised. I am sure you will be very sorry when that day comes, but you will go back to your home life feeling that you have done all that you can to help the soldiers who fought for you in the Great War.

The recipients of cards of honourable service that day were:

Helena J Wilson - Commandant
Mervyn S Wilson, George Laurence - Medical officers
Elizabeth Hulbert - Lady Superintendent
Evelyn Belcher - Quartermaster
Phyllis R Whishaw - Assistant Commandant
Beatrice Houlston - Masseuse
Francis Read - Commandant Wilts 13 (men)
Janet Awdry - Nurse
Nora Collen, Ellen Hardiman, Mabel Tuck, Joan Coventry, Dora Hart, Alice Coward - Staff Nurses
M L Shipp, Ethel Williams - Head cook

[1] *Wiltshire Times* - 28 December 1918

Unity and Loyalty

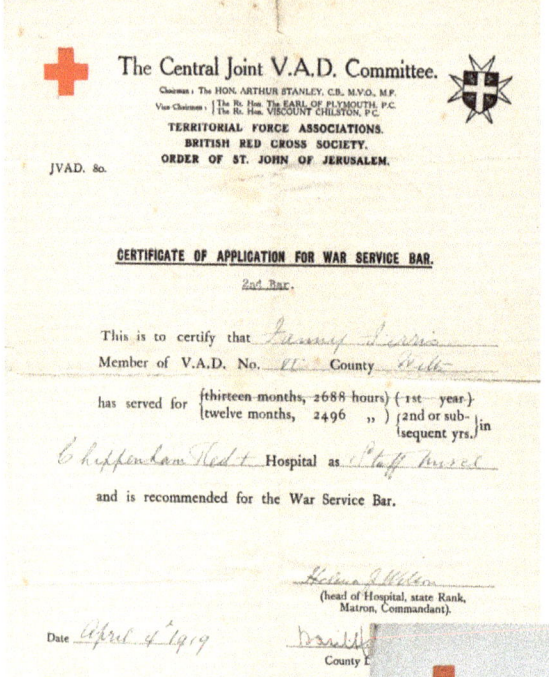

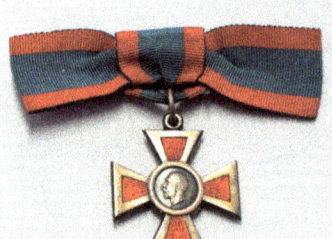

top: War Service Bar awarded to Fanny Ferris in April 1919.

above: Royal Red Cross, 2nd Class, awarded to Ellen Hardiman

right: Ivy Gladstone's Testimonial for her work as a member of the VAD

The Story of Chippenham's Red Cross Hospital

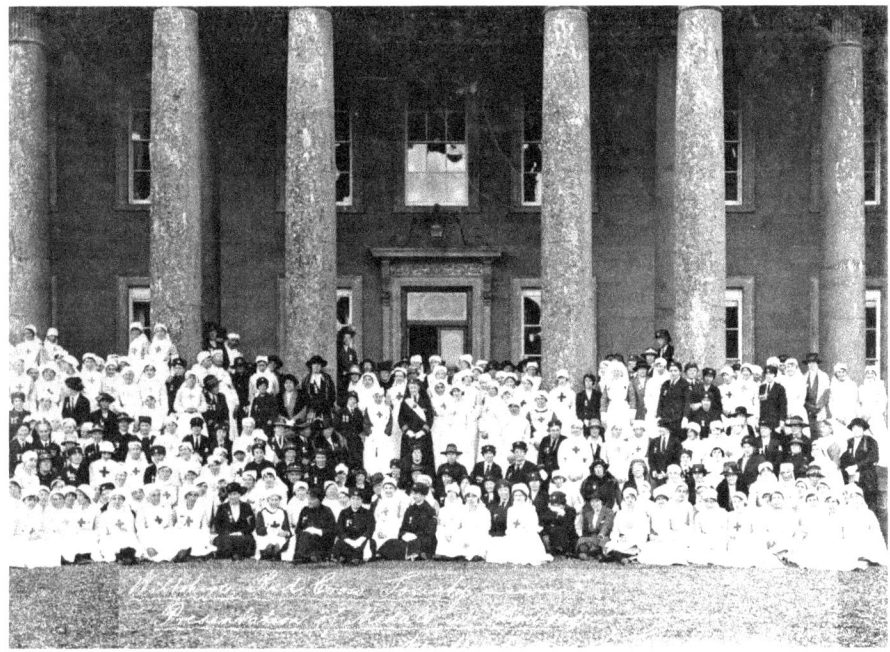

Wiltshire VADs gather at Bowood to receive their medals

Eva Webb, Ivy Gladstone, Elinor Davis - Cooks

Mabel Spinke, Ellen Cornish, Lila Farries, Beryl Wilson - General Service

Mrs Barnes, Mrs Gladstone, Mrs Heath and Miss F L Lane - Red Cross Needlework

The recipients of badges for five-year service:

Olive and Ivy Gladstone, Miss Ferris, Miss Hart, Mrs Shorland, Miss Coventry, Elsie Watts, Mrs Wheeler, Daisy Pope, Mrs Slade and Mrs Malpas.

There were further gatherings where certificates were awarded to VADs, including Mrs Hinton and Mrs Hardiman, who were also mentioned in dispatches.[1]

The Army Council paid a tribute, which was printed and distributed to all members by the Joint VAD Committee.

In August 1919 Eleanor Countess of Suffolk and Ellen Hardiman were awarded the Royal Red Cross second class Medal.[2] Ellen Hardiman was presented with her decoration by the King at Buckingham Palace in July 1920.

Evelyn Belcher, the Quartermaster, was awarded the newly established M.B.E in January 1918 for her services to the Red Cross.[3] On hearing the news Mrs Wilson said:[4]

1   Chippenham Museum – *Ivy Gladstone Scrapbook*
2   *Supplement to the London Gazette* – 6 August 1919. The Countess was described as a nurse at Chippenham Hospital.
3   *Supplement to the London Gazette* – 7 January 1918
4   Chippenham Museum – *Ivy Gladstone Scrapbook*

Unity and Loyalty

Myself, the staff and patients feel proud and delighted that Miss Belcher has received this mark of Royal recognition. She has worked very hard for the Hospital and thoroughly deserves the honour.

A year later Helena Wilson was awarded a well-deserved O.B.E. for her work as Commandant.[1]

In April 1922 over 400 VADs from Wiltshire gathered at Bowood House to receive their Red Cross medals. The medals were awarded to members who had given over 1000 hours service during the War. Chippenham was well represented with 56 ladies from Wilts 6 VAD and 13 men from Wilts 13 VAD receiving awards.[2] Lady Lansdowne also gave a signed a photograph as a mark of her thanks.

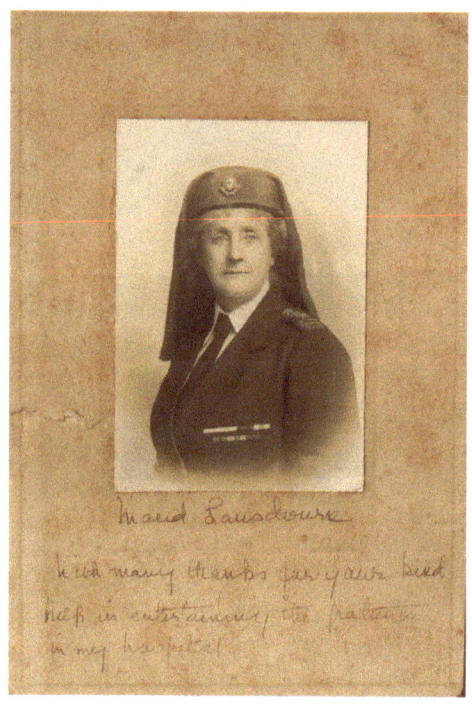

Lady Lansdowne gave signed photos as a personal thanks

1   *Supplement to the London Gazette* – 8 January 1919
2   *Wiltshire Times* – 29 April 1922

Chapter 19
A New World for the VADs

Social Changes

BY THE TIME the hospitals closed their doors the world had become a very different place to that of five years earlier. Many of the traditional society values had been broken.

Unlike the early days of the war VADs came from all social classes. They had shared untold experiences, cried and laughed together, and worked as equals. Close friendships had been made as maids worked next to the gentry. Ivy Gladstone, a member of Wiltshire aristocracy, kept a scrap book of hospital memories. The photos and comments tell of happy times between patients and staff from all backgrounds.

For four years the country had depended on women to keep the wheels of industry turning and the hospitals staffed. As peace returned legislation had been introduced to

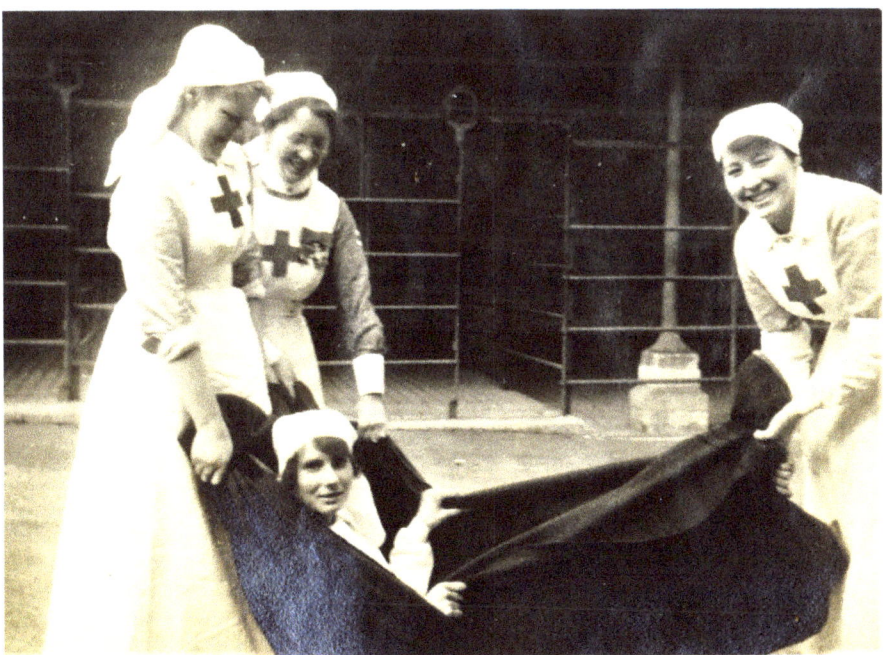

VADs enjoying themselves. The wife of a railway worker, the daughters of a draper, a solicitor and a baronet.

give votes to women and they were reluctant to give up their new found independence, relishing the responsibility they had been trusted with during the War.

A young Wiltshire woman, Winifred Spencer, recalled the attitude: [1]

> The papers were beginning to say we were winning the war and there was talk about what will women want now and reporters praising women's war work saying they could never go back to doing just housework. That idea didn't last long I'm afraid.

At Chippenham, a VAD wrote some years after the War of her experiences. Like most women she was expected to return to her domestic routine, but showed her frustration when she wrote '*I just couldn't go back to my ordinary life.*' [2]

For some who left the VAD in 1919 a future career in medicine seemed inviting. Ladies with VAD experience advertised for positions in the medical profession. The Western Daily Press included the following classifieds under its Dentistry section:

> Doctors daughter, age 30, former VAD seeks post as Dentist's Attendant or similar position.
>
> VAD (nursing) requires position as Dental Attendant.

The Joint War Committee recognised there were many capable VADs who had gained expertise and had a desire to continue their work during peacetime. The Committee financed a Scholarship Scheme in 1919 to train VADs in various areas of medicine.[3] Over 500 scholarships were awarded, but these were not popular with the medical profession as some considered it an easy option.

In Chippenham some of the VADs did continue in the medical profession.

Beatrice Houlston, continuing to work as a masseuse after the War, was eventually employed by the Health Authority in Bath and was still working in 1939.[4]

Phyllis Ramsbottom, a VAD at Chippenham and the daughter of the vicar of Lacock, trained to become a midwife. She emigrated to South Africa where it is thought she continued her work. Perhaps Phyllis felt that something positive needed come out of the War as her brother William had been killed in 1918.

Mary Jones, who grew up in Cardiff, became a VAD in 1915 and worked in a number of auxiliary hospitals between 1915 and 1919. Like Beatrice Houlston and Phyllis Ramsbottom, she decided to continue her medical career at the end of the War and went to the Royal United Hospital in Bath to qualify. After several moves around the country, and gaining further qualifications, she was appointed matron at Chippenham Cottage

---

[1] *Winifred, a Wiltshire working girl* – Sylvia Marlow
[2] Chippenham Museum. An article written by an anonymous writer describing Chippenham, possibly written in 1940s as part of a carnival programme.
[3] *The British Red Cross in Action* – Dame Beryl Oliver.
[4] *1939 Census*

The Story of Chippenham's Red Cross Hospital

Hospital in 1928 where she remained until she retired in 1940.[1]

Romance

IT WAS INEVITABLE that relationships would blossom at the hospitals. Men and women were in daily contact, both as volunteers working together and as patient and nurse.

William King had been a member of the men's Detachment at Chippenham until he left to serve in the Army in 1916. He worked alongside Edith Young, who was a VAD at both Corsham and Chippenham. When he was demobilised in 1919 he returned to Chippenham and the family ironmongers business in New Road. He and Edith married in 1923,[2] settling in St Pauls Street in Chippenham.

Lily Witts, who lived in Parliament Street, was a part time helper. During 1918 Edward Granger, who originally came from Chippenham, arrived at the Hospital having been wounded in Salonika. He had joined the Wiltshire Regiment in 1915 but later transferred to the Royal Dublin Fusiliers.

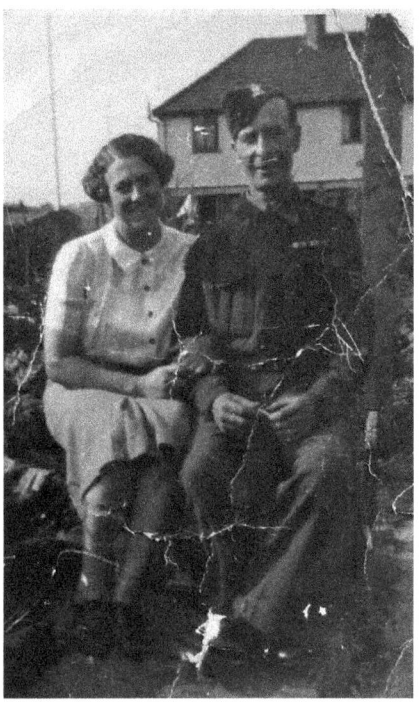

Lily Witts and Edward Granger during the Second World War

Lily Witts and Edward Granger married in 1921 in Chippenham, later moving to Calne.

Hereward Morley was a student at the University of London. In 1915 he joined the 1st London Regiment. Little is known about his service but by 1916 he was a patient in Chippenham and was awarded a Silver War Badge to let the public know the he had given military service but was unfit to continue and was not a shirker. Hereward later joined the Post Office in London.[3]

After leaving the Hospital he remained in touch with Beatrice Houlston, the masseuse, and in 1933 they married. The Wiltshire Times took up the story:[4]

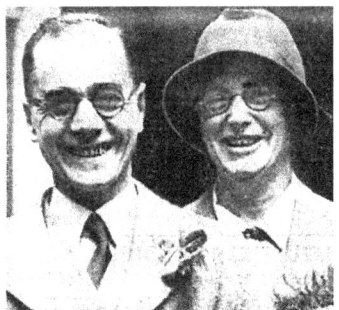

Hereward Morley and Beatrice Houlston on their wedding day in 1933

1   *Wiltshire Times* – 23 November 1940
2   *Wiltshire Times* - 26 May 1923
3   *London Gazette* – 7 January 1927
4   *Wiltshire Times* – 9 December 1933

Unity and Loyalty

The Marriage in London on Saturday of Miss Beatrice Houlston of the Market Place Chippenham and Mr Hereward Morley, a native of London marks the culmination of a war time romance. This started at the Chippenham Red Cross Hospital in 1916 when Mr Morley was a wounded soldier and Miss Houlston was a member of VAD staff at the temporary Hospital.

The newspaper went on to say '*after a short honeymoon Mrs Morley will return to work at Chippenham.*'

The couple settled in Bath, where Hereward remained with the Post Office and Beatrice continued her work as a masseuse.[1]

Gladys Treweke, who lived in Ashfield Road with her parents, worked at Saxby and Farmer making munitions. She was a member of the company's theatrical group, who entertained the men. She also assisted serving teas and meals to the patients in her spare time.

In early 1917 David Bullion, one the first orthopaedic patients from Beaufort Hospital, arrived at Chippenham. During his lengthy convalescence he and Gladys became good friends and when he left to return to his regiment they agreed to keep in touch.

On his demobilisation David Bullion returned to his native Scotland and later emigrated to Canada. David and Gladys continued to correspond and, on his trips back to Britain he visited her in Chippenham. During the summer of 1925 the couple married in Chippenham and they left for a new life in America where they settled in Dearborn, near Detroit.[2]

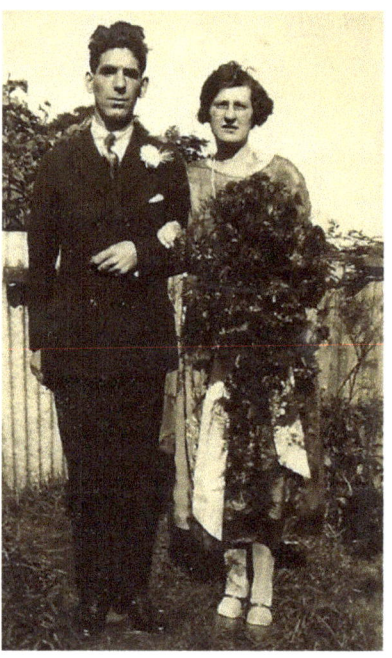

Gladys Treweke and David Bullion married in Chippenham in 1925

As the War ended Olive Gladstone, who had worked tirelessly as a cook at the VAD hospitals, announced her marriage to Major Robert Lindsay Loyd, the son of the former MP for Abingdon. The wedding took place in March 1919 at Bowden Hill Church. It was a 'Society' wedding with Bishop Browne, the former Bishop of Bristol, performing the Ceremony.

Over the three and a half years Olive worked in hospital kitchens she made many friends and, when she announced her marriage, she invited twenty-six of her fellow VADs

---

1   1939 Census
2   Rita Bullion Jackson, daughter of Gladys and David Bullion.

The Story of Chippenham's Red Cross Hospital

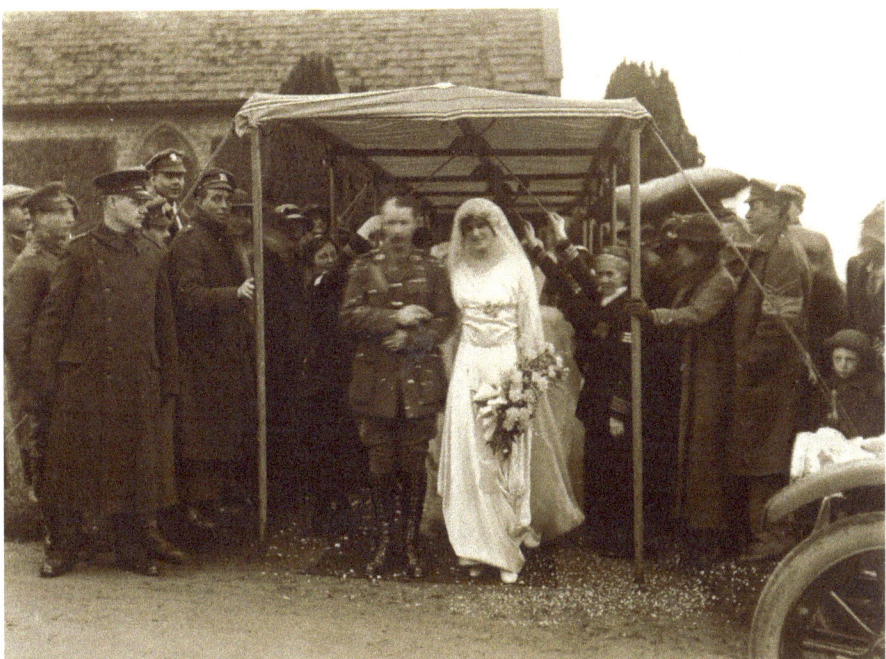

Olive Gladstone's wedding with the VAD Guard of Honour holding soup spoons.

to the wedding:[1] a large number, taking account of the size of the church at Bowden Hill.

Olive had decided she wanted her friends from the hospitals to be part of the ceremony. She got her wish when it was agreed, rather than having a traditional military guard of honour, the VADs would provide the guard of honour carrying crossed spoons to recognise Olives work in the kitchen.[2]

Chippenham wasn't alone in seeing relationships develop between VADs and patients. In Corsham Florence Bishop, who had served at the Hospital in the town and was awarded the Royal Red Cross Medal, married Sergeant David Howells of Cardiff in October 1920. Sergeant Howells was a patient, having been seriously wounded.[3]

The VAD hospitals had also seen relationships break the class divide. Constance Churchill, the daughter of the late Vice Admiral Orford Churchill and a member of Hampshire 'Society', married Gunner Arthur Hulme in January 1919. Constance had served as a VAD in France and with Wiltshire Red Cross at Salisbury where she met Gunner Hulme, who had been an insurance agent before the War.[4]

Caroline Dee, daughter of farmer Charles Dee, of Great Somerford near Chippenham, was a VAD nurse at Malmesbury and later volunteered at London hospitals. One of the patients she nursed was James Fausett, a farmer from Auckland in

1   *The Times* – 20 March 1919
2   *Pall Mall Gazette* - 18 March 1919 and *Western Daily Press* - 19 March 1919
3   *Wiltshire Times* - 9 October 1920
4   *Wiltshire Times* – 4 January 1919

Unity and Loyalty

New Zealand. He had joined the 2nd Battalion Auckland Regiment in February 1916 and served in France. In 1918 he was evacuated to a London hospital.[1]

In December 1920 Caroline Dee married James Fausett at Great Somerford Church a few days later the couple left for a new life in New Zealand.[2]

Peace Day

To mark the end of the War the Government declared a Bank holiday on 19 July 1919, known as Peace Day.

The 11 November 1918 had marked the end of hostilities, but it wasn't until June 1919 that Peace terms were signed, known as the Treaty of Versailles.

Crowds gathered in London. A victory parade took place and a temporary wooden monument was unveiled in Whitehall. A year later it was replaced by the Portland Stone Cenotaph we see today.

Sir Baden Powell, the Chief Scout, had some months earlier asked the Scouts to help organise a chain of bonfires that would stretch across the country to mark the celebrations.[3]

In Chippenham, despite heavy rain, a joint church service was held in the Market Place at 11.30. The Council minutes recorded the following:[4]

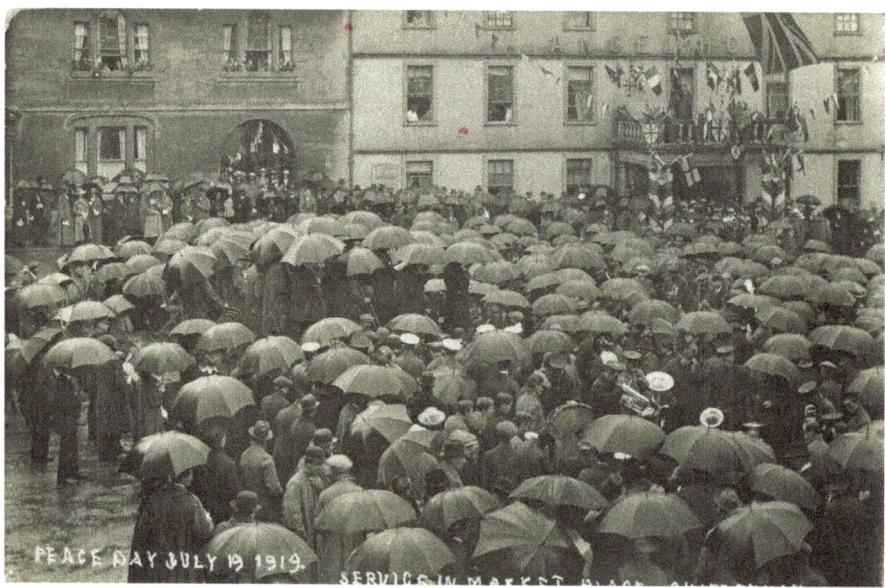

Peace Day service in the Market Place

1 New Zealand service record Pte James Fausett 23997
2 *Wiltshire Times* – 18 December 1920
3 *The Times* – 14 February 1919
4 *Chippenham Council minute book 10*

The Story of Chippenham's Red Cross Hospital

A United Service of thanksgiving for the return of Peace and for the Victory of the Empire and its Allies in the Great War, was held in the Market Place on Saturday, the 19 July 1919, the day appointed for the National Thanksgiving.

The Mayor and Corporation, with the whole of the officers of the Borough attended the service in state.

The men and women of Chippenham Red Cross attended in full uniform led by the Commandants Mrs Wilson and Frank Read. There were celebrations during the afternoon and a meal was held in the Neeld Hall for the ex-servicemen and in the evening the bonfire was lit.

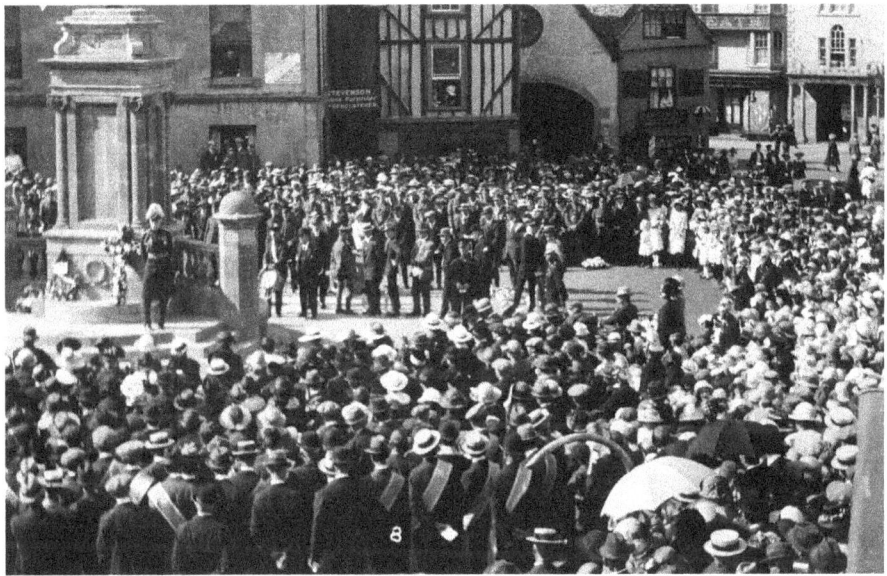

Lord Methuen gives a speech remembering the fallen at the unveiling of the War Memorial

War Memorials

TWO YEARS LATER the VADs were invited to join in commemorating the war dead from the town at the Parish Church. In July 1921 led by Mrs Wilson they attended St Andrew's for the unveiling and dedication of the rood screen. Designed by F E Howard of Oxford it listed 131 Chippenham men who had lost their lives. Lieut-Col Sir Audley Neeld unveiled the screen and asked the Bishop of Bristol for his dedication.[1]

In September 1921 the VADs were at the unveiling of the town's war memorial in the Market Place by Field Marshall Lord Methuen. The Mayor had convened a meeting

1 *Wiltshire Times* - 23 July 1921

Unity and Loyalty

in February 1919 to decide on an appropriate memorial to the fallen of Chippenham and it was decided to form a committee made up of representatives from the Council and various interested organisations, including the Red Cross, who were represented by two VADs.[1]

Families also commissioned their own memorials. Amongst these a brass plaque in the Parish Church to Percival Hunt, son of VAD Matilda Hunt. Alongside Percival Hunt is the memorial to Wallace Rooke, brother of the two Rooke sisters who served at the Hospital and died of influenza in 1918.

In the Baptistery of the church Doctor and Mrs Wilson commissioned a stained-glass window by Christopher Whall to commemorate their three sons killed in action.[2]

Further memorials were erected in churches and clubs throughout the town to remember the fallen.

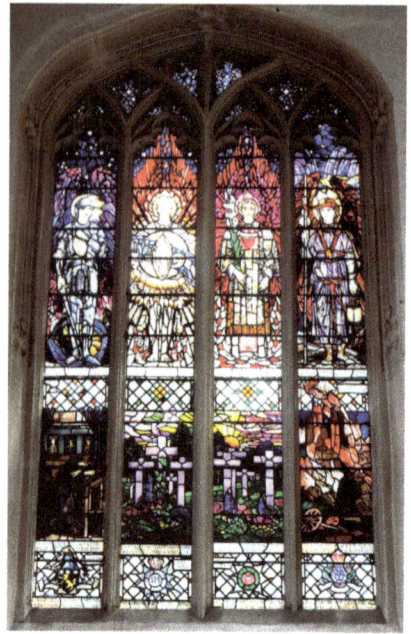

The Wilson Window in St Andrew's Church Chippenham

Remembering the VAD Hospital

THE TOWN HAD commemorated its fallen heroes, but there was no permanent record of the Hospital and VADs. In 1919 much was said about the selfless acts of the VADs and how they had cared so well for those who had suffered in defence of their country. Five years later the memory was fading and it took the local Red Cross Committee to suggest that the Auxiliary Hospital, and the VADs who served it, deserved permanent recognition. The matter was raised in 1924 when the Red Cross approached the Town Council to ask if they could put a memorial tablet on the Town Hall to acknowledge the work done during the War.

The Town Council minutes recorded the request:[3]

> Mr Councillor Bryant moved that this council grant permission to the Chippenham Branch of the Red Cross Society to place a memorial in the form of;
> 1) A small metal tablet to be placed on the outside of the Town Hall and
> 2) A framed certificate granted by the Army Council to be hung inside the building.
> That the permission be on the condition that the whole of the expense is borne

---

1   *Wiltshire Times* - 8 February 1919
2   *Wiltshire Times* - 5 October 1918. The window was dedicated on 29 September 1918
3   *Chippenham Council minute book 11*- 23 June 1924

The Story of Chippenham's Red Cross Hospital

by the Red Cross Society and that the consent of the Neeld Trustees is obtained and further that details of carrying out the proposal be left to the Halls Committee.

The proposition was seconded by Mr Councillor Bowker and agreed to.

It would take almost eighteen months before the tablet was fixed to the Town Hall during which time both Commandant Wilson and Dora Belcher, the Assistant Quartermaster, decided to retire from the Detachment.

To mark their departure there was a gathering of VADs at the Town Hall in January 1925. A number of VADs had moved away from the area but remained in touch and sent both the ladies their best wishes.

Lady Margaret Spicer in making a presentation to the ladies said:

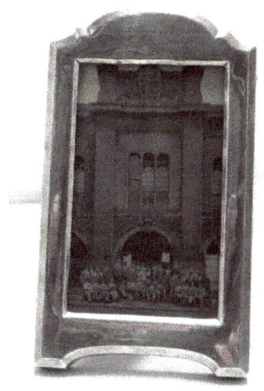

The silver frame presented to Dora Belcher

So much work was carried on during the Great War, work which at times was very nerve-racking and difficult and I know I am only voicing the opinions of the staff of the Red Cross Hospital when I say that the success of the Hospital was largely due to the unremitting efforts of the Commandant and Quartermaster.

Mrs Wilson was presented with a silver bon-bon dish, on which was inscribed: *To Commandant Helena J. Wilson, 1915-1919.*

Dora Belcher was given a silver cabinet photo frame, suitably inscribed.

Mrs Wilson was also given some money that was left over after the gifts were purchased. She put this towards the fund for the planned tablet on the Town Hall.[1]

Later that year, following the Remembrance Day Service on 8 November 1925, Lieut-Col Sir Audley Neeld unveiled the Red Cross tablet on the Town Hall. It said quite simply:

THESE BUILDINGS WERE USED AS A RED CROSS HOSPITAL FROM NOVEMBER 5TH 1915 TO APRIL 8TH 1919. 1,872 SICK AND WOUNDED SOLDIERS WERE TREATED.

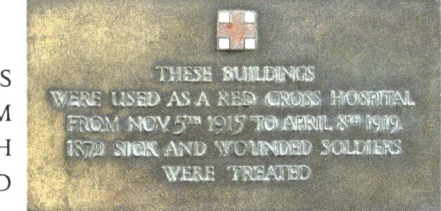

The tablet on the Town Hall

Although she had recently stepped down as Commandant, it was most appropriate for Mrs Wilson to represent the Red Cross at the ceremony as her last official function. She wore her Red Cross medals and the decorations awarded to her sons.

1 *Wiltshire Times* – 17 January 1925

Unity and Loyalty

Before asking Sir Audley Neeld to unveil the tablet, she gave an emotional speech:

We meet today to recall to the memory of everyone present that these Town Hall and Neeld Hall Buildings were used as a Red Cross Hospital during the Great War.

We have just shown in the service at the Cenotaph our continued sympathy for the loss of so many of our townsmen and our undying gratitude to them for their brave endeavour even unto death to defend our country. Now we desire to place on record the fact that these buildings served a very useful part in the war by receiving within their walls 1,872 sick and wounded men to be nursed back to health and made fit to return to their duties. Only two men out of the 1,872 failed to answer again to their roll-call on earth.

These buildings with a few alterations and additions made a beautiful and most satisfactory temporary hospital, beloved and admired by all of us who worked here, and beloved by the patients who carried away with them grateful memories of the treatment received within its walls and of the kindness and hospitality shown to them in various ways by the people of Chippenham and in the villages around.

Our two large wards were called 'Unity and Loyalty' after the arms of this town. Mr Mayor, as Commandant of the hospital, I wish again to express publicly our thanks for the loan of these buildings and my deep gratitude for the help given by the late co-director, the medical officers, the nurses and cooks of each detachment and to all the

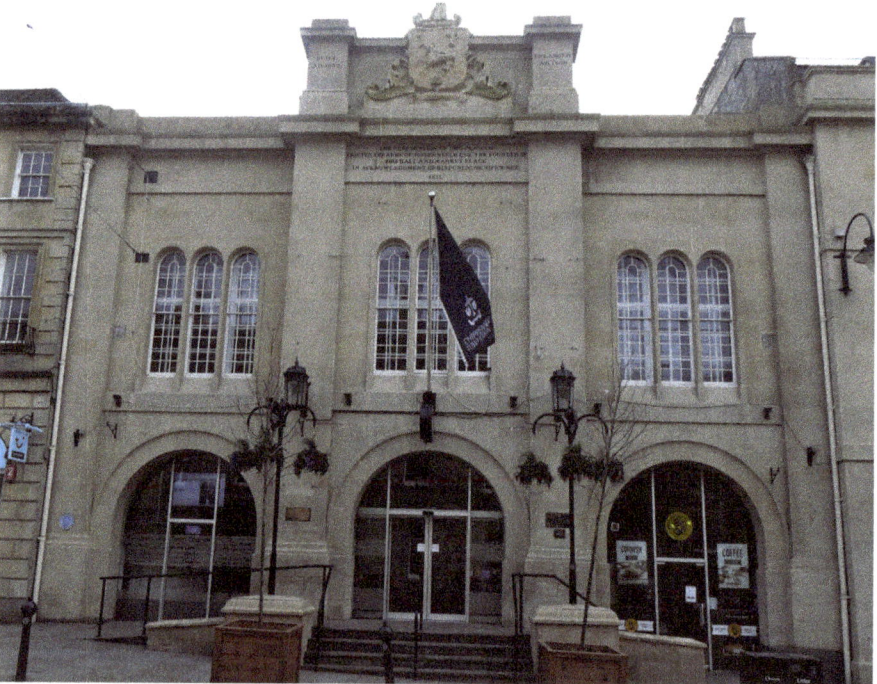

The Town Hall Chippenham in 2019, one hundred years after Unity and Loyalty closed

helpers who so willingly gave their times for 3½ years and for the loyal whole hearted way they performed their duties in every branch of the work.

It was greatly this spirit of unity and loyalty which made the buildings a happy home hospital for our soldier boys. We must not forget the many kind donors of gifts, which helped make the hospital beautiful and health giving.

Now, today we, the members of the British Red Cross Society, and our fellow workers, ask the Mayor and Corporation to accept this small tablet whose words, with the sacred emblem above, will remind them that for the time they too, gave of their best for the use of suffering men.

I will now ask our never-failing friend, Sir Audley Neeld to unveil the memorial tablet.

Following the unveiling Sir Audley Neeld said a few words in praise of Mrs Wilson saying, the work she did was *'heroic and splendid'* and *'she never faltered while facing the greatest trial and sorrow'* (the loss of her sons). He went on to say, *'...the women of Chippenham and district did a noble work.'*

The Mayor, Councillor Swain, who had been a member of the Men's Detachment, responded and gratefully accepted the tablet. The proceedings closed with the playing of the National Anthem.

The unveiling of the tablet finally closed the chapter in Chippenham's history of the Red Cross Hospital during the Great War.

The Final Word

THE FINAL WORD on the Hospital must however go to an Australian soldier. Several of the VADs remarked how many Australians they treated and perhaps, as the men were so far from home, they were made to feel particularly welcome.

One of those patients was Vincent Boreham who served in France with the 7th Field Company Engineers of the Australian Imperial Force. After the War he returned to Australia and settled in New South Wales with his wife Eleanor.

During August 1938 Captain Victor Cazalet, the MP for Chippenham, visited Australia to attend the British Commonwealth Relations Conference. While in Australia he met and received letters from many people who had connections with Chippenham, including one from Vincent Boreham with happy memories of Chippenham during the War. Captain Cazelet was so taken with Vincent's letter that he sent it to the editor of the Wiltshire Times asking that it should be published:

Dear Sir
I notice by the papers that you are the representative of Chippenham in the Houses of Parliament; and because of the district you represent, apart from the pleasure it would

Unity and Loyalty

give me to meet you, I should like you to take back to England my very warm greetings to the people of Chippenham for their kindness to me as an Australian soldier in 1918.

Belonging to the 7th Field Company Engineers, I was invalided to Blighty in 1918 and after a short stay at Rouen and Havre was taken across to dear old England, and from Southampton to the Beaufort Hospital, Bristol. Then later to the Red Cross Hospital at Chippenham; right in the centre of the town.

Dr and Mrs. Wilson (very dear old people, they were) were in charge; and among the nurses I recollect two Miss Gladstones, relatives of England's great Statesmen; also a Mrs Slade (these people owned the brewery etc). There was also a Colonel Neeld, he used to come regularly to see the boys and take them to Bath for a trip; and so I might go on. So you see directly I saw the town of Chippenham mentioned, it awakened in me the old feeling of gratitude for the wonderful time those splendid women gave we boys when we were incapacitated from duty.

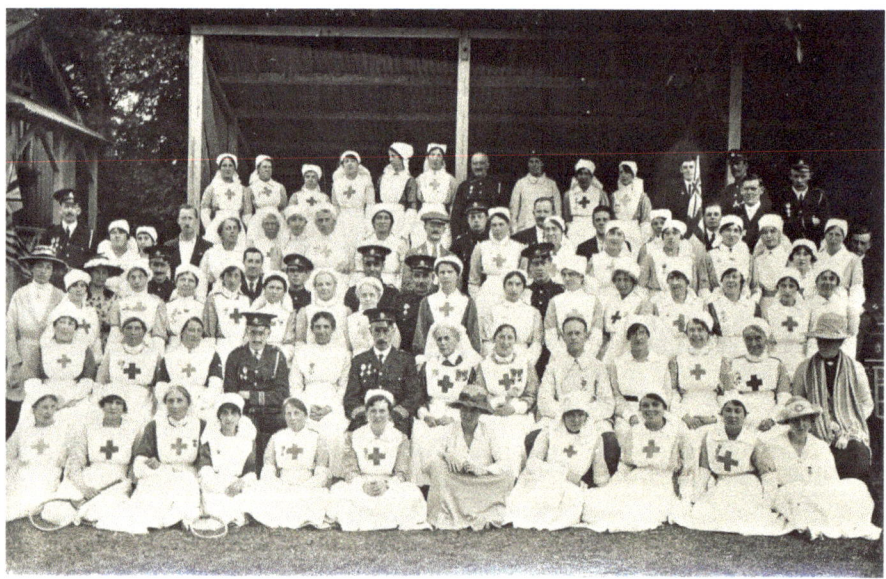

Those splendid women that Vincent Boreham wrote about. The gathering may be to celebrate the award of Mrs Wilson's OBE

Appendix 1
Staff and Volunteers at Chippenham Red Cross Hospital

LISTED BELOW ARE those men and women involved with the Red Cross Hospital in Chippenham, from its opening in November 1915 until it closed in April 1919. The information has been gathered from numerous sources including the Red Cross, newspapers, obituaries, personal papers and family research but inevitably remains incomplete as records and memories have been lost through time.

In April 1919 the newspaper wrote in some detail about the closure of the Hospital and listed those who worked there. The detail is limited, and in some cases the spelling of names is incorrect, therefore several individuals cannot be positively identified. They have however been included in this record.

Olive Adams
In July 1919 Olive gave her address as the Queen Mary Army Auxiliary Corps (QMAAC) Hostel Clarence Barracks Portsmouth. The Red Cross records show she was a kitchen maid at Chippenham Hospital from 1915 until March 1917. It is assumed that Olive left Chippenham during 1917 to join the QMAAC.

Mrs Allen
The only reference to Mrs Allen is that she was mentioned as a volunteer at the closure of the Hospital by the newspaper. It is possible this is Mary Allen who lived in Ladds Lane.

Miss Rachel Doreen Anstee
The daughter of George Anstee of Home Farm Stanton St Quintin, Rachel joined the Wilts 6 VAD in 1916 at the age of 23. Between August 1916 and January 1917 she gave a total of 948 hours as a VAD nurse.

Miss Mary Aps
Little is known about Mary. She gave her address as Greathouse, Kington Langley and was probably in domestic service. Mary is recorded as being a part time mess room helper at Chippenham from November 1917 to April 1919.

Mr Albert E Archard
Albert joined the Wilts 13 VAD in November 1917 at the age of 15 and gave 250 hours service until December 1918. Son of Annie and Walter the family lived on Station Hill in Chippenham.

Mrs Annie Archard
Annie Archard was a member of the Chippenham Red Cross Working Party and an occasional helper in the kitchen serving teas.

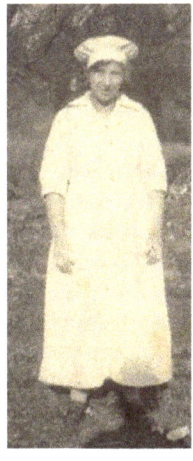

Annie Archard

Unity and Loyalty

Mr Walter Archard
Walter was employed by Great Western Railway as a porter and ticket collector at Chippenham station and qualified in first aid with the St John Ambulance Association. A member of Wilts 13 VAD he died in October 1916.

Mrs Austin
The only references to Mrs Austin is she was mentioned as a nurse at the closure of the Hospital by the newspaper. She was also included in the photograph album of Ivy Gladstone.

Miss Janet Unity Awdry
Born in in 1897 Janet Awdry was the daughter of Chippenham solicitor Edmund Awdry of Rowden Hill who sat on the Management Committee of the Cottage Hospital in the town.
Janet joined the Red Cross Hospital in Chippenham as a probationer nurse and gave 6819 hours service.

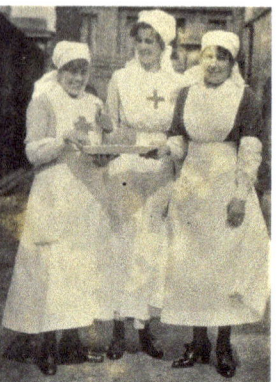

Mrs Austin on the right Olive Gladstone centre and Miss Munday

Reverend Vere Awdry
Vere Awdry was born in 1854 in Notton near Chippenham. In 1886 he was ordained at Chichester Theological College and in 1917 he was living in Box.

In May 1917 he joined Wilts 3 VAD at Corsham and served at Bowood, Corsham and Chippenham Red Cross hospitals as an orderly and ambulance transport. He gave 1000 hours service. His son Carol was killed in action in 1914.

Miss Doris Aylmore
Doris was an accomplished singer and entertainer and took part in concerts for the patients.

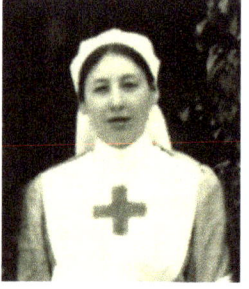

Janet Awdry

Mrs Edith Aylmore
Described as an assistant at the closure of the Hospital Edith was the wife of Charles, who owned a Gentlemen's outfitters in New Road.

Mr Edward Baker
Mr Baker was in his forties when he received his home nursing certificate at Chippenham in December 1916. He was an orderly in the wards. He lived in the Butts and worked at the condensed milk factory.

Mrs H Baker
The only reference to Mrs Baker is that she was mentioned as an assistant nurse at the closure of the Hospital by the newspaper. It is thought she was Susan Baker who lived in St Mary's Place.

Reverend Vere Awdry

Miss Elsie Ball
Elsie Ball was a teacher and lived in New Road Chippenham with her parents. In September 1917, aged 23, she became a part time nurse and gave 700 hours service.

Mrs Ruth Annie Barnes
Ruth, also known as Annie, was the wife of Charles Barnes, the doctor in Sutton Benger. She was a member of Wilts 38 VAD and served at Chippenham Red Cross Hospital from March 1916 until it closed. She became the Assistant Commandant of Wilts 38.

Mr Henry Barsted
Blacksmith and horse dealer Henry Joseph Barsted of Langley Road served with Chippenham

VAD 13 providing his car for ambulance transport. He also arranged transport for outings organised for the wounded patients.

Miss Gwendoline Beaven
Gwendoline Beaven was a daughter of James Beaven a boot maker with a shop in the town. The family lived in St Paul Street. In July 1914 she was a VAD nothing more is known of her service.

Mrs Sarah Beaven
In August 1916, as Loyalty ward opened, 59 year old Sarah Beaven became a member of the kitchen staff. She attended every Sunday and did the washing up and general kitchen duties. She left in April 1919. Sarah and her husband Frank lived in Park Lane in Chippenham.

Miss Dora Belcher
Dora was born in 1885. At the opening of the Red Cross Hospital she was appointed Assistant Quartermaster responsible for the cleaning and mending of clothing and bedding and gave 5170 hours.

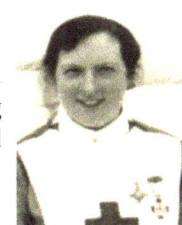

Dora Belcher

Miss Evelyn Belcher
Evelyn was born in 1882 At the opening of the Red Cross Hospital she was appointed full time Quartermaster responsible for the accounts and stores and was assisted by her sister Dora.

Her services were recognised when she was awarded the MBE in January 1918.

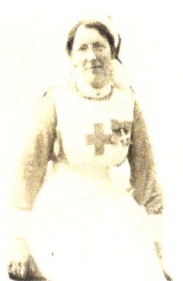

Evelyn Belcher wearing her award

Miss Alice Mary Birkbeck
Alice was a member of the Entertainment Committee and helped in the mess room serving meals. She also repaired hospital uniforms and bedding at home. She served from November 1915 to April 1919 and lived in St Paul Street.

Miss Violet Bessie Bishop
In September 1917 Violet Bishop joined the kitchen staff to peel vegetables, working for 5 hours a month. She lived with her parents at Church Farm at Broughton Gifford near Melksham.

Mrs Elizabeth Jane Blackman
Elizabeth worked part time washing up from January 1918 until the Hospital closed. She lived in Park Lane and was 41 years old.

Mrs Lucy Jane Blake
Lucy Blake registered with Wilts 6 VAD in January 1915 at the age of 55. She immediately went to serve at Corsham Red Cross Hospital as a nurse. During 1916 she transferred to Chippenham where she remained until it closed in 1919. She lived in Biddestone and at the end of the war moved to Bath.

Mrs Lucy Ann Blanchard
Lucy Blanchard, aged 25, was taken on as a cook in 1915. Unusually, she was employed full time and paid £24 a year. She continued her employment until April 1919. Lucy and her husband William, a bricklayer, lived in Downing Street.

Mrs Blanche Bland
In 1916 Blanche Taylor, who lived in Pew Hill with her parents, married William Bland a soldier with the Army Service Corps (ASC). In October 1917 she became a Red Cross VAD at Chippenham and

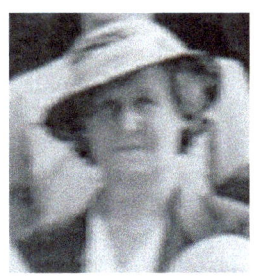

Lucy Blanchard in 1945

joined the kitchen staff to serve teas. She also volunteered in the housekeeping department mending clothing and bedding.

Mrs Ethel Bodman
34 year old Ethel joined the Hospital as a cook in May 1917. She was the wife of farmer William Bodman and they lived at Malford Farm in Christian Malford.

Mr William Bodman
William Bodman worked at Saxby and Farmer as a sawyer. In November 1915, he was an ambulance orderly and was later appointed as section leader of Wilts 13 VAD. He and his wife Kathleen lived in London Road.

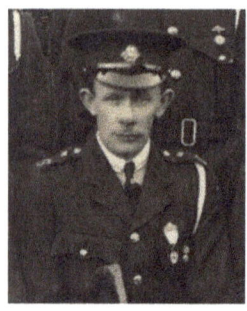
William Bodman

Miss Amy Bolton
Amy Clara Bolton was the daughter of Allan Bolton, the rector at Yatton Keynell. At the outbreak of war Amy became the leader of the Yatton Keynell Work Party: When Chippenham Red Cross Hospital opened she volunteered for work in the kitchens. During the summer of 1916 she decided to apply for Special Service in Salonika and France

Miss Gwendoline Maud Bond
Miss Bond volunteered at both Weybridge and Chippenham Red Cross Hospitals between December 1915 and September 1917. The Red Cross records, dated July 1919, give her address as West Cliff Gardens, Bournemouth however she was born and grew up in nearby Wootton Bassett.

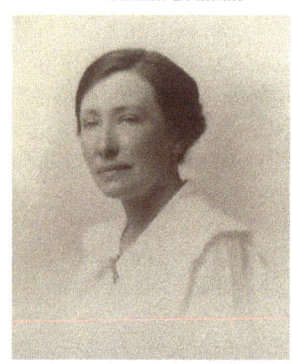
Amy Bolton

Miss Katherine Mary Bond
Katherine lived with her widowed brother and his daughter at Church Farm, Sutton Benger. A member of Wilts 38 VAD, she joined Chippenham Red Cross Hospital in March 1916, aged 43, as a probationer nurse. and gave 1800 hours.

Mrs Minnie Louise Booy
Little is known about Mrs Booy's VAD service. Her obituary in 1932 said 'During the war she did excellent service as a VAD nurse at Chippenham and helped to cheer many a wounded soldier.' Minnie and her family lived at Hans Farm, Upper Castle Combe.

Miss Bower
The only reference to Miss Bower is that she was mentioned as a nurse at the closure of the Hospital in by the newspaper adding that she came from Malmesbury.
It may be that she was Alice Bower who lived at Tetbury Hill in Malmesbury and gave service at Malmesbury and Charlton Park Hospitals. Her work at Chippenham was never formally recorded.

Mrs Brand
The only reference to Mrs Brand is that she was mentioned as an assistant at the closure of the Hospital by the newspaper.

Mrs Alice Clara Brett
Alice was a probationer nurse in November 1915 when the Hospital opened and gave 1500 hours nursing and ward work until April 1919. She lived at Landsend in Chippenham.

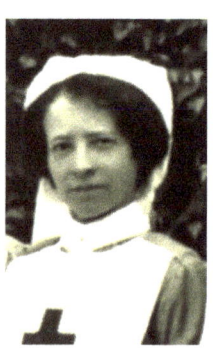
Alice Brett

The Story of Chippenham's Red Cross Hospital

Miss Elsie Brewer
Elsie Brewer was a munitionette at Saxby and Farmer. She was one of the entertainers who performed at the concerts for wounded men and helped at the Hospital serving teas. She lived in Wood Lane with her parents.

Mrs Kate Bright
Mrs Bright lived in Emery Lane. Between January 1916 and January 1917, she worked as a cleaner for two hours every day. Her son George was killed in action in November 1916.

Mrs Jane Brind
69 year old Jane Brind from Langley Burrell joined the Red Cross in October 1914. She regularly took items of bedding and clothing home to mend them.

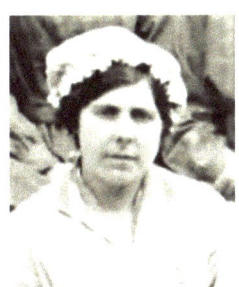

Elsie Brewer

Miss Ethel Matilda Brinkworth
Ethel Brinkworth was born in 1884 in Chippenham and lived with her parents Sarah and George at Frogwell where they farmed. In June 1916 she took the position of full time clerk to the Quartermaster at Chippenham. Within days of joining she was seconded to Dartford War Hospital. On her return to Chippenham in August 1917 she undertook training to become a nurse. During 1918 she also served at the Australian Military Hospital at Harefield and the Royal Naval Hospital in Deal. In June 1918 she received the news her brother Tom had been killed in action.

Jessie Marie Brinkworth
30 year old Jessie lived with her brother who farmed at Peckingell near Langley Burrell.
In November 1915 she was one of the nursing VADs present when the first injured men arrived at Chippenham.

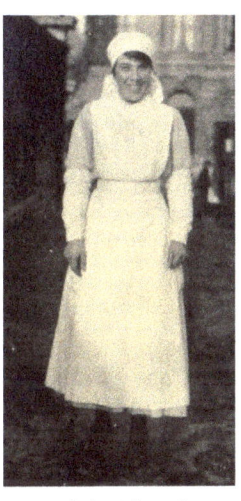

Ethel Brinkworth

Mrs Nancy Briscoe, Doctor Briscoe
Nancy Briscoe was a member of the Red Cross committee at the outbreak of war. In 1914 she mobilised the stretcher bearers to prepare to receive patients at Chippenham. She was the wife of Doctor William Briscoe and they lived in the Market Place, where William had his surgery.

Miss Mary Elizabeth Brockway
Mary was an elementary school teacher and lived at 33 Park Lane with her parents. In August 1917 she volunteered as a nursing probationer and gave 1500 hours service. The Red Cross records said 'She did duty in spare time eg Evenings, Weekends and Holidays.'

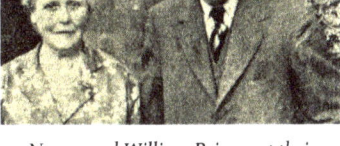

Nancy and William Briscoe at their Golden Wedding in 1960

Miss Brotherhood
The only reference to Miss Brotherhood is that she was mentioned by the newspaper as an assistant when it reported on the closure of the Hospital.

Miss Bessie Browning
Little is known about Bessie. She gave her address as Greathouse, Kington Langley and was probably in domestic service. She is recorded as being a part time messroom helper at Chippenham from November 1917 to April 1919.

Unity and Loyalty

Mrs Agnes Bryant
In September 1914 Agnes, aged 43, joined the Red Cross. When the Hospital opened in Chippenham Town Hall, she became a probationer nurse and continued to serve until it closed giving 2600 hours. She and her husband, a head teacher, lived at 22 Marshfield Road.

Miss Bessie (Elizabeth) Bryant
Bessie helped serve meals in the mess room. She attended for 2 hours, two days a week from October 1916 to April 1918. She lived at the Beeches, East Tytherton with her parents.
Bessie's sisters Eva and Lily also worked at the Hospital.

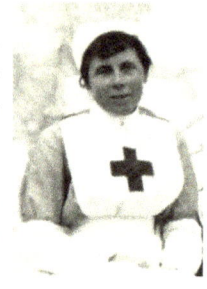
Agnes Bryant

Miss Eva May Bryant
Eva helped serve meals in the mess room. She attended for 2 hours, two days a week from October 1916 to November 1918. She was joined by her sisters Bessie and Lily and lived at the Beeches, East Tytherton.

Miss Lily Rose Bryant
Lily helped serve meals in the mess room. She attended for 2 hours, two days a week from October 1916 to April 1918 and worked with her sisters Bessie and Eva. She lived at the Beeches, East Tytherton.

Mr Frank Henry Buckland
Frank and his wife Rose had many years' experience in the catering trade. They put their experience to good use at the Hospital. From August 1916, Frank regularly supervised at meal times and officiated at the dining table to carve the joint of meat and propose the toast to the King.

Mrs Rose Elizabeth Buckland
Wife of Frank, Rose put her hotelier skills to good use in the kitchen. She also prepared the vegetables and served teas to the patients. Rose and Frank Buckland lived in Audley Road.

Mrs Rosa Mary Buckland
Farmers wife Rosa lived at New Priory Farm in Kington St Michael. She attended the Hospital for a few hours each week to help in the kitchen and prepare vegetables. She served between October 1917 and April 1919.

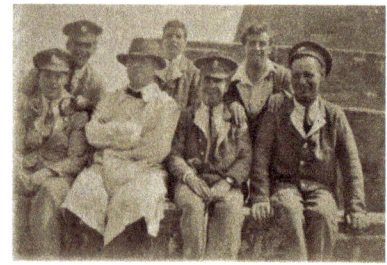
Joe Buckle with a group of patients at Cherhill monument near Calne

Mr Joseph Buckle
Joe Buckle was a well-known figure in Chippenham. He was the Captain of the town Fire Brigade and a game and poultry dealer with a shop on the High Street. He was a regular helper at the Hospital and like Frank Buckland he officiated at the dining table. He was a member of the Entertainment Committee and helped arrange day trips for the patients.

Mrs Phyllis Burgess
Phyllis lived at 36 Park Lane. From 1916 to 1919 she gave 400 hours service preparing vegetables in the Hospital kitchen.

Mr William Burridge (Jnr)
William Millman Burridge was the proprietor of motor

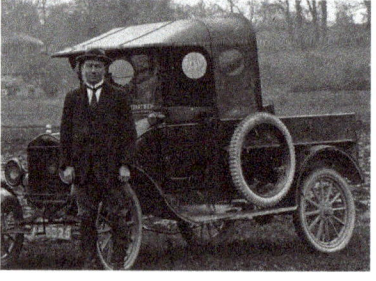
William Burridge Jnr with one of his vehicles

The Story of Chippenham's Red Cross Hospital

garages at the Angel Hotel and Station Hill. His father was the proprietor of the Angel Hotel. When the injured men arrived at the station he provided motor cars to transport the 'walking wounded' to Bowood and Chippenham hospitals.

He was also a member of the Entertainment Committee and arranged day trips for the patients, often supplying the vehicles and drivers.

Mr William Burridge (Snr)

William was in his fifties at the outbreak of war and the proprietor of the Angel Hotel in the Market Place. He was a member of the Entertainment Committee and helped organise shows for the patients. Visiting performers would stay at his hotel and he provided transport for them to visit other hospitals in the district.

Mrs Lilian Butler

From August 1918 until April 1919 Lilian, who lived in Sheldon Road with her husband William, worked every Saturday afternoon. The Red Cross records described her as a "men's room lady."

Mr William Butler

William was a clerk at Saxby and Farmer and a part time ambulance orderly with Wilts 13 VAD. He served at Chippenham from August 1916. His wife Lilian was also a volunteer.

Miss Mary S Buy

Mary was a member of Wilts 38 VAD. She lived in Sutton Benger with her father.

In March 1916, aged 47, she became a probationer at Chippenham and continued until the Hospital closed.

Miss Capel

The only reference to Miss Capel is that she was mentioned by the newspaper as an assistant when it reported on the closure of the Hospital.

Miss Evelyn Carnley

Evelyn Carnley lived at the Chestnuts in Upper Seagry, near Chippenham. During 1915, aged 26, she became a member of Wilts 38 VAD. She transferred to Devonport Military Hospital and later served on the hospital ship Aquitania. In 1917 she was serving at military hospitals in France.

Mrs Fanny Charles

Mrs Charles, who lived in Bayntons Lane, Chippenham, helped part time in the hospital kitchens from July 1916 to March 1917.

Mrs M Chesterton

The only reference to Mrs Chesterton is that she was mentioned by the newspaper as a nurse at the closure of the Hospital.

Miss D Clarke

The only reference to Miss Clarke is that she was mentioned by the newspaper as a nurse at the closure of the Hospital. The newspaper also said she came from Sutton Benger.

Miss Ethel Mary Clements

27 year old Ethel spent every Monday afternoon from September 1916 to June 1917 with the patients serving drinks and clearing the mess room.

The Red Cross records give her address as Hawthorn Road in Chippenham. Before the war she was living with her widowed mother at Jacksoms Farm, Langley Burrell, and worked as a dairymaid.

Mr George Clifford

Thought to be Isaac George Clifford an engineer, employed by Saxby and Farmer, who lived in Wood Lane and later London Road. He served part time with the Ambulance Detachment until December 1918. After the war he and his family emigrated to Canada.

Unity and Loyalty

Miss Clutterbuck
The only reference to Miss Clutterbuck is that she was mentioned by the newspaper as a nurse at the closure of the Hospital. It is thought the report refers to either Miss Hope Joan Clutterbuck or Miss Phyllis Clutterbuck who both lived at Dicketts in Corsham and served at Corsham Hospital as VAD nurses. One or both of them may have served temporarily at Chippenham.

Miss Minnie Coates
According to the Red Cross records Minnie lived in High Street Corsham. In November 1915 she joined Chippenham Hospital as a part time nursing probationer. In May 1917 she left due to ill health.

Mrs Ethel May Codrington
Mrs Codrington, of Lowden Avenue in Chippenham, volunteered at the Hospital from June 1917 until March 1918. She came in for 2 hours every week to serve tea to the patients.

Miss Nora Sybil Collen
In September 1915 Nora joined Bowood Red Cross Hospital as a probationer nurse and transferred to the newly opened Hospital in Chippenham in November where she remained until the it closed in 1919. She was promoted to VAD Staff Nurse and gave a total of 5284 hours. In April 1918 she was honoured by being Mentioned in Despatches. Nora was the daughter of George Collen, a retired mill owner, and lived in Cote House in Chippenham.

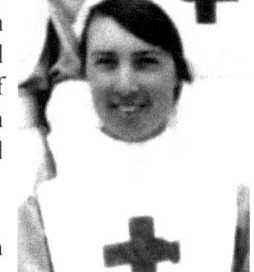

Nora Collen

Mrs Florence Collen
Wife of Daniel Collen. The Collen family owned the mill in the town and lived in New Road. Florence volunteered at the Hospital from September 1916 until it closed in 1919. She gave 2 hours a week serving teas.

Miss Comerford
The only reference to Miss Comerford is that she was mentioned by the newspaper as a nurse at the closure of the Hospital. The newspaper also said she came from Sutton Benger.

Mr Stewart A Cook
Mr Cook, who lived in St Mary Street, joined the Wilts 13 VAD in September 1916 as a hospital and ambulance orderly. He continued in this role until April 1919 and gave 1300 hours.

Miss Coombs
The only reference to Miss Coombs is that she was named as an assistant by the newspaper when it reported on the closure of the Hospital.

Miss Cooper
The only reference to Miss Cooper is that she was named as a nurse by the newspaper when it reported on the closure of the Hospital.

Miss Eileen Mabel Cordner
Eileen Cordner was employed as a full-time qualified nursing sister in October 1917. She was paid a Guinea (£1. 1s) a week and did both day and night duties until the Hospital closed in 1919. Little else is known about Eileen, although it is thought she came from Dublin.

Miss Ellen Susannah Cornish
In February 1916 Ellen joined Wilts 38 VAD at Sutton Benger and served at Chippenham Hospital. She was included in the roll of Honourable Service. Ellen lived at the Comedy, in Christian Malford and was described as having a private income.

Mrs Isabella Emily Cotes

The Story of Chippenham's Red Cross Hospital

Isobella, who lived at Rowden House, was the sister of John Dickson-Poyndor, an MP for Chippenham. In October 1916 she and some of her staff joined the Red Cross Hospital. Isabella volunteered two and a half hours a week as a mess room attendant serving teas and meals continuing until it closed in 1919.

Miss Muriel Coventry
Muriel, also known as Joan, joined Wilts 6 VAD as a probationer in 1916 aged 18. She gave 6065 hours. Muriel was the granddaughter of Eleanor Countess of Suffolk who was also a VAD. Muriel lived with her family at Monkton Park House in Chippenham.

Mrs Rachael Alice Coward
Rachael was the wife of Frederick Coward, the Manager of the Chippenham branch of the Union of London and Smiths Bank. She was a supporter of the Belgian Relief Fund and helped the refugees when they arrived in Chippenham. In November 1915 she was a probationer at the Hospital and was later promoted to VAD Staff Nurse. She gave 5115 hours.

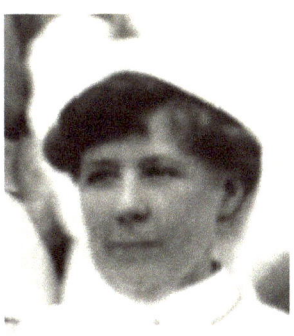

Countess Clare Cowley
Clare Cowley took on the role of Commandant of Wilts 38, the Sutton Detachment, during the last year of the war. The Earl and Countess moved to their property, Draycot House, during 1916. Prior to their occupation the property had been used as a Red Cross hospital.

Rachael Coward

Mrs E Craig
There are very few details of Mrs Craig. She was a member of the Chippenham Detachment that won the Division competition at the Neeld Hall in July 1914. She was named as an assistant by the newspaper when it reported on the closure of the Hospital.

Miss Olive Croker
Olive lived at Bridge House Lacock. In October 1918 she joined Wilts 6 VAD but went to serve in a number of Military hospitals in London.

Miss Ethel Daniels
The daughter of Emma and Henry Daniels. Ethel was a draper's assistant and lived with her parents in Lowden. In August 1916 she volunteered as a part time cook giving 600 hours service.

Mrs Elinor Davis
The wife of William Davis, the town's postmaster. Elinor lived at The Hayes in Malmesbury Road, Chippenham. She served as a part time cook and organised and performed at many of the concerts for the wounded soldiers.

Miss M Davison
In January 1918 the British Nursing Journal reported that Miss Davison was appointed as a qualified Sister at the Red Cross Hospital in Chippenham. Nothing more is known about her.

Miss Day
The only reference to Miss Day is that she was named as an assistant by the newspaper when it reported on the closure of the Hospital.

Mrs Dowding
The only reference to Mrs Dowding is that she was named as an

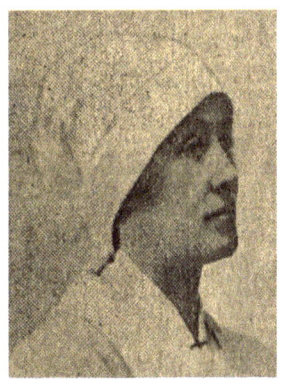

Elinor Davis

Unity and Loyalty

assistant by the newspaper when it reported on the closure of the Hospital.

Mr Edwin Duck
Edwin Duck lived in Park Lane and was a foreman working for Great Western Railway at Chippenham Station. He was an ambulance orderly with Wilts 13 VAD transporting patients from the station. His son George was killed in Mesopotamia.

Miss Eddolls
Miss Eddolls was named as an assistant by the newspaper when it reported on the closure of the Hospital. It is thought she was Florence Kate Eddolls the housekeeper for Mrs Minnie Booy of Hans Farm, Castle Combe Mrs Booy was also a VAD at Chippenham.

Mr William Thomas Edwards
William Edwards was discharged from the army as unfit for further military service. In September 1916 he was employed as caretaker and handyman at Chippenham Red Cross Hospital at a wage of £1.5s a week and continued until April 1919. After the war he was employed by Doctor and Mrs Wilson as their driver. He lived in St Mary Street.

Mrs Escott
The only reference to Mrs Escott is that she was named as an assistant by the newspaper when it reported on the closure of the Hospital.

Miss Alice Ellery
Alice lived with her uncle, William Bray, the village blacksmith, in Sutton Benger. She was a member of Wilts 38 VAD and in March 1916, aged 40, she became a probationer at Chippenham. She gave 1404 hours until she left in June 1918.

Mrs May Ennis
Mrs Ennis lived in the High Street and was one of the first ladies to join the Chippenham VAD in 1910, rising to the post of Quartermaster. She left the Detachment when her husband, William, a bank manager, was transferred to Bristol in 1915.

Mrs Caroline Everard
Caroline Everard was the housekeeper at Greathouse at Kington Langley. From November 1917 until the Hospital closed, Caroline worked 2 hours a week as a mess room helper.

Miss Violet Mary Faithfull-Davies
In November 1916 the British Nursing Journal reported that Violet was appointed as a qualified Sister at the Red Cross Hospital in Chippenham. She also served at hospitals in Kent, Nottingham and Isle of Wight. Violet was born in 1874 in Lancashire the daughter of a clergyman.

Miss Lila Farries
Lila volunteered at the Hospital from June 1916 to December 1918 as the Quartermaster's orderly giving 3200 hours. She was lodging with the Belcher family in Marshfield Road, nothing further is known about Lila.

Miss Fanny Ferris
Fanny Ferris was born in 1897 and grew up in Tytherton. She joined the Red Cross in 1913 and in 1914 became a probationer nurse at Bowood Hospital. She transferred to the newly opened Chippenham Red Cross Hospital in November 1915 and remained there until it closed, giving 5184 hours service. She attained the rank of Staff Nurse.

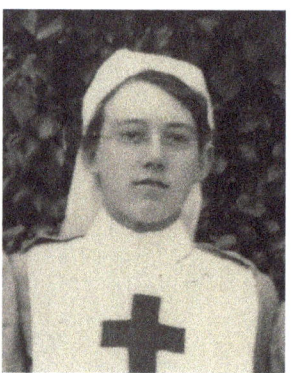

Fanny Ferris

Mr Reginald Fields
In September 1916 Reginald, who lived in Wood Lane, joined

The Story of Chippenham's Red Cross Hospital

Wilts 13 VAD as an ambulance assistant and hospital orderly.

Mrs Emmie Finn
Mrs Finn was employed as hospital cleaner and general assistant. She worked 4 hours a day and earned 6s 6d a week between November 1916 and July 1917. She lived in Marshfield Road with her husband and young family, later moving to St Mary Street.

Miss Elsie Kate Fortune
Elsie was born in October 1894. She grew up in Foghamshire in Chippenham and was employed as Mrs Garnett's lady's maid at Greathouse in Kington Langley. At the outbreak of war, she was asked to convert rooms in the house to receive wounded men from the hospitals. It is thought she also volunteered at Chippenham Hospital.

Miss Mollie Lavinia Fowler
Miss Fowler was a trained nurse and had served at a number of hospitals around the country. On 31 March 1919 she arrived at Chippenham and remained for ten days, until the Hospital finally closed.
It is thought she came to Chippenham for the sole purpose of helping to arrange the transfer of the remaining patients. After leaving Chippenham she went to Grove Park Hospital in Chiswick.

Miss Alice Fox
Alice Fox lived in London Road, Devizes. She joined Wilts 2 VAD, Devizes Detachment in January 1915 as a nurse and later took on cooking duties. In October 1917 she transferred to Chippenham as a nurse and remained there until July 1918. In September 1918 she transferred again to Ryde on the Isle of Wight where she was an assistant cook at a hospital.

Mrs Elizabeth Maud Fox
Mrs Fox served at the Hospital between 1915 and 1916. She worked 5 hours a week washing up and preparing vegetables. She lived in Downing Street in Chippenham.

Miss Fry
The only reference to Miss Fry is that she was named as an assistant by the newspaper when it reported on the closure of the Hospital.

Miss Fudge
The only reference to Miss Fudge is a group photograph of VADs belonging to Wilts 6 VAD that included her name.

Miss M Gale
The only reference to Miss Gale is that she came from Castle Combe and was named as a nurse by the newspaper when it reported on the closure of the Hospital.

Mr Percy James Gane
Percy Gane was Commandant of Corsham Men's Detachment, VAD 3, and helped organise the transport for Chippenham Hospital until Chippenham Detachment, VAD 13 was established in 1916.

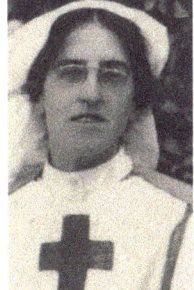
Miss Fudge

Mr Henry Gardner
Between November 1916 and January 1919 Henry Gardner drove his pony and cart from Lower Stanton, where a laundry work party had been established, to Chippenham twice a week to collect and deliver laundry for the Hospital.

Mrs Garne
The only reference to Mrs Garne is that she was named as a nurse by the newspaper when it reported on the closure of the Hospital. It is possible that the person referred to was Mrs Isobel Garne who also served at Corsham Hospital, but her service at Chippenham is not recorded.

Mr Charles Garnett

Charles Garnett was a successful barrister and owned Greathouse in Kington Langley.

At the beginning of the war Charles Garnett went to France with the Red Cross and drove his own ambulance behind the lines. He was attached to the Red Cross Headquarters at Ypres until May 1915.

On his return to Kington Langley he continued his ambulance work and assisted with ambulance convoys to Bowood and Chippenham hospitals until 1919. He was the Honorary Commandant of Wilts 13 VAD.

Mrs Claire Garnett

Claire Garnett was the wife of Charles Garnett. She was the Red Cross Finance Chairman for Chippenham Division. She also helped organise musical evenings at Chippenham Hospital and entertained patients at her home Greathouse.

Mrs Janet Blanche Gibbs

Mrs Gibbs lived at Sheldon Manor. In February 1918 she joined Wilts 6 VAD as the Assistant Commandant. She had previously been a member of Somerset 64 VAD.

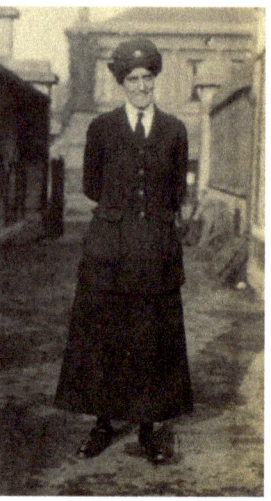

Janet Gibbs

Mrs Ginn

The only reference to Mrs Ginn is that she was named as an assistant by the newspaper when it reported on the closure of the Hospital.

Miss Muriel Ivy Gladstone

Murial, better known as Ivy joined the Red Cross in 1913. She was awarded her five year service badge in December 1918. When the Red Cross Hospital opened in Chippenham she trained as a nurse and also deputed as a staff nurse. She gave a total of 5300 hours and was included in the Roll of Honourable Service. Her sister, Olive, also served at Chippenham.

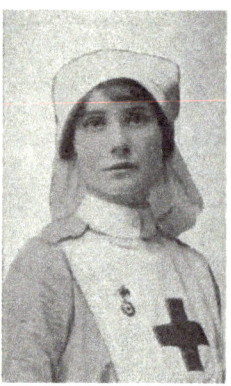

Ivy Gladstone

Miss Olive Mary Gladstone

Olive joined the Red Cross in 1913 aged 19. In December 1918 she was awarded her five year badge. She served at Chippenham Red Cross Hospital as a third and second cook, occasionally deputising as head cook. She gave 1688 hours and left the hospital in December 1918. Her sister, Ivy, also served at Chippenham.

Miss Ivy Beatrice Glass

Ivy Glass lived at New Leaze Farm at Pewsham. She joined the VAD in April 1917 as a mess room attendant and gave half a day a week. She continued at the Hospital until it closed in 1919.

Miss Edith Rachel Godwin

Edith was a farmer's daughter living at Manor Farm, North Wraxall. She joined the Red Cross Hospital in September 1916 as a VAD nurse and gave 1500 hours until April 1919. She served with her sister Margaret. A further sister, Lydia, was a Cook at a VAD hospital in Yorkshire.

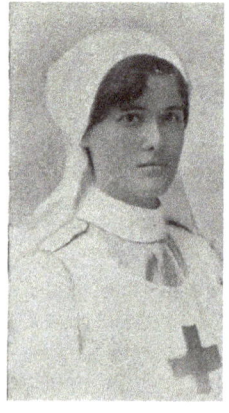

Olive Gladstone

The Story of Chippenham's Red Cross Hospital

Miss Margaret Elizabeth Godwin
Margaret joined the Red Cross Hospital in September 1916 with her sister Edith. She was a VAD nurse and gave 1500 hours.

Mademoiselle Lucie Golaz
Lucie Golaz was lady's maid to Isabella Cotes of Rowden House. Lucie was a Swiss national, but had worked for Mrs Cotes for some years. In October 1916, aged 49, she joined the VAD as a part time mess room attendant and worked alongside Mrs Cotes. She continued until April 1919.

Lady Alice Goldney
Alice lived at Monks Park in Corsham. She was the Assistant Commandant at Corsham Hospital and a member of the Red Cross Central Work Rooms headquarters in Piccadilly. She organised sewing groups in Chippenham Division and would have been involved in the organisation of the depot in Chippenham that distributed donations. She was awarded an OBE for her work with the Red Cross.

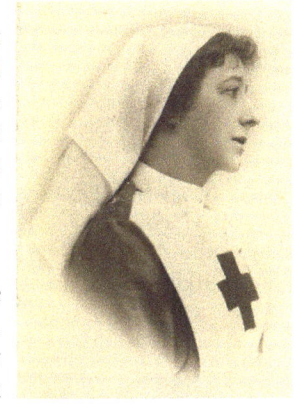

Miss Alice Kathleen Granger
Alice. or as she was better known, Kathleen was one of the munitionettes at Saxby and Farmer who helped at the Hospital. In 1917 she was a member of the women's football team to play the men from the Hospital. Kathleen lived with parents in Park Lane.

Alice Goldney

Miss Mary P Green
Mary Green was the District nurse in Chippenham. When the Hospital opened in November 1915, she was the Lady Superintendent: a post that needed a medically qualified person.

Miss Queenie Green
Queenie was a member of Chippenham Detachment in July 1914 and was on duty when the first patients arrived in November 1915. Nothing else is known about Miss Green.

Mrs M Greig
The only reference to Mrs Greig is that she was named as a nurse by the newspaper when it reported on the closure of the Hospital.

Mrs Grey
The only reference to Mrs Grey is that she came from Sutton Benger and was named as a nurse by the newspaper when it reported on the closure of the Hospital.

Miss Louisa Annie Grimshaw
25 year old Louisa was one of the VAD nurses present when Chippenham Red Cross Hospital opened.
In June 1916 she transferred to the Red Cross Hospital at Brighton. Known as the Pavilion Hospital for Limbless Men it specialised in treating and rehabilitating amputees. She remained there until 1920.
In July 1919 she was awarded the Royal Red Cross for her work at Chippenham and Brighton. Louisa came from Langley Burrell and her father was a navvy on the railway.

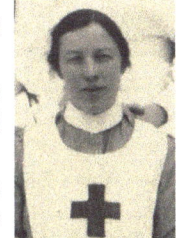

Louisa Grimshaw

Miss Elsie Ellen Hamlin
23 year old Elsie lived with her parents in Wood Lane. In April 1916 she was
engaged as a charwoman (cleaner) for 12 hours per week. She remained at the Hospital until it closed in 1919.

Unity and Loyalty

Mr Basil Howard Alers Hankey
Throughout the war Basil Hankey was director of the Wiltshire Branch of the British Red Cross Society. He lived at Stanton Manor near Chippenham and worked closely with Chippenham Division, often representing the Red Cross when meeting with Chippenham Town Authorities.

Mrs Ellen Hardiman
In August 1914 Ellen Hardiman joined the Chippenham, Wilts 6 VAD, as a probationer nurse and by the early part of 1915 she was serving at Corsham Red Cross Hospital. She returned to Chippenham when the Hospital in the town hall opened. She gave 7311 hours service and became a VAD staff nurse.

Ellen Hardiman lived at Elmfield Villa, 74 London Road, Chippenham with her husband Tom a telegraph inspector with Great Western Railway.

Miss Elsie Hardiman
Daughter of Ellen Hardiman. It is understood she volunteered at the Hospital with her mother but there is no information to confirm her role.

Miss Maud Hardiman
Daughter of Ellen Hardiman. It is understood she volunteered at the Hospital with her mother but there is no information to confirm her role.

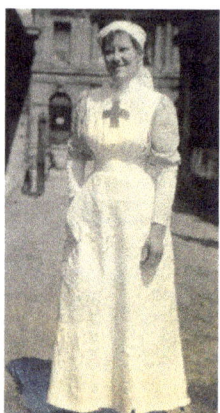

Ellen Hardiman

Mrs Matilda Harding
Matilda Harding called at the Hospital for a few hours every weekend between April 1917 and July 1918 to help with the washing up. She lived in London Road.

Mrs Katherine Harrison
In 1916 Katherine Harrison was the temporary Commandant of Wilts 38 VAD at Sutton Benger. She and her husband lived at Park View in Sutton Benger. It is thought in 1914 Katherine was instrumental in arranging the opening of the wards at Draycot House.

Mrs Margaret Hathaway
From June 1916, until the Hospital closed, Margaret Hathaway, the wife of George Hathaway the Chippenham butter churn manufacturer, visited one morning a week to help in the mess room serving tea and meals. She lived at Shottery in Langley Road.

Miss Dora Beatrice Hart
Dora Hart joined the Red Cross in 1913. She lived at Rooks Nest Farm at Pewsham with her parents. In February 1915 she joined Bowood Hospital, transferred to Corsham and finally joined Chippenham in November. She gave a total of 4000 hours and was a staff nurse when she left the Hospital.

Miss Ada Havell
56 year old Ada Havell volunteered in the kitchens as a part time vegetable peeler and preparer. She continued this work until April 1919, usually giving six hours a week. She lived in Marshfield Road.

Miss Anna Blanche Hayman
Anna, known as Blanche, was a housemaid in the household of Mrs Isobella Cotes at Rowden House. In October 1916 Blanche joined Mrs Cotes and two other servants from the household, as part time mess room assistants.

Mrs Margaret Hayward
Margaret Hayward worked in the kitchen peeling vegetables. She joined the Hospital in January 1916 and left in November 1918. She lived at 20 St Paul Street, Chippenham.

The Story of Chippenham's Red Cross Hospital

Mrs Beatrice Lilian Hetherington.
27 year old Beatrice volunteered at the Hospital in November 1915 and continued until it closed in 1919. She worked in the kitchen for four hours each week. She was also a member of the Chippenham Concert Party that entertained at hospitals around the district.
Beatrice worked alongside Sarah and Norah Hetherington: her mother in law and sister in law.

Miss Norah Hetherington
Norah lived in the High Street in Chippenham. Apart from being described as a nurse in a newspaper article and being included in a group photograph of VADs, nothing is known about Norah's service at the hospital. Her sister in law Beatrice and Mother Sarah also worked at the hospital. In 1924 Norah married Sydney W H Dann at Chippenham.

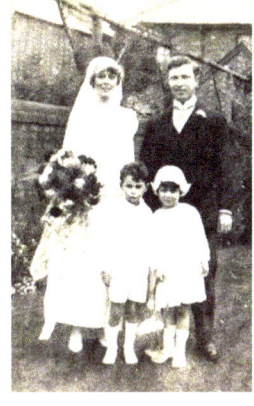
Wedding of Norah Hetherington in 1924

Mrs Sarah Ann Hetherington
Sarah, also known as Ann, was the mother of Norah and mother in law of Beatrice.
Like Norah, apart from being described as a nurse in a newspaper article and being included in a group photograph of VADs, nothing is known about Sarah's service at the Hospital. She lived in the High Street above the family tailoring business.

Mrs Kathleen Highmore
Kathleen Highmore lived in Marshfield Road. In November 1917 she joined the Hospital as a part time cook. She normally worked two mornings a week and continued until it closed in 1919.

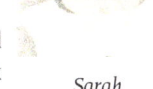
Sarah Hetherington

Mrs Hill
The only reference to Mrs Hill is that she was named as an assistant by the newspaper when it reported on the closure of the Hospital.

Mrs Kate Hinton
Kate Hinton joined the Red Cross VAD in 1910. When the Hospital opened in November 1915 she was appointed as a Staff Nurse. She served until March 1917. The Hinton family lived in New Road and Kate's husband Frederick was the headmaster of Ivy Lane School.

Mrs Ada Hiscock
Ada Hiscock regularly visited the Hospital and worked as a general assistant. Known as "Happy Ada" due to her cheery nature she would entertain the patients and help organise outings.
Ada was the wife of Walter Hiscock, a linen draper and they lived in the Market Place in Chippenham.

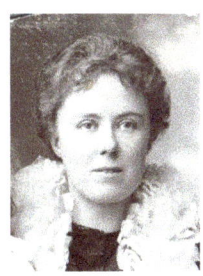
Ada Hiscock

Miss Dorothy Hiscock
Born in 1898 Dorothy was an assistant at the Hospital. She was an accomplished musician being an Associate of the Royal College of Music and joined her mother Ada Hiscock entertaining the patients and organising outings.

Miss Edith Hiscock
Edith was an assistant at the Hospital and helped serve teas. She

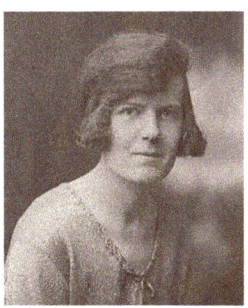
Dorothy Hiscock

joined her mother Ada when organising outings for the patients. In May 1917 Edith asked that her coming of age party, at the sports club, included all the wounded patients. She married Ludlow Tayler, a chemist in the town in 1927. Ludlow Tayler regularly donated medical supplies to the Hospital.

Mr Walter Hiscock
Walter owned a linen draper shop in the Market Place. In 1916 he became the mayor of Chippenham. Walter was one of the organisers of the Christmas meals for the patients. His wife Ada and daughters were regular helpers at the Hospital.

Miss Gladys Mary Hobbs
Gladys Hobbs was born in 1892 and lived St Mary Street. In July 1918 she married Major Scott Watson. She is shown on a group photograph of VADs otherwise nothing is known about Gladys's service at the Hospital.

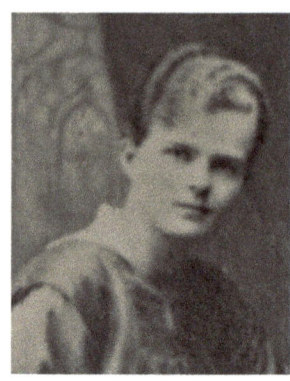
Edith Hiscock

Miss Olive May Holland
16 year old Olive started volunteering in the kitchen at the Hospital in January 1916. She went on to become a nurse probationer and served until January 1919. She lived at Cleveland House in New Road, Chippenham with her parents Francis and Ella Holland who were tobacconists.

Mrs Daisy Maud Hodges
Daisy Hodges joined the Hospital as a part time mess room worker in August 1916 and volunteered 7 hours a week. She left in October 1917 and went to live in Swindon.

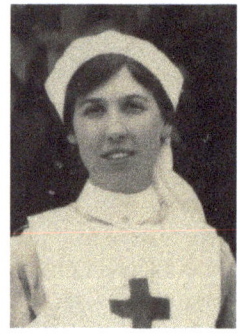
Gladys Hobbs

Miss Louisa Hosey
Louisa was a member of Wilts 32 VAD, Derry Hill Detachment. Between August 1914 and January 1918 she served as a part time assistant at both Bowood and Chippenham Red Cross hospitals. She was employed as housekeeper at Pewsham House.

Miss Beatrice Houlston
Beatrice was the daughter of Robert Houlston a stationer and printer who had a shop in the High Street in Chippenham. She was a member of Chippenham Wilts 6 VAD. When war broke out Beatrice volunteered at Corsham Red Cross Hospital. She trained in Swedish and Electrical massage to treat orthopaedic patients including amputation cases. She travelled around the district and treated patients at hospitals in Corsham, Calne, Bowood, Chippenham, Bath and Warminster.

Mrs Alice Hulbert
In May 1916 58 year old widow Alice Hulbert, who lived at 33 Timber Street, volunteered her services, washing up for a few hours every week. She continued until the Hospital closed.

Mrs Annie Brown Hulbert
Annie lived in Myrtle Villa, Lowden Avenue, Chippenham. Between September 1917 and November 1918, she volunteered a number of hours each week to prepare vegetables for the Hospital kitchen. During this time one of the patients was her son Charles.

Mrs Emma Elizabeth Hulbert
Emma, also known as Elizabeth, lived in New Road in Chippenham. She and her family later moved to the Causeway. Her husband Francis ran his own building and plumbing company. It

The Story of Chippenham's Red Cross Hospital

was Mr Hulbert's company that converted the town hall to a hospital in November 1915.

Emma was a trained nurse. In 1891 she was working at Sussex County Hospital in Brighton and 10 years later she was a District Nurse in Chippenham. In August 1914 with her experience of nursing she joined Wilts 6 VAD. She was appointed Assistant Superintendent and Sister in charge of a ward of 40 beds. The British Journal of Nursing confirmed her appointment on 20 May 1916.

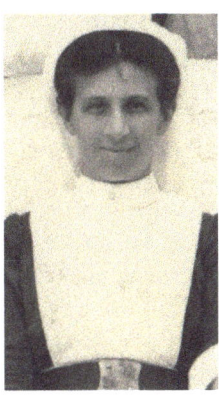

Emma Hulbert

Mrs Bessie Humphries
Bessie lived in Sutton Benger and was a member of Wilts 38 VAD. She joined Chippenham Hospital in March 1916, as a probationer nurse, and gave 1800 hours. She left in April 1919.

. In March 1919 Bessie received news that her son Leonard had died of Pneumonia in France.

Miss Ellen Humphries
Ellen came from Corsham but was in service, at Rowden House in Chippenham, employed as a cook. In October 1916, she volunteered part time at the Hospital helping in the mess room until April 1917.

Mrs Matilda Emma Hunt
Matilda Hunt served meals in the Hospital and helped in the wards. She volunteered from November 1915 until April 1919. She was also a member of the Entertainment Committee and helped organise excursions for the patients.

Matilda and her husband George lived in Albany House in Chippenham, later moving to New Road. In November 1917 Matilda and her husband received the news that their son Percival had been killed in action.

Miss Hurley
The only reference to Miss Hurley is that she came from Castle Combe and was named as a nurse by the newspaper when it reported the closure of the Hospital.

Miss Eva Hutton
Eva Hutton became a full-time probationer VAD nurse at Chippenham in December 1916. She went on to serve at a number of military hospital around the country and in France . In July 1919 she gave her home address as 20, The Brittox, Devizes.

Mrs Alice Ellen Isaacs
54 year old widow Alice Isaacs was employed at the Red Cross Hospital soon after it opened. She was a cleaner and worked 16 hours a week. She was paid 6s 9d and continued until it closed in April 1919. She lived in the Butts in Chippenham.

Mr Herbert James
Herbert James of Park Lane, Chippenham joined Wilts 13 VAD in January 1917 to assist with ambulance transport and gave 100 hours part time service.

Miss Frances Marion Jefferys
Frances Jefferys gave her address as The Girls' School at Tytherton. She joined the Red Cross Hospital in August 1916 as a part time cleaner and continued this work until she left in January 1918. She was a member of Wilts 38 VAD.

Mr Lewis Arthur Jessop
Lewis Jessop was a clerk at Saxby and Farmer and was well known in the town as a performer with the Chippenham Amateur Operatic and Dramatic Society. He lived in St Paul Street and

Unity and Loyalty

joined the Wilts 13 VAD in November 1915 as an ambulance orderly. He gave a total of 1700 hours service.

Mrs Sarah Jane Johnson
Mrs Johnson volunteered at the Hospital between December 1915 and November 1917. She was a part time kitchen worker. She gave her address as The Dairy in Parkfields, Chippenham.

Mrs Jukes
The only reference to Mrs Jukes is that she was named as an assistant by the newspaper when it reported the closure of the Hospital.

Mrs Keel
The only reference to Mrs Keel is that she was named as a volunteer by the newspaper when it reported the closure of the Hospital.

Mr William Charles King
William King worked in his father's ironmongers in New Road Chippenham. In January 1916 he joined the men's Detachment, as an ambulance orderly but left in May when he joined the military. He gave 150 hours service as an ambulance orderly in Chippenham. His sister Winifred also served as a VAD.

Miss Winifred Agnes King
Winifred was an assistant in her father's ironmongers in New Road, Chippenham. In January 1915 she joined Wilts 6 VAD and served at Corsham Red Cross Hospital as a nurse. In November 1915 she transferred to the newly opened Chippenham Red Cross Hospital, where she remained until it closed in 1919.

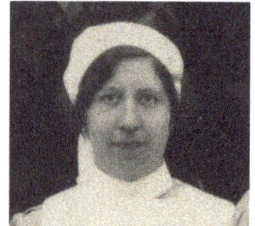
Winifred King

Dr George Laurence
George Laurence qualified as a doctor in 1904. He joined Dr Briscoe's practice in the Market Place and when the Red Cross Hospital opened he took on additional duties as one of its medical officers. He visited two days a week and was on call for emergencies at both Chippenham and Bowood.

Dr Laurence lived in Marshfield Road, Chippenham. In 1953 he married one of the VADS, Minnie Pike.

Miss Grace Day Lavington
Grace lived with her parents, John and Grace Lavington in Christian Malford. She was an assistant in her father's bakery and grocery shop in the village. In March 1916, aged 36, she joined Chippenham Hospital as a part time probationer. She was a member of Wilts 38 VAD and gave 1032 hours service.

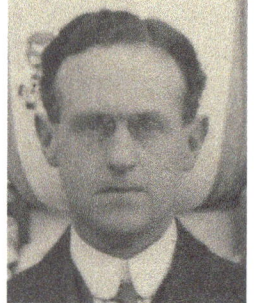
Dr Laurence

Miss Helena Gertrude Lawrence
31 year old Helena Lawrence joined Chippenham Red Cross Hospital as a trained nurse in September 1916. The British Nursing Journal confirmed her appointment as a Sister. She had previously been a nurse at Tetbury Union Workhouse. Helena was the daughter of Alfred Lawrence who was the Sergeant Major for the Yeomanry in Chippenham. The family lived at Churchdown in Bath Road, Chippenham.

Miss Mary Louisa Lea
Mary was the daughter of John Lea who farmed in Sutton Benger. She was a member of Wilts 38 VAD and joined Chippenham Hospital in March 1916 as a probationer giving 1189 hours. Her

The Story of Chippenham's Red Cross Hospital

brother John died at Gallipoli in October 1915.

Mrs Bertha Lewis
From June 1918 until the Hospital closed Bertha assisted by mending bedding and patients clothing. She lived at Jays Farm at Stanley.

Mrs Margaret Edith Little
Margaret, who lived in the Causeway, Chippenham, joined the Hospital in July 1918. She gave two hours a week and helped in the mess room, serving teas and meals.

Mrs Mary E Lodder
Mary, who lived in Audley Road, Chippenham, joined the Hospital in October 1916. She visited every Monday and helped in the mess room, serving teas and meals. She continued to volunteer until July 1917.

Miss Kathleen Jean Mackay
Miss Mackay joined Wilts 6 VAD at Chippenham Hospital as a probationer nurse in November 1915. By October 1917 she had transferred to London and served at several military hospitals in the city. Her home was The Firs, Kington Langley.

Mrs Sarah Ann Mackness
Sarah Mackness was one of the first recruits to join Chippenham VAD in 1910. In February 1915 she reported to Corsham Red Cross Hospital for duty as a staff nurse, but after a short time was forced to leave due to ill health. When she recovered, she continued her VAD duties at Chippenham Red Cross Hospital. Sarah was the wife of Frederick Mackness who owned a wagon making business in the Causeway.

Mrs Lily Maloney
Lily, who lived at Clift Cottage in Chippenham, joined the Hospital in August 1916. She visited one day a week to help in the mess room and do the washing up. She continued to volunteer until 1919.

Miss Phyllis Malpas
Phyllis served at Chippenham Red Cross Hospital between August 1917 and April 1919 as a probationer nurse. Her address was 17 St Mary Street and it is thought she was the daughter in law of Sarah Malpas, who also volunteered at the Hospital.

Mrs Sarah Ann Malpas
Sarah was a certified nurse and for many years midwife in the town. Her home at 17 St Mary Street, Chippenham, was used as a 'Nursing Home for mother and baby'. She volunteered as a part time nurse at Chippenham Red Cross Hospital in October 1916 and continued until the Hospital closed in 1919.

She joined the Red Cross in 1913 being awarded her five-year badge in 1918.

Mr Albert Edwin Mann
Albert Mann was a builder and lived in Stanton St Quintin with his wife Ellen and family. It is thought before the war he was a member of the local St John Ambulance Association and at the outbreak of war he joined Malmesbury Red Cross Detachment. In March 1915 he became a full time orderly at Netley Military Hospital near Southampton where he remained until June 1916. He returned to Stanton St Quintin and gave further service at Chippenham Red Cross Hospital, where he was listed as a member of Chippenham,

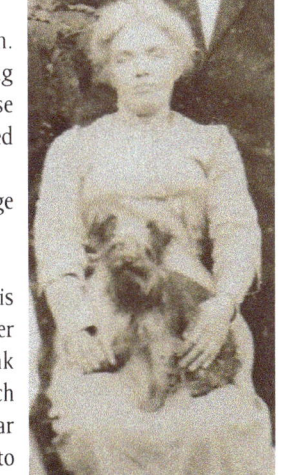

Sarah Malpas

Wilts 13 VAD.

Mr Albert Maslen

Albert Maslen lived in Parkfields in Chippenham and worked for Great Western Railway as a locomotive foreman. He joined Wilts 13 VAD and attended the wounded men arriving at the railway station.

Mr Ernest Maslen

Ernest Maslen lived at Townsend in Box. In May 1917 he joined Wilts 3 VAD at Corsham and served at Bowood, Corsham and Chippenham Red Cross Hospitals as an orderly. He gave 1000 hours service.

Mr Arthur George Mattingly

Arthur Mattingly lived in the High Street where he traded as a fishmonger. He gave 200 hours helping to transport the walking wounded from the station using private cars.

Mr Harry Maynard

Harry Maynard was a member of Wilts 3 VAD and volunteered as a Red Cross Orderly. He gave 300 hours service including work at Chippenham. He lived in the High Street in Colerne and was a boot and shoe maker.

Miss Ada Merchant

Ada was employed as a full-time kitchen assistant between March and September 1917. She lived in The Gardens, London Road, Chippenham.

Mrs Elsie Mary Miller

Elsie lived in the High Street in Chippenham. She was a relief sister at Bowood Hospital and also served at Chippenham as a nurse.

Mrs Ethel Mills

Between 1917 and 1919 Ethel helped in the mess room at the Hospital. She lived at Bayntun House in London Road, Chippenham. Her husband was an Accountant at the condensed milk factory.

Mrs Minty

The only reference to Mrs Minty is that she was named as an assistant by the newspaper when it reported the closure of the Hospital.

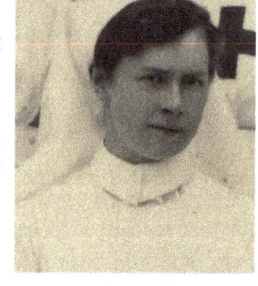

Elsie Miller

Mrs Julie Morgan

Mrs Morgan was registered with Wilts 44 VAD in Swindon. She lived in Priory Cottage in Wootton Bassett. During 1916 she served at Chippenham for several months as a nurse. She was 64 years old, a widow and had a private income.

Miss K Morgan

The only reference to Miss Morgan is that she was named as an assistant by the newspaper when it reported the closure of the Hospital.

Miss Alice Munday

25 year old school teacher Alice joined Wilts 6 VAD in November 1915. She was a part time cook and continued to volunteer at the Red Cross Hospital until it closed in April 1919. She gave 3200 hours. She lived in Landsend, Chippenham.

Miss Neale

The only reference to Miss Neale is that she was named as an assistant by the newspaper when it reported the closure of the Hospital. It is possible she was Phyllis, the daughter of Edgar Neale, who had a chemist shop in the town and donated supplies to the Hospital.

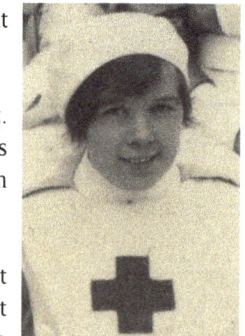

Alice Munday

The Story of Chippenham's Red Cross Hospital

Lt Col Sir Audley Dallas Neeld
Colonel Neeld was a great friend to the Hospital. He frequently visited the patients and invited them to his home, Grittleton House to play bowls in the garden. He also arranged day trips for the patients and VADs in his car. His wife Lady Edith headed the Work Party in Grittleton.

Mrs Ogilvie
The only reference to Mrs Ogilvie is that she was named as an assistant by the newspaper when it reported the closure of the Hospital.

Miss Oliver
The only reference to Miss Oliver is that she was named as an assistant by the newspaper when it reported the closure of the Hospital.

Mrs Edith Pannell
Edith lived in St Paul Street, Chippenham with her husband William, an inspector at Saxby and Farmer. She joined Wilts 6 VAD when the Hospital opened in 1915, but left after a few months due to poor health. She did ward work and sewing and gave 100 hours.

Miss Alfreda Maud Parry
41 year old Alfreda joined Wilts 6 VAD in October 1915 and volunteered as a part time night nurse giving a total of 5031 hours. She was a school teacher and lived with her widowed mother at the Woodhouse in St Mary Street, Chippenham.

Mrs Gertrude Violet Paterson
From October 1917 until the Hospital closed Gertrude Paterson was a part time helper in the mess room. She lived in Park Lane, Chippenham.

Miss Sarah Payne
Sarah Payne was in domestic service in Great Somerford. In August 1916, aged 23, she joined Malmesbury Hospital (Wilts 28 VAD) as a part time nurse. She later served as a nurse at Chippenham and was still working when the Hospital closed. She gave a total of 1200 hours service.

Miss Winifred Pearce
16 year old Winifred, from Langley Burrell, joined the Chippenham Red Cross Hospital as an assistant cook in March 1916 giving 1300 hours until she left in September 1918. It is thought she was the daughter of Ralph Pearce who owned the Langley Brewery.

Arthur J Phillips
After being declared unfit for war service 25 year old Arthur joined the men's VAD, Wilts 13, in November 1916. He worked at Hinders the cycle shop and made wheeled stretchers using bicycle wheels to help move patients. He was still serving at the Hospital in April 1919 when it closed and gave a total of 1220 hours service. Arthur lived in Sandbrook Place in Chippenham with his parents.

Mrs Phillips
The only reference to Mrs Phillips is that she was named as an assistant by the newspaper when it reported the closure of the Hospital.

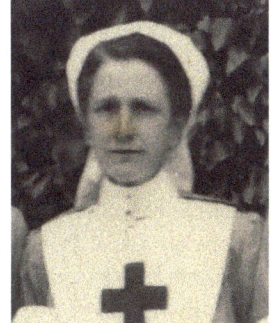
Edith Pannell

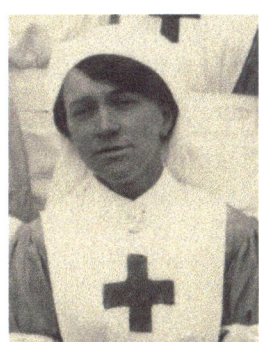
Alfreda Parry

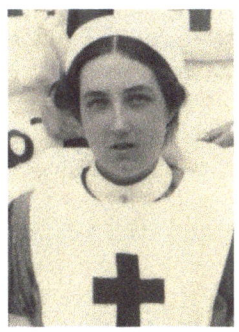
Winifred Pearce

Unity and Loyalty

Miss Minnie Pike
20 year old Minnie Pike joined Chippenham Red Cross Hospital in 1915 as a staff nurse. She lived at 2 Greenway Park, Chippenham and remained an active member of the Red Cross in Chippenham after the war. In 1936 she was appointed Commandant of Wilts 6 VAD and was awarded the long service medal. In 1953 Minnie married Doctor George Laurence, one of the medical officers during the war.

Mrs Annie Letitia Pinfield
Annie was the wife of Bernard Pinfield, son of Henry and Emily Pinfield. It is not known what duties Annie carried out but she was listed as a VAD by the newspaper when the Hospital closed. Her husband, Bernard, enlisted in the 28th London Regiment and was wounded in December 1917 and again in May 1918.

Mrs Emily Pinfield
55 year old Emily Pinfield volunteered at the Red Cross Hospital as an assistant in the kitchen preparing vegetables and serving in the mess room. She gave 9 hours every week from 1915 until 1919. She lived in Audley Road with her husband Henry.

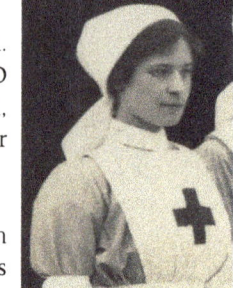
Annie Pinfield

Their son Bert was killed in action in France while another son was wounded.

Mrs Rosa Gertrude Pinfield.
Rosa, known as Gertie, was the daughter of Frank and Rose Buckland, who also served at the Hospital. In her obituary she was described as working hard with the VAD, although it is not known what her duties were. Rosa was married to Bert Pinfield. In September 1917 Rosa received the news that her husband had been killed in France.

Mrs Selina Pinniger
Mrs Pinniger lived in Wood Lane Chippenham. From May 1916 until the Hospital closed she attended for 3 hours each week to help with washing up.

Mrs Elsie Pocock
The only reference to Mrs Pocock is that she was named as an assistant by the newspaper when it reported on the closure of the Hospital.

Mrs Louise Jane Pocock
From March 1916 until the Hospital closed Mrs Pocock, who lived in Malmesbury Road, collected bedding and clothing that needed repairing and worked on them at home. She gave 1892 hours service.

Miss Daisy E Pope
Daisy Pope was a schoolteacher. She taught at Ivy Lane School in Chippenham and went on to teach at East Tytherton and Lacock schools. In May 1916, aged 26, she volunteered as a part time nursing probationer and served at the Hospital until it closed in April 1919. She lived in Hawthorn Road in Chippenham.

Miss Eugenia Grace Pope
Eugenia, known as Grace, was the daughter of the Rector of Langley Burrell. She joined Chippenham Red Cross Hospital when it opened in 1915 and worked as an assistant in the wards and the mess room. She also served at Bath and Carlisle hospitals and volunteered a total of 4248 hours.

Miss Lilian Porter
Lilian Porter joined the Hospital in August 1917 as a probationer. She

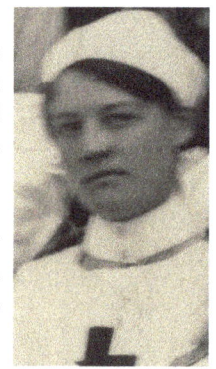
Daisy Pope

The Story of Chippenham's Red Cross Hospital

continued until it closed and gave 625 hours service. She lived at Greenway Park in Chippenham.

Mrs Lilian Alice May Pound
Mrs Pound lived at 12 St Mary's Place. From June 1918 until the Hospital closed she volunteered as a part time mess room assistant. She gave 155 hours service. Her husband Sidney was a part time orderly.

Mr Sidney Eric Pound
30 year old Sidney joined Wilts 13 VAD in February 1918 as a part time ambulance orderly and gave 350 hours service. He worked at Saxby and Farmer and he and his wife lived in St Mary's Place.

Mrs Bessie Powell
Bessie lived in Rural Gardens in Chippenham. In March 1917 she started to volunteer 2 hours a week at the Hospital doing the washing up which she continued until 1919.

Mr Henry D Powell
Henry Powell lived in Sheldon Road. He joined Wilts 13 VAD in September 1916 as a part time ambulance orderly and gave 1340 hours service.

Miss Phyllis Ramsbottom
Phyllis was the daughter of William Ramsbottom the Vicar of Lacock. She joined Chippenham Red Cross Hospital in September 1916 as a probationer nurse. Phyllis ended her engagement in May 1917. It is not known why she left, but she continued in the medical profession and by 1922 she was working as a midwife.

Mrs Rawle
The only reference to Mrs Rawle is that she was named as an assistant by the newspaper when it reported the closure of the Hospital.

Mr Francis Read
Frank Read was employed as an engineer at Saxby and Farmer. He was appointed Commandant of the Chippenham men's Detachment in 1916, a role he retained for the remainder of the war. He gave 2150 hours to the Detachment. Frank and his wife Lily, who also served at the Hospital, lived at 25, Parkfields, Chippenham.

Mrs Lily Read
Lily was the wife of Frank Read the Commandant of Wilts 13 VAD. She volunteered at Chippenham Red Cross Hospital as a mess room assistant and mended sheets and clothing.

Sister Reed
Sister Reed was working at the Hospital in February 1917 when Private Stubbert died. She sent a wreath with other staff. Nothing else is known about her.

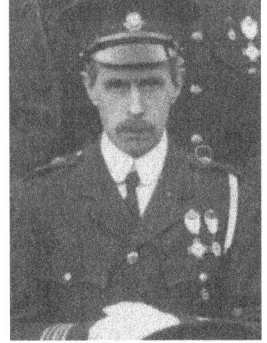

Frank Read

Miss Ellen Kathleen Reeves
21 Year old Ellen joined as a probationer in July 1918. Her home was in Bromham near Devizes. She had taken lodgings in Park Lane, Chippenham. In January 1919 she appeared before the magistrates accused of stealing bedding, tea towels and aprons from the wards. The magistrates dealt with her leniently because she said it was an oversight as she had been on duty a lot and suffered from want of sleep.

Miss Ethel Margaret Rich
From November 1916 Ethel Rich volunteered two days a week helping in the mess room. She was the daughter of the late Canon Rich, who had been Vicar of Chippenham for 43 years. Ethel lived

at Lowden Lodge with her sister Gertrude. Ethel was also member of the Management Committee of Chippenham Division.

Miss Eva Leslie Rich
Eva lived with her parents at Loxwell Farm, Pewsham. In June 1915, when she was 19, she volunteered as a cook at Bowood Red Cross Hospital. In November 1915 she joined the newly opened Chippenham, as a part time nursing probationer. She remained at Chippenham until December 1918 and gave a total of 2458 hours service, of which 196 were at Bowood.

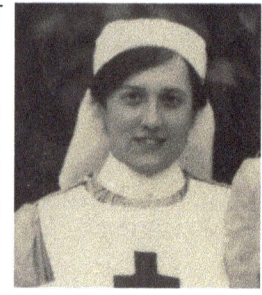

Eva Rich

Miss Roach
The only reference to Miss Roach is that she was named as an assistant by the newspaper when it reported the closure of the Hospital.

Mrs Alice Maude Rogers
Mrs Rogers, who lived in Ivy Road, Chippenham helped in the kitchen preparing vegetables for two and a half hours each week. She worked from September 1917 until the Hospital closed in 1919.

Miss Doris Rooke
Doris helped at the VAD Hospital in Chippenham but there is no record of her duties. She lived with her family at The Ivy in Chippenham. In October 1918 Doris and her sister became victims of the flu pandemic and died within days of each other.

Miss Ellen Rooke
Ellen helped at the VAD Hospital in Chippenham but there is no record of her duties.
She lived with her family at The Ivy in Chippenham. In October 1918 Ellen and her sister became victims of the flu pandemic and died within days of each other.

Mr James William Reginald Royle
James Royle lived in Park Lane, Chippenham, and joined Wilts 13 VAD as an orderly in September 1916. He was about 18 years old and an apprentice at Saxby and Farmer; his family home being in Reading. In January 1917 he left the Detachment to join the Stafford Regiment. Within weeks of arriving in France he was shot in the leg by a sniper and was invalided home. He was awarded the Military Medal for his wartime actions.

Miss Phillis Violet Rudler
19 year old Phillis volunteered in October 1917 as a probationer. She gave 980 hours service. Phillis lived at Hither Farm at Stanley, with her parents but by the end of the war was living in the village of Grittleton.

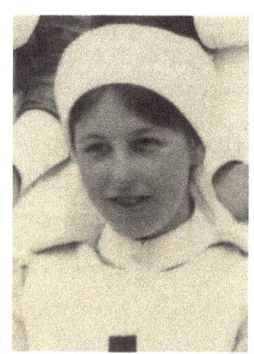

Mary Rudman

Miss Alice Mary Rudman
Alice, or Mary as she was better known, was 16 years old when she volunteered to work in the kitchen in November 1915. She worked for 8 hours a week until she left in March 1917. She lived in New Road, Chippenham, with her parents Robert and Alice. Robert Rudman was a building contractor.

Mrs Alice Rudman
Alice Rudman helped at the Hospital to organise social events for the wounded men. She was involved in arranging outings and afternoon

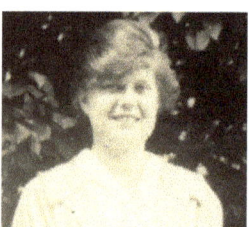

Alice Rudman

The Story of Chippenham's Red Cross Hospital

tea parties. Alice lived in New Road and was married to Robert Rudman, a building contractor. Her daughter Mary was a VAD.

Miss Edith Russ
Edith was born in 1891 she was the daughter of butcher Henry Russ of Sutton Benger. She joined the Detachment in her home village, Wilts 38 VAD, but soon left the area to serve at a number of military hospitals. In 1917 she was nursing at the Military Hospital at Fovant, near Salisbury, and by the end of the year was at the Military Hospital Alexandria in Egypt. Her brother Albert was killed at Gallipoli in August 1915

Mr Lionel Sanders
Lionel Sanders lived with his parents John and Rose in Malmesbury Road. In 1917 at the age of 16 he joined Wilts 13 VAD. He was an orderly at the Hospital and assisted with the transport of patients. He gave 150 hours service.

Miss Miriam Irene Scott
Miss Scott was a full time qualified nurse paid a salary of £20 per year. During 1915 and 1916 she served at a number of VAD hospitals in Wiltshire. In June 1915 she joined Bowood Red Cross Hospital, transferring to Chippenham in April 1916 and to Devizes at the end of the year. She was the daughter of the vicar of Derry Hill and gave her address as Derry Hill Vicarage.

Miss Mary Agnes Selman
Mary was a member of the Chippenham Detachment that won the Division competition at the Neeld Hall in July 1914 and is also included in a group photograph of VADs taken in Chippenham about 1916. She was born in 1887 the daughter of Jacob Selman a retired farmer who lived at Kington Langley.

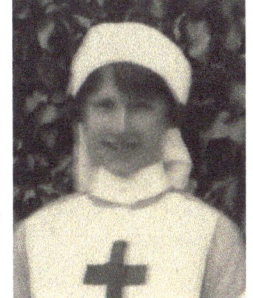
Mary Selman

Mrs Florence Selman
Florence lived at 67 Marshfield Road, Chippenham, with her husband Thomas. In May 1916, aged 58, she volunteered 7 hours a week in the kitchen of the Hospital preparing vegetables. She left in September 1918.

Mrs Elizabeth Shave
Elizabeth was a part time mess room assistant from April 1918 until the Hospital closed. She was the wife of Frederick who was member of Wilts 13 VAD.

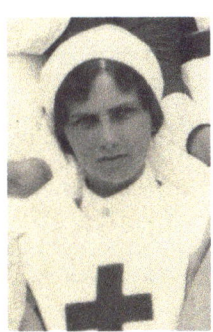
Ivy Shipp

Mr Frederick Shave
Born in 1880 Frederick, also known as George, worked at Saxby and Farmer and was a member of the company First Aid unit. He joined Wilts 13 VAD in September 1916 and gave 1400 hours service. He lived in St Paul Street with his wife Elizabeth who also served at the Hospital.

Miss Ivy Shipp
16 year old Ivy joined the kitchen staff in November 1915 as a part time cook. She was the daughter of one of the head cooks, Minnie Shipp. Ivy lived with her family at Cadenham Manor, near Foxham.

Mrs Minnie Shipp
Minnie and her husband Edgar Shipp farmed at Cadenham Manor,

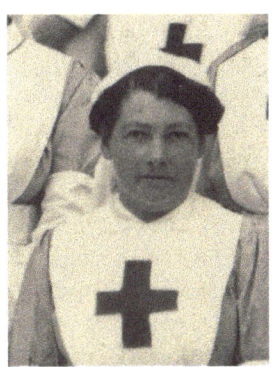
Minnie Shipp

near Foxham. When Chippenham Hospital opened in November 1915 Minnie was engaged as one of the head cooks. She worked part time and gave 5088 hours.

Miss Vera Shipp
20 year old Vera joined her mother Minnie and sister Ivy in the kitchen at the Hospital in January 1917. After a year working in the kitchen she became a probationer nurse in the wards. She worked part time and gave 3024 hours.

Mrs Annie Elizabeth Shorland
Annie Shorland joined the Red Cross in 1913 and became a probationer nurse when Loyalty ward opened in August 1916. She gave 3282 hours. In December 1918 she was awarded her 5 year Red Cross badge. She and her husband Edward lived in Malmesbury Road, Chippenham.

Herbert James Sidnell
Herbert Sidnell lived with his parents Ada and William in Lowden, Chippenham. In January 1916, aged 18, he joined Wilts 13 VAD as an orderly and assisted with ambulance transport giving 150 hours service. In September 1916 he left the Detachment to join the Wiltshire Regiment and saw action in France.

Miss Simmond
The only reference to Miss Simmond is that she came from Sutton Benger and was named as a nurse by the newspaper when it reported the closure of the Hospital.

Mrs Simpson
The only reference to Mrs Simpson is that she was named as an assistant by the newspaper when it reported the closure of the Hospital.

Mrs Skipp
The only reference to Mrs Skipp is that she was named as a nurse by the newspaper when it reported the closure of the Hospital.

Mrs Sara Slade
Sara Slade lived at Ferfoot on Bristol Road. She volunteered as a cook at the Hospital for 10 hours every week from November 1916 until April 1919.

Miss Ida Christabel Small
Ida, known as Chrissie, joined Wilts 6 VAD in October 1916 as a probationer nurse and continued until May 1917. She lived at 19 Market Place with her parents, William and Kate Small. She was also a Sunday School teacher at St Pauls Church. Her father William was mayor of Chippenham in 1910 and 1917.

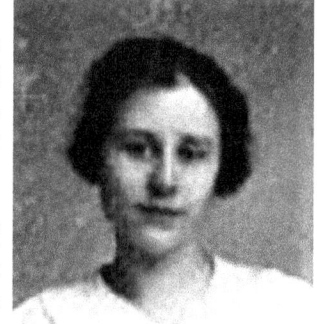

Chrissie Small

Miss Alice Smith
According to the newspaper report on the closure of the Hospital a Miss Smith from Malmesbury served at Chippenham. It is thought this was Alice Smith who also served at Charlton Park and Malmesbury hospitals. She lived in Gloucester Road, Malmesbury.

Mr Charles Edward Smith
Charles Smith worked for the Great Western Railway. In October 1916, aged 45, he joined Wilts 3 VAD, the Corsham men's Detachment, as a part-time orderly. He gave 1750 hours and saw service at Corsham, Chippenham, Devizes and Bath hospitals. He lived in Mill Lane Box.

Mrs Dorothy Marriott Smith
Dorothy lived in Calne. In June 1915 she was appointed Quartermaster at Bowood Hospital. From February 1917 until August 1917 she was a part time cook at Chippenham.

The Story of Chippenham's Red Cross Hospital

Mrs Emma Jane Smith
Emma Smith lived in Langley Road. From July 1916 she helped in the kitchens 1 day every fortnight preparing vegetables.

Miss Dorothy Spencer
Dorothy was the daughter of Kate and Arthur Spencer who owned the music shop in the Market Place. In 1916 Dorothy, who was only 13, was an accomplished singer and took part in some musical productions for the wounded men.

Mrs Kate Spencer
Kate Spencer lived in the Market Place in Chippenham with her husband Arthur. They lived above their shop known as The Music Warehouse.
She volunteered at Corsham Red Cross Hospital in October 1914. A year later she helped establish the VAD Hospital in Chippenham and was appointed staff nurse. She remained at Chippenham until December 1917 and volunteered 2500 hours.

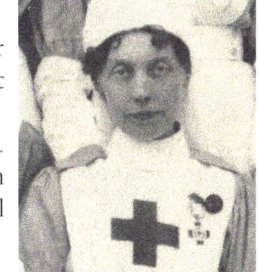

Katherine Spencer

Miss Joan Spicer
Joan was the daughter of Lady Margaret Spicer, the Vice President of Chippenham Division. She lived at Spye Park and from 1915 volunteered at Bowood and Chippenham hospitals doing ward work. She gave a total of 2688 hours. In 1919 she died aged 23: a victim of the flu pandemic.

Mrs Katherine Sophia Spicer
Katherine, the wife of Julian Spicer, the brother in law of Lady Margaret Spicer, was Quartermaster of Wilts 38 VAD and lived in Sutton Benger. She joined Chippenham Red Cross Hospital in May 1916 and gave 984 hours.

Lady Margaret Spicer
Margaret Spicer was born in 1870, the daughter of the Earl of Westmorland. In 1888 she married John Spicer of Spye Park near Chippenham. During 1914 she was appointed the Vice President of Chippenham Division. After the war she continued her work with the Red Cross retiring in the 1940s.

Miss M Spiers
The only reference to Miss Spiers is that she was named as an assistant by the newspaper when it reported the closure of the Hospital.

Miss Daisy Spinke
27 year old Daisy Spinke was one of the VADs to receive the first patients at Chippenham in 1915. She lived with her parents at Kingston House in the Causeway. She left the Hospital in 1917 having given 1000 hours in the kitchen.

Miss Mabel Spinke
From 1915, 25 year old Mabel worked with her sister Daisy in the kitchen as a cook and gave 2189 hours service continuing to work at the Hospital until 1919. After the war she remained in the Red Cross and in 1936 she was appointed Assistant Commandant of the Detachment.

Mr Arthur Zebedee Stanley
Arthur Stanley was born in 1891. He lived in Lowden and worked at Saxby and Farmer where he was an active member of the First

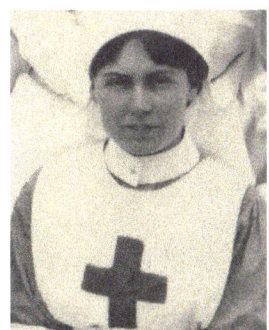

Mabel Spinke

Aid unit. He was the Quartermaster for Wilts 13 VAD and served at Chippenham Hospital from November 1915 until the end of the war. He served alongside his brother Francis.

Mr Francis C Stanley.
Francis Stanley was a foreman at the condensed milk factory in Bath Road. In 1916 he was a member of Wilts 13 VAD initially as an ambulance orderly and later promoted to section leader. He gave 1600 hours service. His brother, Arthur was also a member of Wilts 13 VAD.

Francis, and his wife Emily, lived in Lowden Terrace in Sheldon Road, Chippenham.

Mr William Stanley Stephens
William was a hairdresser with premises in Market Place. He would regularly call at the Hospital to give haircuts and shave the patients.

Mrs Lilian A Stevens
Lilian, with her sisters Mabel and Daisy Spinke, were amongst the VADs in attendance when the Hospital opened. In December 1918 she became a victim of the flu epidemic. Aged 43, she was buried at St Paul's Church. Amongst the mourners were many of her friends from the Detachment.

Mr Ernest Stevenson
Mr Stevenson was an upholsterer with premises in the Market Place. He was the Secretary of the Military Entertainments Committee and in 1918 became the Secretary of the Club for Wounded Soldiers. He also volunteered 2 days every week at the Hospital helping at mealtimes.

Miss Lilian Amy Stewart
35 year old Miss Stewart became a part time probationer nurse during 1917. She was also a member of the Chippenham Sewing Work Party with her mother Lucy.

They lived at the Old Palace in the Market Place in Chippenham. Lilian was the daughter of Archdeacon Stewart.

Eleanor Countess of Suffolk
Eleanor Countess of Suffolk, the widow of 18th Earl of Suffolk was a member of the County Red Cross Committee.

In October 1914, aged 67, she became Commandant of Charlton Park VAD Hospital near Malmesbury. She then became nurse in charge at Malmesbury until November 1917 when she transferred to Devizes and Chippenham hospitals. In August 1919 she was described as a nurse at Chippenham in the London Gazette when it was announced she had been awarded the Royal Red Cross for her services. It is thought that while serving at Chippenham Eleanor lived with her relations, the Coventry family, at Monkton Park House. Her granddaughter Muriel was also a VAD.

Eleanor's son Henry Howard, 19th Earl of Suffolk, was killed in action in April 1917.

Mrs Georgina Sutton
Mrs Sutton lived at Rookery Farm House in Seagry. She was a member of Wilts 38 VAD. In December 1914 she left Wiltshire for France, where she worked as a cook at the military hospitals. She returned to Seagry in April 1915. In 1917 she joined Chippenham Hospital and volunteered for night duty until 1919.

Mrs Swain
The only reference to Mrs Swain is a newspaper article report on the closure of the Hospital when she is described as an assistant. It is thought she may be Annie Swain wife of Edward Swain.

Mr Edward Swain
Mr Swain, who lived in Marshfield Road, had been a member of St John's Ambulance for some years. When the Hospital opened, he served as an orderly and maintained the rotas, ensuring men and vehicles were available to meet the trains at the station. He was also a member of the

The Story of Chippenham's Red Cross Hospital

Entertainment Committee. In 1925 he was the Mayor present at the unveiling of the Tablet to the Red Cross at the Town Hall. Colonel Neeld said at the ceremony 'I cannot stand here without referring to the splendid work done by the present Mayor of Chippenham, Councillor Swain, who was one of the regular workers at the Hospital'.

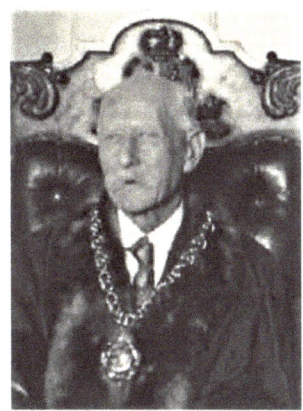

Edward Swain

Mr Ernest Swaffield
Ernest Swaffield was an ambulance orderly in 1916; he went on to became a section leader. In March 1917 his employer, Stevens the bootmaker in the High Street, appealed to the tribunal against Swaffield's military conscription. Stevens said the business relied on Swaffield and in the evenings he did essential work at the Red Cross Hospital. The tribunal agreed to exempt Swaffield and he continued to work part time at the Hospital until it closed in 1919. He gave 1050 hours service. Ada and Ernest Swaffield lived in the Market Place in Chippenham.

Mrs Annie Maria Tanner
Mrs Tanner attended the Hospital 2 hours a week to wash dishes. Aged 61 she started volunteering in December 1915 and left in July 1918. She lived at 8 Timber Street with her husband Eli, who was coal carter.

Mr Percival Ernest Tanner
Percy Tanner joined Wilts 13 VAD in September 1916 aged 16. He was an apprentice pattern maker and lived with his parents in Parliament Street. He was awarded his home nursing certificate in December 1916. He gave 650 hours service and left in April 1918 to enlist in the Machine Gun Corps.

Mrs Alice Taylor
Alice lived at Pew Hill and volunteered at the Hospital from October 1917 until April 1918 for two hours a week to serve teas and do mending.

Mrs Eliza Taylor
Eliza Taylor volunteered at the Hospital between April and November 1916, serving teas for the patients. She moved to Stroud but it is not known if she continued to volunteer with the Red Cross it that area.

Miss Marjory Taylor
From January 1918 to January 1919 Marjory Taylor volunteered at Chippenham Red Cross Hospital as a cook. In January 1919 she left Chippenham and went to Yorkshire where she served at the Red Cross Hospital in Barnsley. While in Chippenham she lived at Steinbrook House at Kington Langley.

Mrs Mary Jane Taylor
Mrs Taylor lived at the Butts in Chippenham. She was a general helper and worked five hours a month from September 1916 until November 1917.

Miss Teagle
The only reference to Miss Teagle is that she came from Sutton Benger and was named as a nurse by the newspaper when it reported the closure of the Hospital.

Miss Gladys Treweke
In 1916 Gladys Treweke started work at Saxby and Farmer the railway engineering company in Chippenham making munitions. She was one of a number of factory workers who took part in

Unity and Loyalty

variety shows to entertain the patients. They would also meet the patients when helping serve teas at the Hospital.

Mrs Mabel Tuck

Mabel Tuck was the wife of Edward Newell Tuck, the Principal of the Secondary School. They lived in St Paul Street, Chippenham. In March 1915 She volunteered at Corsham Red Cross Hospital and transferred to Chippenham in November where she remained until April 1919. Mabel served as a staff nurse and gave 4410 hours.

Mr Victor Tucker

Victor Tucker joined Wilts 13 VAD in January 1916 aged 18. He lived with his parents in Sheldon Road, Chippenham, and worked for Bussell and Wheeler as a seedsman.

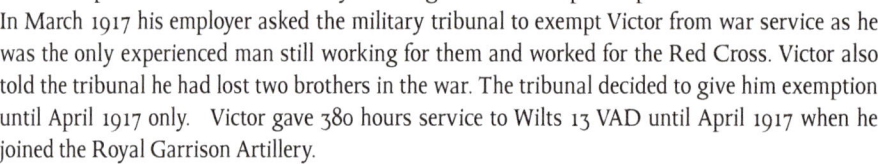

Mabel Tuck

He was awarded his home nursing certificate in December 1916 and was a part time ambulance orderly assisting with the transport of patients.

In March 1917 his employer asked the military tribunal to exempt Victor from war service as he was the only experienced man still working for them and worked for the Red Cross. Victor also told the tribunal he had lost two brothers in the war. The tribunal decided to give him exemption until April 1917 only. Victor gave 380 hours service to Wilts 13 VAD until April 1917 when he joined the Royal Garrison Artillery.

Mr Albert Tyler

Albert Tyler was one of the orderlies to receive the first wounded at Chippenham station. Aged 41, he worked for Saxby and Farmer as a tool fitter. He lived in Lowden Avenue in Chippenham with his wife and family.

Mrs Ethel Louise Vicborn

Ethel Vicborn was born in 1881 and trained at Paddington Infirmary as a nurse. In 1915 Ethel and her daughter, Evelyn, were living with her father, Francis Crook and his wife at 42 Park Lane in Chippenham and she offered her services as a trained sister to the Red Cross Hospital.

She was paid a guinea a week and later transferred to Avoncliff, Bradford on Avon Hospital.

Ethel was very popular with the staff and patients and when she left Chippenham she was presented with a silver cruet set. Ethel collected cap badges from her patients as a keepsake of their stay. She displayed them on a blanket in the ward.

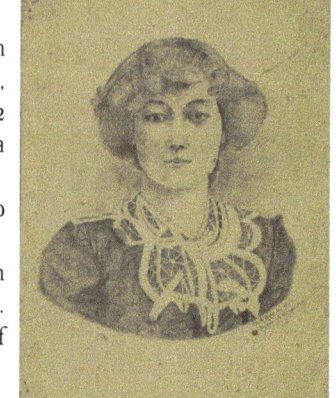

Thought to be Ethel Vicborn drawn by Rifleman Dodd in 1917

Mrs Elizabeth Margaret Waters

Elizabeth Waters volunteered for the Red Cross and was awarded the VAD First Aid Certificate and Home Nursing Certificate in September 1914 a month after the outbreak of war. Nothing is known about her Red Cross service following her training. She and her family lived at Steinbrook Cottage in Kington Langley.

Miss Elsie Watts

Elsie Watts was a VAD at Chippenham. In December 1918 she was awarded her five-year Red Cross badge. She was also a member of the Chippenham Concert Party that entertained at hospitals around the district.

The Story of Chippenham's Red Cross Hospital

Mr Albert Webb
Albert Webb joined Wilts 13 VAD in January 1916 as a hospital orderly. He continued in that role until December 1917 and gave 400 hours service. He lived in the Englands area of Chippenham.

Miss Eva Webb
Eva Webb was born in 1897 in West Kington. She was the daughter of Frederick Webb a farmer in the village. She joined the Red Cross in 1912. In August 1916, when Loyalty ward opened she joined Wilts 6 VAD as a probationer. She stayed at Chippenham Red Cross Hospital doing ward work until August 1918 when she transferred to nearby Malmesbury where she remained until March 1919. In total she gave 5492 hours service. Eva's sister Sybil also became a member of the Chippenham Detachment.

Miss Sybil Webb
Sybil Webb was born in 1899 in West Kington. She was the daughter of Frederick Webb a farmer in the village. In August 1917 she joined Wilts 6 VAD as a probationer doing ward work until June 1918. In September 1918 she joined her sister Eva at Malmesbury Red Cross Hospital where she remained until February 1919. In total she gave 3324 hours service.

Miss Christine Weissenbruch
Christine Weissenbruch joined Chippenham Red Cross Hospital in March 1917 and worked one day a week, as a ward maid, until August 1918. When the Red Cross records were compiled in 1919 she gave her address as 193 Chaussee de Vleurgat, Brussels. It is likely she was a Belgian refugee living in Chippenham during the war.

Miss Dora Westlake
Dora was the daughter of the Rector of Sutton Benger. She was a member of the local Red Cross Detachment, Wilts 38 VAD, and in January 1916 she became a probationer at Chippenham. It is not known why she left after only 3 months in March 1916.

Mrs Johanna Weston
Widow, Johanna Weston was 69 years old when the Hospital opened in 1915. She volunteered for general duties as and when she could. She lived in River Street, Chippenham.

Mr William H Weston
William Weston joined Wilts 13 VAD in November 1917 as a part time ambulance orderly and continued until the Hospital closed giving 300 hours service. He lived in London Road in Chippenham.

Mrs Wheeler
Mrs Wheeler was listed amongst the recipients of the five year Red Cross certificate awarded at Chippenham in December 1918. It is thought she was Kate Wheeler wife of Frederick Ernest Wheeler a confectioner. They lived in Marshfield Road.

Mr Frederick James Wheeler
Frederick Wheeler joined Wilts 13 VAD in January 1919 aged 40. He served as an ambulance orderly until the Hospital closed in April 1919 giving 100 hours service. He lived in Tugela Road in Chippenham and was employed by Saxby and Farmer.

Mons. Charles Wellens
Charles (Karel) Wellens was one of the Belgian refugees to settle in Chippenham during the war. After arriving in Chippenham and living in temporary accommodation he started work at Saxby and Farmer and moved to Park Cottages in Chippenham.

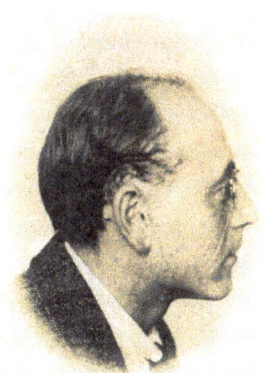
Charles Wellens

Unity and Loyalty

Before the war he was a well-known artist and when he arrived in Chippenham he advertised painting lessons and exhibited his work. He held exhibitions of his and his students work at St Paul's parish hall. The admission fee was donated to the Red Cross Hospital. He was a great supporter of the Red Cross and would volunteer his time giving painting lessons to the patients and VADs at no charge.

Mr James Whishaw

James Whishaw was born in 1853, and lived in St Petersburg until the first decade of the twentieth century when he and his family moved to Britain and settled near Bath. In 1913 they moved to Chippenham and lived at Rowden Hill House until the early 1920s.

James Wishaw was a supporter of the Red Cross Hospital in Chippenham. He regularly gave donations, both financial and practical and loaned his car to transport walking wounded to the Hospital. His daughter Phyllis was the Assistant Commandant.

Miss Phyllis Ruth Whishaw

Phyllis was born in 1888 in St Petersburg in Russia. She was appointed Assistant Commandant of the Hospital and gave 4688 hours until May 1918 when she left Chippenham. Phyllis continued in the Red Cross until May 1919 but it is thought she took up driving duties with the Red Cross and the military.

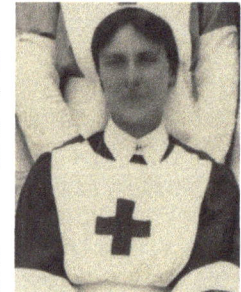

Phyllis Whishaw

Mr George H White

George White was a solicitor in Chippenham, he lived in the High Street almost opposite the Town Hall. Soon after the Red Cross Hospital opened Mr White and his wife started to invite wounded men to their home and enjoy their gardens. The gardens were a peaceful retreat where men could sit quietly or enjoy a game of bowls.

Miss Winifred Wilks

Miss Wilks lived in Timber Street, Chippenham. In September 1916, aged 28, she joined the Hospital as a probationer and was on duty on alternate Sunday afternoons until April 1919. Her sister Marie carried out similar duties.

Miss Marie Wilks

Music Teacher Marie Wilks lived in Timber Street. In December 1916, aged 29, she joined the Hospital as a probationer and was on duty on alternate Sunday mornings. She left in April 1918. Her sister Winifred carried out similar duties.

Mrs Ethel Gertrude Williams

Ethel Williams was born in Chippenham in 1878 the wife of George Herbert Williams, a local Veterinary Surgeon. They lived at Clift House in Langley Road. When the Belgian refugees arrived in Chippenham in 1914 Ethel was part of the committee to provide them with food and accommodation. With the opening of the Red Cross Hospital in Chippenham she was appointed as one of the head cooks. It was said she was quite a formidable woman, an organiser, who ensured the patients received the best treatment the town could offer. She was also a leading member of the Entertainment Committee.

Miss Henrietta Williams

Henrietta Williams was the head mistress at Sutton Benger school. She lived at Ross Cottage in the village with her sister Millicent and was a member of the local Red Cross Detachment, Wilts 38 VAD. In July 1916 she volunteered for general work at Chippenham Red Cross Hospital. She gave part time service until October 1918 and the Assistant Commandant said about Miss Williams 'This member has been a splendid worker'.

The Story of Chippenham's Red Cross Hospital

Miss Millicent Williams
Millicent lived with her sister Henrietta at Ross Cottage in Sutton Benger. She was a member of Wilts 38 VAD and volunteered as a probationer at Chippenham Red Cross Hospital in June 1916. She gave 1270 hours service.

Miss Beryl Mary Wilson
Beryl Wilson was the daughter of Doctor Wilson and Mrs Helena Wilson the Chippenham Commandant. Despite her disability 17 year old Beryl volunteered from November 1915 to April 1919, 20 hours every week preparing vegetables.

Mrs Helena Wilson
Helena Wilson was the Commandant of Wilts 6 VAD and the Red Cross Hospital. Her devotion was repeated time after time in the press and by the patients. Colonel Audley Neeld, at the unveiling of the Red Cross plaque on the Town Hall, said about Mrs Wilson 'I must refer to the heroic and splendid work done by the Commandant of this Hospital' referring particularly how she continued her work despite the loss of her 3 sons in action. She was included in the Red Cross Roll of Honourable Service and was mentioned in Dispatches and awarded the OBE for her service at the Hospital. She retired as Commandant of the Detachment in 1925 and died in Chippenham in 1934.

Dr Mervyn Seppings Wilson
Mervyn Wilson was born in Kings Lynn in 1855. In 1885 he was a surgeon at Salisbury Infirmary. A few years later he moved to Chippenham where he went into private practice. His surgery and home were in St Mary Street. He was also the medical officer for Chippenham District and a surgeon at the Cottage Hospital. In November 1915 he became the Principal Medical Officer to the Chippenham Red Cross Hospital and continued this work until April 1919.

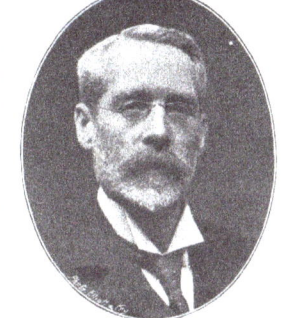

Dr Mervyn Wilson the husband of Commandant Helena Wilson

Lily Witts
Lily Witts lived in Parliament Street and was a part time helper. She met her future husband, Edward Granger at the Hospital when he was a patient.

Mrs Elizabeth Wren
Mrs Wren lived in Hawthorn Road in Chippenham and volunteered as a mess room helper from September 1916 until the Hospital closed. She went in for three hours on alternate Thursdays.

Miss Edith Hilda Young
24 year old Edith Young, lived with her parents in Park Lane, Chippenham and joined the VAD in early 1915 as a probationer nurse. She served at Corsham Hospital and at Wells in Somerset. In March 1916 she joined Chippenham Red Cross Hospital and remained until it closed giving a total of 100 hours. Edith was a teacher at Westmead School.

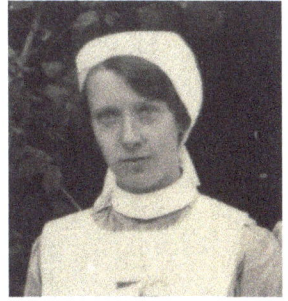

Edith Young

Appendix 2
Work parties in Chippenham Division

THE RED CROSS organised sewing and knitting work parties to make hospital supplies including pyjamas, blankets, sheets, bandages, splints and swabs and warm clothing, known as comforts, for the troops at the front. Each work party registered with the Red Cross and were assigned to a County Division. The Chippenham Divisional Needlework Association were responsible for administering the workers in Chippenham Division. Some of the members of the work parties were also volunteers in the Red Cross hospitals.

Many of the records were compiled after the war and addresses were recorded at that time. This accounts for some workers appearing to live outside the area.

Work Party 1404, Derry Hill.
Work Party Leader, Lady Hervey.

Miss	Ethel	Allen	58 Rockliffe Road Bath
Mrs	Eveleigh	Baines	Buckhill House, Bowood
Mrs	Emily	Chaytor	Studley Calne
Mrs	Ann	Cleverly	Buckhill Cottages, Calne
Mrs	Ada	Crocker	82 Studley, Calne
Lady	Hilda	Hervey	Rumsey House, Studley Calne Wilts
Mrs	Ada	Hillier	33 Wyke Road Trowbridge
Miss	Louisa	Hosey	10 Bakers Cottage, Limpley Stoke, Bath
Mrs	Elizabeth	Jefferies	Norley Lane Studley
Mrs	Frances	Lewis	6 Derry Hill
Miss	Joan	Money-Kyrle	Whetham, Calne
Mrs	Florence	Money-Kyrle	Whetham, Calne
Mrs	Miriam	Scott	Derry Hill Vicarage
Miss	Doris	Way	Keepers Lodge, Bowood

Work Party 1614, Grittleton.
Work Party Leader, Lady Edith Neeld

Miss	Emma	Broome	Grittleton, Chippenham,
Miss	Carrie	Brown	Grittleton House, Chippenham
Mrs	Jane	Childs	Grittleton House, Chippenham
Mrs	Mary	Gale	Grittleton, Chippenham

Mrs	Lilian	Gowring	Grittleton Vicarage, Chippenham
Mrs	Annie	Gumbrell	Grittleton, Chippenham
Miss	Ada	Holbrow	Grittleton, Chippenham
Miss	Annie	Morris	The Stables, Grittleton, Chippenham
Miss	Elizabeth	Morris	The Stables, Grittleton, Chippenham
Lady	Edith	Neeld	Grittleton House, Chippenham
Mrs	Laura	Pearson	Grittleton, Chippenham
Mrs	Ellen	Seasell	Grittleton House, Chippenham
Mrs	Florence	Sumbler	Grittleton

Work Party 1625 Corsham, (Hartham and Biddestone)

Work Party Leader Hon Mrs Eva Talbot

Miss	Annie	Abbott	Hartham Park, Corsham
Mrs	Elizabeth	Baker	Biddestone
Mrs	Lily	Barrow	Hartham Cottages, Hartham
Mrs	Anna	Beazer	Biddestone
Mrs	Rosa	Beazer	Biddestone
Mrs	Sarah	Beazer	Biddestone
Mrs	Kate	Bird	Hartham Cottages, Hartham
Mrs	Sarah	Bishop	Hartham Cottages, Hartham
Miss	Mary	Brazer	Biddestone
Lady	Frances	Briggs	Biddestone
Mrs	Anne	Brookes	Biddestone
Mrs	Elizabeth	Careless	Elm Lodge, Biddestone
Mrs	Mary	Coates	Biddestone
Mrs	Edith	Cullimore	Biddestone
Mrs	Jessima	Davis	Hartham Park Cottages, Hartham
Mrs	Louisa	Elliott	Biddestone
Mrs	Mary	Elliott	Biddestone
Miss	Lily	Francis	Pickwick Lodge, Corsham
Mrs	Mary	Francis	Pickwick Lodge, Corsham
Mrs	Eliza	Funnell	Hartham Cottages, Hartham
Mrs	Annie	Gorton	Biddestone
Mrs	Kate	Haddrall	Biddestone
Miss	May	Haddrall	Biddestone
Mrs	Bella	Hand	Biddestone
Mrs	Clara	Hart	Home Farm, Biddestone
Mrs	Alice	Hazell	Hartham Cottages, Hartham
Miss	Edith	Honour	Hartham Park
Mrs	Maria	Hulbert	Biddestone
Mrs	Rosetta	Mackland	The Old Vicarage, Corsham
Miss	Violet	Marfitt	Hartham Park
Miss	Elizabeth	Mills	Hartham Park
Mrs	Mary	Morley	Biddestone Manor
Mrs	Elizabeth	Neale	Biddestone
Mrs	Catharine	Orchard	Biddestone

Mrs	Elixabeth	Paget	Hartham Park
Miss	Anne	Pullen	Biddestone
Mrs	Agnes	Robertson	Hartham Park
Miss	Alice	Sainsbury	High Street, Corsham
Mrs	Mary	Summers	Biddestone
Hon	Eva	Talbot	Hartham Park
Mrs	Elizabeth	Taylor	Biddestone
Mrs	Alice	Wait	Biddestone
Mrs	Edith	West	Rudloe Lodge, Box
Mrs	Margaret	Wills	Hartham Park

Work Party 1628 Bradenstoke
Work Party Leader Miss E F Wiltshire
There are no records of the members for this Work Party.

Work Party 1672 Chippenham Divisional Red Cross Association
Leader Lady Margaret Spicer, Honorary Secretary, Mrs G T Gladstone.
It is thought this was the organising committee for the Work Parties administered by Chippenham Division. It is not known who the other members of the committee were.

Work Party 1686, Spye Park
Work Party Leader, Lady Margaret Spicer

Miss	Nellie	Amor	Westbrook
Mrs	Eliza	Breach	Chittoe
Mrs	Louise	Carter	Manor Farm, Chittoe,
Miss	Ethel	Davis	Spye Park
Miss	Mabel	Davis	Spye Park
Mrs	Mary	Davis	The Stables, Spye Park
Mrs	Sophia	Dolman	Westbrook
Mrs	Mary	Duck	Sandy Lane
Mrs	Nellie	Fennell	Westbrook
Mrs	Jane	Gee	Chittoe
Mrs	Lottie	Gee	Chittoe
Miss	Annie	Gregory	Spye Arch, Lacock,
Miss	Alethea	Harmsworth	Home Farm, Spye Park,
Mrs	Bessie	Hunt	White Lodge, Spye Park,
Miss	Winnie	Hunt	White Lodge, Spye Park,
Mrs	Daisy	King	Sandy Lane
Mrs	Mary	Knapp	St Edith's Marsh, Bromham
Mrs	Celia	Laverton	Chittoe
Mrs	Mary	Maynard	School House, Chittoe
Mrs	Alice	Miles	Chittoe
Miss	Annie	Odell	Tedworth Square, Chelsea,
Mrs	Alice	Pearce	Chittoe
Mrs	Annie	Pearce	Chittoe
Mrs	Sarah	Reeves	Devizes Road, Chittoe

The Story of Chippenham's Red Cross Hospital

Mrs	Anna	Robins	Chittoe
Mrs	Emily	Rudman	Westbrook
Mrs	May	Sleightholme	Chittoe
Lady	Margaret	Spicer	Spye Park
Mrs	Jane	Weston	Westbrook
Mrs	Elizabeth	Whatmore	Chittoe

Work Party 1701, Sutton Benger
Work Party Leader, Countess Cowley

Mrs	Ruth	Barnes	Sutton Benger
Mrs	Annie	Beaulands	Sutton Benger
Miss	Katherine	Bond	Church Farm, Sutton Benger
Miss	Emily	Brind	Draycot Cerne
Mrs	Kate	Bryant	Sutton Benger
Mrs	Annie	Butler	Sutton Benger
Miss	Mary	Buy	Sutton Benger
Lady	Clare	Cowley	Draycot Park
Miss	Mildred	Dunford	Draycot Cerne
Miss	Belinda	Frogley	Sutton Benger
Miss	Alice	Gregory	Box Villa, Sutton Benger
Miss	Florence	Henden	Sutton Benger
Mrs	Bessie	Humphries	Sutton Benger
Mrs	Lucy	Lea	Sutton Benger
Miss	Mary	Lea	Sutton Benger
Mrs	Harriet	Teagle	The Laurels, Kington Langley
Miss	Millicent	Williams	Ross Cottage, Sutton Benger,
Mrs	Lilian	Wright	Sutton Benger

Work Party 1702, Box
Work Party Leader, Mrs Adelaide Langton

Miss	Lilian	Andrews	Mead Villas Box
Mrs	Louisa	Coles	The Clift Box Hill
Miss	Mary	Deane	Ditteridge
Miss	Gladys	Freegard	Sherbrooke, Box
Mrs	Mary	Goulstone	Hill Farm Box.
Miss	Florence	Guy	Newport, Isle of Wight
Miss	Edith	Hickman	Sherbrooke, Box
Miss	Beatrice	Hignett	Sherbrooke, Box
Mrs	Sarah	Hignett	Sherbrooke, Box
Mrs	Adelaide	Langton	Sherbrooke, Box
Miss	Alice	LeFevre	Sherbrooke, Box.
Mrs	Edith	Luttrell	Ben Mead, Box
Mrs	Hellena	Manfield	Ingolls Cottages, Box
Miss	Jessie	Rutherford	Halt House Cottage, Box
Mrs	Ethel	Shallcross	The Hermitage, Box
Mrs	Annie	Slade	22 Farm head Box

Unity and Loyalty

| Hon | Dora | Twisleton | Heleigh House, Box |
| Miss | Alice | Vezey | Mead Villas Box. |

Work party 1703, Slaughterford
Work Party Leader, Mrs A E Bolwell

Mrs	Annie	Bartlett	Slaughterford
Mrs	Alice	Bolwell	Slaughterford
Mrs	Margaret	Corsen	Manor Farm, Slaughterford,
Miss	Gladys	Griffin	Ford
Miss	Evelyn	Hillier	Slaughterford
Miss	Rose	Hillier	Slaughterford
Mrs	Marianne	Rawlings	Slaugnterford

Work Party 1725, Middlewick, Corsham
Work Party Leader, Mrs C H Williamson

Miss	Florence	Ayling	The Old House, Westrop,
Miss	Barbara	Dancer	Spa House, Middle Hill, Box.
Mrs	W	Dillon	Brewery Cottage Batheaston
Mrs	Alice	Gardner	Middlewick Cottages
Mrs	Maud	Grimston	Brewery Cottage Batheaston
Miss	Amy	Harris	Middlewick
Miss	Mary	James	Pickwick Rd, Corsham
Mrs	Emily	Morley	Shockerwick, Bath
Mrs	Charlotte	Williamson	Middlewick House

Work Party 1731 Chippenham
Work Party Leaders Mrs Newton Heath and Miss Florence Lane

Mrs	Annie	Archard	Station Hill, Chippenham
Mrs	Susan	Baker	St Mary's Place, Chippenham
Mrs	Louise	Bowker	Marshfield Rd, Chippenham
Mrs	Sarah	Bradbury	Marshfield Rd, Chippenham
Mrs	Rose	Brinkworth	Lowden, Chippenham
Mrs	Georgiana	Clarke	The Vicarage Langley Fitzurse
Miss	Alice	Collen	Rowden Hill, Chippenham
Mrs	Elizabeth	Collen	Rowden Hill, Chippenham
Mrs	Isabella	Cotes	Rowden House, Chippenham
Mrs	Emily	Devonald	Market Place, Chippenham
Mrs	Constance	Edwards	Park Lane, Chippenham
Mrs	Florence	Edwards	The Causeway, Chippenham
Mrs	Nancy	Fox	Audley Avenue, Chippenham
Mrs	Elsie	Gardner	Park Lane, Chippenham
Mdlle	Lucie	Golaz	Rowden House, Chippenham
Miss	Annie	Goldsworthy	Lowden, Chippenham
Mrs	Margaret	Hathaway	Langley Road, Chippenham
Miss	Blanche	Hayman	Rowden House, Chippenham
Mrs	Helen	Heath	Market Place, Chippenham

The Story of Chippenham's Red Cross Hospital

Miss	Bessie	Humphries	London Rd, Chippenham
Mrs	Harriette	Humphries	London Rd, Chippenham
Miss	Hilda	Jay	St Mary Street, Chippenham
Mrs	Louisa	King	Audley Rd. Chippenham
Mrs	Annie	Lane	Pickwick, Corsham
Miss	Florence	Lane	St Mary Street, Chippenham
Mrs	Emily	Light	Audley Road, Chippenham
Mrs	Jane	Liminton	Sheldon Road Chippenham
Mrs	Sarah	Markwick	Lowden, Chippenham
Miss	Mary	Neville	St Mary Street, Chippenham
Mrs	Hilda	Nixon	Bath Rd, Chippenham
Mrs	Ann	Palmer	Audley Road, Chippenham
Mrs	Harriette	Purser	Princes Rd, Felixstowe
Mrs	Hester	Ramsay	Hullavington Vicarage
Mrs	Rosine	Raymond	Parliament St, Chippenham
Mrs	Ada	Sidnell	Lowden Chippenham
Mrs	Emily	Stanley	Lowden Terrace Chippenham
Miss	Lilian	Stewart	The Palace, Chippenham
Mrs	Lucy	Stewart	The Palace Chippenham
Miss	Sophie	Summers	St Mary Street, Chippenham
Mrs	Georgina	Tanner	Moseley Terrace Chippenham
Miss	Gertrude	Tanner	Moseley Terrace Chippenham
Mrs	Pheobe	Tidmarsh	Sheldon Road, Chippenham
Mrs	Lucy	Weston	St Mary Street, Chippenham
Mrs	Alice	White	Woodlands, Chippenham
Mrs	Ellen	Woods	High Street, Chippenham

Work Party 1771, Lacock
Work Party Leader, Mrs Annie Ramsbottom

Miss	Bessie	Banks	Nethercote Hill, Lacock
Mrs	Mary	Edmunds	East Street Lacock
Mrs	Louisa	Latham	Lacock
Mrs	Annie	Ramsbottom	The Vicarage Lacock
Miss		Westcott	Lacock
Miss		Wiltshire	Lacock

Work Party 1784 and 1786 Corsham
Work Party Leaders, Miss Katherine Goldney and Lady Goldney

Miss	Mary	Barton	Easton House Corsham
Miss	Lilian	Brakespear	Corsham
Mrs	Maryann	Breach	Hastings Road Corsham
Miss	Alice	Butt	High Street Corsham
Mrs	Emmie	Cole	Church St Corsham
Mrs	Fanny	Flower	Easton Corsham
Mrs	Isobel	Garne	Landsend, Chippenham
Lady	Alice	Goldney	Monks Park, Corsham

Unity and Loyalty

Miss	Ethel	Goldney	Beechfield, Corsham
Miss	Katherine	Goldney	Beechfield, Corsham
Mrs	Eugenia	Gooding	Roseleigh, Corsham
Mrs	Ursula	Halhed	Warden's House, Corsham
Miss	Charlotte	Hart	Wimbledon, London
Miss	Mabel	Hart	Wimbledon, London
Miss	Blanche	Kirkpatrick	Lindfield, Corsham
Miss	Daisy	Large	Prospect, Corsham
Mrs	Mary	Luchford	Woodbine Villa, Corsham
Miss	Ida	McGlaughlin	Lockingarth, Corsham
Mrs	Selina	Mildmay	Westrop House, Corsham
Mrs	Isolde	Parker	Lindisfarne, Corsham
Hon	Rosamund	Parker	The Grove Corsham
Miss	Winifred	Rogers	Mosley House, Corsham
Mrs	Sarah	Salisbury	The Grove, Corsham
Mrs	Ethel	Shepherd	Beechfield, Corsham
Mr	Ruth	Sheppard	Hastings Road, Corsham
Mrs	Helen	Simons	Pickwick House Corsham

Work Party 1883, North Wraxall
Work Party Leader, Mrs B C Langley
There are no records of the members for this Work Party.

Work Party 1893, Bowden Park
Work Party Leader, Mrs G T Gladstone

Mrs	Charlotte	Chivers	Nash Hill, Lacock
Mrs	Fanny	Crook	Bowden Common, Lacock
Mrs	Selina	Dewey	Bowden Hill, Lacock
Miss	Frances	Donaldson	Bowden Park
Mrs	Sarah	Dummer	Bowden Hill, Lacock
Mrs	Amelia	Dunn	Church Lodge, Bowden Park
Mrs	Gertrude	Gladstone	Bowden Park
Miss	Olive	Gladstone	Bowden Park
Miss	Ivy	Gladstone	Bowden Park
Miss	Elsie	Jenner	Bowden Park
Mrs	Mary	Slade	Bowden Park Farm, Lacock,
Mrs	Emily	Tucker	The Bell, Bowden Hill, Lacock
Mrs	Minnie	Webb	Bowden Hill, Chippenham

Work Party 1916, Yatton Keynell
Work Party Leader, Miss Amy Bolton, Yatton Keynell Rectory
There are no records of the members for this Work Party.

Work Party 1917, Colerne
Work Party Leader, Mrs Stephens, Colerne Rectory
There are no records of the members for this Work Party.

The Story of Chippenham's Red Cross Hospital

Work Party 4914, Chippenham
Work Party Leader, Hon. Mrs Allfrey, Greenways, Chippenham
There are no records of the members for this Work Party.

Work Party 4933, Tytherton
Work Party Leader, Mrs Alice Collett and Mrs Myra Ferris

Miss	Lily	Andrews	East Tytherton
Mrs	Fanny	Andrews	Underdown, Charlcutt, Calne
Mrs	Anna	Bailey	East Tytherton
Mrs	Margery	Bailey	East Tytherton
Mrs	Charlotte	Birtill	East Tytherton
Mrs	Bessie	Boas	East Tytherton
Mrs	Emma	Brewer	East Tytherton
Miss	Lily	Brewer	West Tytherton
Mrs	Clara	Bryant	West Tytherton
Mrs	Jane	Budge	East Tytherton
Mrs	Hannah	Budge	East Tytherton
Mrs	Mary	Bull	East Tytherton
Mrs	Elizabeth	Cleverly	East Tytherton
Mrs	Emma	Coaten	East Tytherton
Mrs	Lucie	Collett	East Tytherton
Mrs	Alice	Collett	East Tytherton
Miss	Olive	Collett	East Tytherton
Miss	Hilda	Cripps	West Tytherton
Miss	Ethel	Eatwell	East Tytherton
Mrs	Myra	Ferris	West Tytherton
Miss	Nellie	Freeth	West Tytherton
Mrs	Sarah	Gale	East Tytherton
Miss	Gussie	Goodway	East Tytherton
Mrs	Rose	Grimshaw	East Tytherton
Miss	Hope	Heath	West Tytherton
Miss	Elizabeth	Hollis	East Tytherton
Mrs	Emily	Jefferys	Malmesbury
Miss	Nellie	Jefferys	East Tytherton
Mrs	Mary	Lewis	Wick, Calne
Mrs	Fanny	Matthews	East Tytherton
Miss	Edith	Newman	East Tytherton
Mrs	Rose	Newman	East Tytherton
Mrs	Sarah	Newman	East Tytherton
Mrs	Sarah	Rumming	East Tytherton
Mrs	Sophy	Rumming	Studley, Calne
Mrs	Annie	White	Cheverill, Devizes
Mrs	Frances	Wright	West Tytherton

Work party 5774, Lacock
Work party leader, Mrs Taylor

Mrs	Emily	Barker	Bowden Hill, Lacock
Mrs	Phoebe	Bath	Bowden Hill, Lacock
Mrs	Alice	Blanchard	Bowden Hill, Lacock
Miss	Ida	Butcher	Bowden Hill, Lacock
Miss	Helen	Daniels	Bowden Hill, Lacock
Miss	Laura	Eggleton	Bowden Hill, Lacock
Miss	Alice	Fountain	Park Mead, Spye Park,
Miss	Florence	Goodwin	Bowden Cottage, Lacock
Mrs	Edith	Hunt	Bowden Hill, Lacock
Mrs	Louisa	Reed	Griffin Cottages Bowden Hill, Lacock
Miss	Mary	Sawyer	Bowden Lacock
Mrs		Taylor	

Work party 5679, Dauntsey

Work party leader, Mrs W Winwood, Idover House, Dauntsey

There are no records of the members for this Work Party.

Bibliography

Arnold, Catherine, 2018, *Pandemic 1918*, Michael O'Mara Books

Barrett, Geoffrey, & Jefferies, Sally,1985 *100 Pictures of Chippenham* Past, Chippenham Civic Society

Belsey, James, 1986, *Forgotten Front: Bristol at War, 1914-18*, Redcliffe Press

Bowman, Gerald, 1967, *The Lamp and the Book*, Queen Anne Press,

Bowser, Thekla, 1917, *The Story of British VAD work in the Great War*, Melrose

Broadhead, Richard, 2010, *The Great War Chippenham Soldiers*, O&B Services

Chippenham Borough Council, *Minute books 8,9 and 10*, Now held at The Wiltshire and Swindon History Centre

Clarke, Kate, 2001, *The Royal United Hospital 1747-1947*, Mushroom Publishing

Cohan, Susan, 2014, *Medical Services in the First World War*, Shire Publications

Davies, Mavis, 2006, *Valiant & Determined*, Salisbury British Red Cross

Drury, Jill and Peter,1980, *A Tisbury History*, Tisbury Books

Farris, Nellie,1991, *The Downs and then Upps*, Wincanton Press

Fincham, Henry, 1933, *The Order of the Hospital of St. John of Jerusalem and Its Grand Priory of England*, Order of the Hospital of St John

Gosling, Lucinda, 2014, *Great War Britain, The First World War at Home*, The History Press

Heath Armstrong, Lucie, 1913, *Etiquette and Entertaining*, John Long Ltd

Hird, Ernest, 2008, *A Life Revealed, The Diaries of Herbert Spackman*, Ernest Hird

Hurst, Arthur, 1940, *Medical Diseases of the War*, Arnold

Lloyd George, David, 1938, *War Memoirs of David Lloyd George*, Odhams Press

Lovett, Maureen, 2013, *Hullavington Memories: Maurice Wicks (1914-1967) with Mary Clark*, Applefire Press

Makin, William, 1935, *The Story of Twenty-Five Years: Celebrating the Royal Silver Jubilee 1910-1935*, C. Arthur Pearson

Marlow, Joyce, 1999, *Women and the Great War*, Virago Press

Marlow, Sylvia, 1991, *Winifred, a Wiltshire working girl*, Ex Libris Press

Nock, O.S, 2006, *A Hundred Years of Speed with Safety*, Hobnob Press

Oliver, Dame Beryl, 1966, *The British Red Cross in Action*, Faber

Paddock, W.J, 1984, *A Country Boy*, C J Hall

Platts, Arnold, 1947, *A History of Chippenham AD 853-1946*, Wiltshire Gazette

Smith, Cecil, 1977, *Chippenham Walkabout*, Chippenham Civic Society

Stone, George F, and Wells, Charles, 1920, *Bristol and the Great War 1914-1919*, Arrowsmith

Stone, Mike, 2003, *Images of England – Chippenham*, Tempus

Stone, Mike, 2011, *Chippenham Then & Now*, The History Press

Talbot, Matilda, 1956, *My life at Lacock Abbey*, George Allen and Unwin

Van Emden, Richard and Humphries, Steve, 2003, *All Quiet on the Home Front*, Headline Books

Ward, Muir, 1917, *Observations of an Orderly -Some glimpses of Life and work in an English War Hospital*, Simpkin, Marshall Hamilton & Kent

Wiltshire Federation of Women's Institutes, 1993, *Wiltshire Within Living Memory*, Countryside Books

Internet sources

The National Archives, Spotlights on History series, www.nationalarchives.gov.uk

British Red Cross Society, WW1 Information sheets series and VAD card index, www.vad.redcross.org.uk/en/What-we-did-during-the-war

House of Commons, Historic Hansard 1803-2005, www.parliament.uk/business/publications/hansard

The British Newspaper Archive, www.britishnewspaperarchive.co.uk/.

Further reading

Anon, 2014, *Diary of a Nursing Sister*, Amberley

Brittain Vera, 1933, *Testament of Youth*, Victor Gollancz

Crewdson, Dorothea, 2014, *Dorothea's War*, Phoenix

Index

Admiralty, The, 34, 153
Affleck, Mr, 173
Ainsworth, Captain, RAMC, 46
Aldbourne, 23
Aldrich, Second Lieutenant Leo Edwin, 206-7
Allfrey, Captain and Hon Mrs, 88, 96, 127
Allsop, Mrs Emma, 131
Almeric Paget Military Massage Corps, 223
Alsop, Miss, 179
Ambulance, 36, 78, 99, 100, 122, 137, 189, 191-5, 207, 228
Ambulance Detachments and Sections, 6, 34-5, 37, 46, 71, 78, 98, 100, 122, 127, 138, 140, 149, 153, 181-2, 187, 189, 193-5, 228
Ambulance, St John; see St John
Ambulance Training, 20, 35, 37, 42, 140
Angel Hotel, 5, 101, 172, 203-4
Angling Club, 113, 139, 178
Anstee, Rachel, 189
Anstis, Miss, 179
Archard, Family, 35, 98, 177, 187
Army Nursing Service, later The Queen Alexandra's Imperial Military Service, 13
Ashby, Mrs W, 169
Ashe, Miss, 127
Ashford Litter, 36-7, 191
Ashley House, Box, 192
Ashmead, Arthur, 219, 220
Asquith, H H, 50, 93, 128, 138
Asquith, Raymond, 128
Atkinson, Trooper, 169
Awdry, Edmund, 111
Awdry, Janet Unity, 103, 111, 173, 231
Aylmore, Miss G, 82

Baden-Powell, Sir Robert (Chief Scout), 22, 240
Badminton House, Gloucestershire, 16
Bailey, Mrs, 127
Baker, Miss G, 177
Balfour, Arthur, 27, 31
Ball, Mr W, 173
Bands
    Chippenham Town Silver Band, 58
    Salvation Army Band, 144, 202-3
    Saxby and Farmer Ladies Band, 176-7
    Wiltshire Regiment Band, 188
Barnes, George, 154-5
Barnes, Mrs Ruth, 120, 233
Barsted, Mr, 65, 100
Beamish, Mr, 179
Beaufort Hospital, Bristol; see Hospitals
Beaven, Sarah, 117
Beaven, Mr T, 82
Beechfield, Corsham, 88
Belcher, Frank, 20, 26
Belcher, Sisters (Evelyn and Dora), 26, 44, 54, 96, 102, 127, 130, 170, 228, 231, 233-4, 243
Belgian Refugees, 80, 81-3 92, 118, 225
Beltwood Dalling; see Hospitals
Bergstrom, Mr, 127
Biddestone, 119
Bishop, Miss (Kington St Michael), 147
Bishop, Miss Florence (Corsham), 239
Bodman, Mrs Ethel, 120, 139
Bodman, Miss, 177
Bodman, William, 122, 138
Bolton, Reverend Allan, 87, 127
Bolton, Miss Amy, 63, 69, 87-8, 103, 115
Bolwell, Mrs, 88
Boreham, Vincent, 219, 245-6
Bosmere Farm, Tytherton, 96
Bowden Park, 27, 70-1, 87-8, 193
Bowker, Edwin, 229, 243
Bowood, 12, 19, 43, 45-8, 79-80, 91-2, 104, 108, 120, 142, 173-4, 186, 193, 209, 224, 234
Bowsher, Mrs Sarah, 131
Box, 87-8, 119, 189, 192, 197
Bradenstoke, 87
Bradford on Avon, 54, 153
Braeside; see Hospitals, Beltwood Dalling
Brett, Mrs Alice, 103
Brewer, Miss Elsie, 115, 177
Brewer, William, 66-8
Bright, Mrs Kate, 118, 129
Brinkworth, Miss Dorothy, 47
Brinkworth, Miss Ethel, 27, 105, 115, 163
Brinkworth, Miss Jessie, 103

Briscoe, Dr William and Mrs Nancy, 19, 30, 35-6, 38, 71
Bristol Royal Infirmary; *see* Hospitals
British Red Cross Society, The, 15-7, 24, 28-9, 31, 37, 54, 69, 76. 80, 85, 115, 154
British Red Cross Society, Wiltshire Branch; *see* Wiltshire Branch, Red Cross
Brock, Mr, 96
Brook, Norman, 160
Brotherhood, Mrs, 147
Brown, Mrs Louise (Louis), 127
Brown, George, 15
Buckland, Mrs E, 147
Buckland, Frank, 182
Buckle, Joe, 111, 139-40, 172-3, 199, 203
Bullion, Private David, 140-1, 143, 238
Burden, Mr F J, 113, 203
Burderop Park, 52
Burridge, William (Father and Son), 20, 100, 146, 172, 182, 199
Burridge, Miss H, 189
Bush, Colonel James Paul, Surgeon, 17, 18, 97, 126

Cadenham Manor, Foxham, 47
Calley, Emily, 52
Calne, 17, 25, 27, 45, 48, 51, 53, 81, 89, 135, 189, 194-5, 224
Carnley, Mr, 121
Cazalet, Captain Victor, MP, 245
Charlton House and Park, 31, 52-3, 77, 80
Cherhill, 199
Chesterton, Mrs, 127
Chippenham Sanitary Laundry, 26, 99-100, 130
Chivers, William, 216, 220
Christian Malford, 47, 79, 119-20, 139, 147
Churchill, Constance, 239
Clark, Mr E M, 194
Clevedon, 135
Clutterbuck, Mrs, 18
Cole, John (Mayor), 90
Cole, Sergeant, 170
Coleman, Mr, 96
Colerne, 88
Colston, Edward, 52
Combe Park, Bath, 124
Comforts, 62, 70, 83-5, 97, 108, 134, 173, 185
Cooke, Mrs, 139
Coombs, Sergeant, 170
Cornish, Ellen, 47, 120, 127, 233
Corsham, 22, 27, 32, 47, 52-3, 58, 68, 75, 80-4, 87-8, 91, 95, 104, 119, 122, 124, 126, 141-2, 149, 165, 173-4, 180-1, 189, 192-3, 195-7, 207, 224, 228, 237, 239
Cottrell, Mrs Mabel, 132
County Territorial Association, 12, 15, 17, 34, 37
Couzens, Mrs Harriet, 132
Coventry, Miss Joan, 231, 233
Coventry, Lady Muriel, 36, 82
Coventry, Miss Joan, 231, 233
Coward, Alice, 231
Coward, Frederic and Mrs Rachael, 82, 103
Cowley, Earl and Countess,. 80, 88, 121, 127
Cox, Corporal James, 187
Craig, Mrs, 54
Cricket, 180-1, 183-4
Cripps, William and Mrs Ellen, 132
Crofts, William, 18, 169
Crudwell, 53

Daniels, Mrs H, 169
Dauntsey, 88
Davis, Mrs Elinor, 44, 82, 145, 174, 182, 233
Davis, Fanny, 130
Davis, Miss, 177, 179
Dee, Miss Caroline, 239-40
Dempsey, Joseph C, 102, 106-7
Devizes, 18-19, 25, 45-6, 52, 53-4, 73, 91, 149, 188
Devonshire House, 38, 84
Dickson Poynder, Family, 18, 20-21, 23
Dickson, Miss, 127
Dickson, Mrs, 127, 136, 147
DORA (The Defence of the Realm Act), 65
Dorwell, Miss, 179
Draycot House, Draycot Cerne, 79-80, 88, 119-20, 191
Dunford, Mr, 127
Dutton, John and Mrs Louisa, 189

Easton, 84
Eldridge, Mr H, 82
Ellerton, Private William, 145
Ellery, Alice, 120
Elliott, Mrs, 127
Ennis, William and Mrs May, 26, 54, 68, 70, 96
Evans, Fred, 218

Farries, Lila, 130, 233
Farris, Miss, 127
Fausett, Private James, 239-40
Ferris, Miss Fanny, 91, 103, 207, 229, 232-3

Ferris, Mrs Myra, 186
Ferris, Walter, 96, 186
Finn, Emmie, 129
Fogg, Mr T H, 82
Football, 109-10, 179-80, 184
Forgan, Mrs, 127
Foxham, 47, 147
Freegard, Mr and Mrs, 147
Freeth, George, 82
Fry, Miss Dorothy, 173
Fry, Mrs Emma, 132
Fuller, Mrs Robert (Mabel), 66, 68, 75
Fuller, Major William Fleetwood, 66

Gallipoli, 94, 105-7, 114
Gardner, Henry and Mrs Maria, 130-2
Garnett, Charles and Mrs Claire, 77-8, 96, 108, 121-3, 127, 147, 169, 173, 178, 181, 192, 195
Giffard, Henry, May and Walter, 42
Gillett, George, 18
Gillman, Mrs Elizabeth, 132
Gladstone, Mrs Gertrude, 71, 85, 87-8, 97, 127
Gladstone, Miss Ivy, 27, 121, 148, 152, 193, 232-3, 235, 239
Gladstone, Sir John, 27
Gladstone, Miss Olive, 27, 233, 238
Goldney, Sir John and Lady, 88, 124, 192
Goldney, Miss K L, 88
Gorst, Miss, 38, 147
Goulding, Miss, 175
Grainger, Miss, 127
Granger, Miss Alice (Kathleen), 115, 179-80
Granger, Edward, 237
Granger, Lieutenant William, 180
Great Somerford, 191, 239-40
Greathouse, Kington Langley, 77-9, 96, 108, 121
Greenman, Miss, 127
Grimshaw, Miss Louisa, 103, 134
Grittleton House, 17, 77, 83, 87, 96, 198-9

Hadzfeldt, Princess, 79
Hague, The (Peace Conference), 56
Haldane, Richard (Secretary of State for War), 11-13,
Haldane, Miss Elizabeth, 13, 31
Hamlin, Elsie, 129
Hamlyn, Mrs, 127
Hancock, Miss Florence May, 50
Hankey, Basil and Mrs E, 17, 68-70, 76, 95, 115, 117, 126-7, 129, 132, 148, 157, 189, 222, 224-5

Hardenhuish House and Park, 18, 58, 188
Hardiman, Mrs Ellen, 32, 103, 147, 231, 233
Hardiman, Miss Maud, 32
Harrison, Mrs Katherine, 120
Hart, Miss Dora, 2, 103, 106, 189, 231, 233
Hart, Mr, 96
Hartham, Park, 23, 87
Hathaway, Mr and Mrs Margaret, 18, 181, 183
Heath, Newton and Mrs Helen, 88-9, 233
Heddington, 71, 82
Helme, Sir George and Lady, 18, 20-1, 23, 127, 183
Hervey, Lord Walter and Lady, 52, 70-1, 87, 108
Hetherington, Mrs Beatrice, 103, 173-174
Hetherington, Mrs Sarah, 47
Hetherington, Miss Norah, 103
Hibberd, Henry, 215-6
Hickling, Elsie, 27
Hinders Cycle Shop, 191
Hinton, Frederick and Mrs Kate, 26, 30, 54, 76, 103, 233
Hiscock, Sisters, 44, 119, 170
Hiscock, Walter and Mrs Ada, 111, 119, 136, 138-139
Holland, Sergeant, 170
Hooper, Mr, 172
Hospitals
    Beaufort, Bristol 94, 101, 124, 130, 134-5, 140-1, 216, 219, 226, 238, 246
    Beltwood Dalling (Braeside) 91
    Bristol Royal Infirmary 17, 73-5, 94, 124, 135, 222
    St Andrews, Chippenham (Later Chippenham Community Hospital) 157
    Southmead, Bristol 74, 94, 98, 106-7, 124, 191
Houlston, Miss Beatrice, 145, 171, 223-4, 231, 236-8
Howells, Sergeant David, 239
Hulbert, Francis and Mrs Elizabeth Emma, 30, 96, 102, 104, 128, 228, 231
Hulbert, Miss, 136
Hullavington, 63, 191, 216
Humphries, Mrs, 127
Hunt, George and Mrs Matilda, 182, 184, 242
Hunt, Percival, 184, 242
Hunt, Sisters (Calne), 27
Hutton, Eva, 115
Hyatt, Councillor, 231

Infirmary, Bristol Royal; see Hospitals
Isaacs, Alice, 129

JCITMP (Joint Committee of the Ministry of Pensions on Institutional Treatment), 154
Jefferys, Frances, 129
Jenning, Miss, 177
Jessop, Lewis, 122
Jones, Mrs Gladys Stafford, 84
Jones, Mary, 236
Jones, Miss, 179

Keogh, Sir Alfred, 15
Kington Langley, 74, 77-8, 83, 108, 147, 183
Kinnear, Corporal Alexander, 106
Kinneir, Mr A C (JP), 192
Kirkham, Miss, 177
Knight, Miss, 179
Kyrle; see Money-Kyrle

Lackham House, 172
Lacock, 40, 73, 82, 87-8, 110, 187, 218, 236 88
Langley, Mrs B C, 88
Langley Burrell, 134, 147
Langton, Mrs Stephen, 88
Lansdowne, Lord and Lady, 12, 17, 19, 25, 43, 45-7, 51, 53-4, 68, 80, 143, 174, 234
Laurence, Doctor George, 123, 144, 207, 211, 224, 231
Lavington, Grace, 120
Leatham, Captain and Mrs, 110, 147
Lessiter, Miss, 177
Lethbridge, Ralph, 160
Limbrick, Miss, 127
Livingstone, Reverend, 18
Llewellyn, Mrs, 127
Lloyd, Mr H V, 173
Lloyd George, David, 22, 58, 62, 93, 138, 158
Longleat, 80, 135
Lowden School, 148
Loyd, Major Robert Lindsay, 238
Luce, Ursula (Evelyn), 187
Ludlow Tayler, Mr, 96, 136
Lysley, Mrs, 127
Lysley, Miss Joan, 147

Mackness, Mrs Sarah, 26, 54, 91, 127, 174
Maddock, Miss, 54
Malmesbury, 31, 51, 53, 80, 172, 187, 191, 224, 239
Malpas, Mrs, 233
Marlborough, 45, 52-4
Marshall, Lionel, 18-20, 25, 34, 36, 45, 213-4
Maslen, Albert, 122

Massage Treatment, 141-2, 221-4
Maxwell-Gumbleton; see Smith, Reverend Maxwell H
McDougall, Second Lieutenant Edward John, 206-7
Melksham, 54, 58, 66, 68, 75, 91, 149, 164, 173-4, 211, 219, 220, 226
Mercer-Nairne, Lord Charles, 68
Merriman, Mr, 177
Methuen, Lord George and Lady Mary Ethel, 22, 52-3, 58, 68, 81, 241
Methuen, The Hon Christian, 52
Milford, Miss, 179
Millard, Mrs Rhoda, 132
Miller, Sister, 145
Military Service Act 1916, 114
Ministry of Pensions; see Pensions
Ministry of Pensions Act 1916, 154
Money-Kyrle, Mrs Florence, 17, 71, 82
Money-Kyrle, Miss Joan, 40, 63, 71, 73, 82, 89, 91, 104
Monks Park, Corsham, 88, 124
Morgan, Miss, 174
Morley, Hereward, 237-8
Morse, Mrs Kate, 132
Munday, Miss Alice, 103
Munday, Private Walter, 171
Munitions of War Act 1915, 93, 112, 115
Mustoe, Miss, 179

Naval and Military War Pensions, &c. Act 1915, 153-4
Neale, Edgar, 56, 96-7, 225
Neate, Ambrose, 64
Neate, Miss, 179
Neate, Richard, 145
Needlework Association, Red Cross, 85-6, 87, 97, 233
Needlework Guild, North Wilts, 83-4, 87, 96
Neston Park, 66
Nettleton, 84
Newman, Mrs, 136

Olivier, Miss Edith, 65
Orthopaedic Treatment, 134-5, 140-1, 221-3, 238

Palace Theatre, Station Hill, Chippenham, 172, 187
Palmer, Mr and Mrs Llewellyn, 172
Parkinson, Sergeant J E, 106
Parry, Miss Alfreda, 174
Parry, Miss Maud, 182

The Story of Chippenham's Red Cross Hospital

Parry, Mrs, 147
Pearce, Oliver, 218
Pearce, Mrs, 127, 173
Pearn, Mr F J, 82
Pecher, Mr M, 176
Pennez, Miss B, 177
Penniniez, Mademoiselle, 225
Pensions, 132, 150, 153-8, 156-7, 214, 220-225
Perrott, Sir Herbert, 15, 37
Perry, Miss, 177, 179
Pewsey, 45-6
Phillips, Arthur, 191
Phillips, Captain Ashley, 18
Phillips, Nora, 83
Pickwick, 84
Pike, Nellie, 44
Pinfield, Frederick (Bert) and Mrs Rosa (Gertie), 184
Pinfield, George and Mrs Emily, 103, 180, 182-3
Pocock's Cloth Factory, 66-8
Portman, Reverend, 191
Powell, Sir Robert Baden-; see Baden-Powell, Sir Robert
Poynder; see Dickson Poynder

Radnor, Lord and Lady, 12, 17, 34, 221
RAMC (Royal Army Medical Corps), 45-6, 53-4
Ramsbottom, Mrs Annie, 87-8
Ramsbottom, Miss Phyllis, 236
Red Cross Ambulance; see Ambulance Detachments and Sections
Red Cross Society; see British Red Cross Society
Red Cross, Wiltshire Branch; see Wiltshire Branch, Red Cross
Reed, Sister, 145
Refugees, 11, 13, 15, 40, 80-82, 118
Rich, Miss, 108
Richardson, Mr, 173
Richmond, Mr, 96
Ridsdale, Sir Edward, 37
Rogers, Louisa Newman, 52
Rogers, Mr, 123
Rooke, Mortimer, 208
Rooke, Sisters, 127, 208, 242
Rooke, Captain Wallace, 208, 242
Roundway Park, 52
Rowden Hill House, 96
Rowden House, 121

St Andrew's Church, 91, 144, 150, 241-2

St Andrew's Hospital; see Hospitals
St Dunstan's, 87, 154
St John (Order of St John, St John Ambulance Association and Brigade), 3, 15, 24, 29, 34-8, 69, 71-80, 119, 122, 185, 193-4
St Paul's Church, 87, 97, 118, 150-1, 198, 208
Salisbury, 18, 25, 34, 41, 52-3, 63-6, 68, 84, 107, 115, 208, 214, 222, 239
Savin, Mrs Mary, 132
Savin, Edith (Smith), 132
Saxby and Farmer, 23, 34, 66, 82, 93, 98, 114-5, 122, 136, 161, 167, 174-7, 179-80, 182-3, 204, 213, 218, 225, 238
Scammell, Ernest Charles, 176-7
Schomberg, Mr and Mrs E C, 77
Scout Movement, 22, 39, 41, 43, 46, 54, 91, 96, 102, 152-3, 203, 240
Seagry, 79, 120-1
Seend House, 77
Seeney, Lance Corporal Frank, 171
Selman, Florence, 118
Sewing, 19, 39, 62, 71, 81, 84-7, 154; see also Needlework Association, Work Groups and Parties
Sharpe, Private, 17
Shipp, Family (Foxham), 44, 47, 54, 103, 111, 147, 171, 231
Shorland, Miss, 179
Shorland, Mrs, 233
Slade, Edith Greta, 183
Slade, William Goold and Mrs Sara, 96, 182-3, 233, 246
Smallcombe, Mr, 96
Smith, Mrs Edith, 132
Smith, Henry Herbert, 19, 25, 45, 48
Smith, Reverend Maxwell H, (also known as Maxwell-Gumbleton), 18, 20, 91-2, 97, 128
Somerford; see Great Somerford
Somme, 112, 123-4, 140, 191, 123-4, 140, 191
Sopworth, 53
Souter, Private and Mrs, 197
Southern Military Hospital Command, 17, 70, 74, 95, 97, 128, 135, 140, 225
Southmead Hospital; see Hospitals
Spackman, Family, 83, 173
Spencely, Lieutenant Colonel, 192
Spencer, Arthur (The Music Warehouse), 26, 167-8
Spencer, Miss Dorothy, 174
Spencer, Mrs Katherine (Kate), 26, 174
Spicer, Mrs Frank, 127

Spicer, Miss Joan, 187-8, 209
Spicer, Julian, 183
Spicer, Lady Margaret, 17, 53, 71, 85, 88, 97, 128, 133, 148, 157, 209, 211, 231, 243
Spinke Family, 27, 46, 103, 126, 128, 173, 189, 208, 224, 228, 233
SpyePark, 17, 53, 71, 88
Stanley, Arthur - Chairman, Central Joint VAD Committee, 115, 146
Stanley, Arthur, 122-3
Stanton (including Stanton St Quintin and Upper & Lower Stanton), 130-2, 147
Stanton Manor, 17, 68, 132
Star and Garter Home; see St Dunstan's
Steinbrook House and Cottage, 74, 183
Stephens, Mrs, 88
Stephens, Sergeant, 167
Stephens, William, 118
Stevens, Mr, 55, 127
Stevens, Private, 173
Stevens, William and Mrs Annie, 208
Stevenson, Mrs, 127
Stewart, Mrs, 127
Stubbert, Private Raymond, 143-4
Suffolk, Earl and Countess of, 31, 52-3, 77, 80, 233
Sutton Benger, 79, 119-21, 127, 147-9
Sutton, Bertie, 121
Sutton, Georgina, 120
Swain, Councillor Edward, 245
Swindon, 18, 52, 222, 224

Talbot, Miss E, 87
Talbot, Matilda, 40, 82
Tanner, Miss Margaret, 30, 177
Tayler; see Ludlow Tayler
Taylor, Dr, 73
Taylor, Mrs Hilda, 127, 183-4
Taylor, Mrs John, 88
Terrell, George (MP) and Mrs, 35, 127, 197
Territorial and Reserve Forces Act 1907, 12-3
Territorial Association; see County Territorial Association
Territorial Force, 12-4, 19-20, 27, 34, 41,48,60
Territorial Force General Hospital, 14, 73
Territorial Force Nursing Service, 14-5
Theatre; see Palace Theatre, Station Hill, Chippenham
Thomas, Mrs Annie, 132
Thompson, William, 218
Tisbury, 53, 124

Titcombe, Henry and daughter Mary, 14
Tofts, Sergeant, 202
Tomlin, Miss E, 104
Tompkins, Miss, 179
Townsend, Alderman, 112, 128
Tribunals, 112, 121, 153
Troughton, H, 82
Trowbridge, 12, 38, 49-55, 57, 68, 75, 89, 104, 153, 156, 172
Tyler, Albert, 122, 177
Tytherton, 88, 96, 147, 186, 218

Venables, Private, 165
Vicborn, Mrs Ethel, 145, 161, 197
Voluntary Aid Scheme, 4, 9-10, 14-17, 37-9, 58, 115

Wallace, Mrs Ellen, 132, 147
Wallace, Mrs Jenny, 132
Walters, Mrs, 127
Warminster, 53
Warrilow, Miss, 179
Watts, Miss Elsie, 174, 233
Webb, Ernest, 218
Webb, Eva, 233
Wellens, Charles (Carolus Clemens Eugenius), 82, 118
Westmead, 41, 130, 148, 218
Westoby, Mrs, 127
Whall, Christopher, 242
Whetham House, 17, 40, 63, 71
Whishaw, James, 96-7, 100-1,
Whishaw, Miss Phyllis R, 97, 101,183 231
Williams, Mrs Ethel, 81, 100-4, 111, 118, 136, 147-8, 169-70, 188, 197, 231
Williams, Miss, 127
Williamson, Mrs C H, 88
Wilson, Miss Beryl, 233
Wilson, Mrs Helena, 4, 30, 45, 47, 52, 55-6, 68, 70-1, 75, 95, 98, 101, 128, 130, 136, 139, 143, 148, 152, 160, 211, 218, 226, 228, 230-1, 233-4, 241-3, 245-6
Wilson, Dr Mervyn, 19, 38, 45, 82, 133, 143, 218, 231, 242
Wilson, Sergeant, 145
Wilts County Association; see County Territorial Association
Wilts Joint Voluntary Aid Committee, 17, 18, 38, 156-7, 200-4
Wilts War Pensions Committee, 156-7, 220-4
Wiltshire Branch, Red Cross, 17, 19, 45, 48, 50-2,

68, 75, 94-5, 157, 234
Wiltshire Farmers, 123, 128, 185-6, 188-90, 194-5
Wiltshire Regiment, 12, 63, 66, 68, 180, 188, 237
Wiltshire Territorial Force, 12, 48
Wiltshire Yeomanry, 12-13, 60, 63, 66-67, 92, 108-10, 169, 208, 218
Winwood, Mrs W, 88
Witts, Miss Lily, 237
Wood, Mrs R B, 127
Woods, Mrs, 127
Work Groups and Parties, 70, 71, 81, 85-9, 97, 130-2, 154, 186
Workhouse, 14, 46, 157, 228
Wyld, Canon Edwin, 58

X-Ray, 189

Yatesbury, 206-7
Yatton Keynell, 77, 87-8, 127
Yeomanry, Wiltshire; *see* Wiltshire Yeomanry
Young, Edith, 237
Ypres, 68, 78, 106, 180

Unity and Loyalty

www.ingramcontent.com/pod-product-compliance
Lightning Source LLC
Chambersburg PA
CBHW061138230426

43662CB00023B/2460